CONQUERING ATHLETIC INJURIES

American Running and Fitness Association

Paul M. Taylor, D.P.M.
Diane K. Taylor, B.A.
Editors

Leisure Press
Champaign, Illinois

The following articles were previously published by the American Running and Fitness Association in the *Running and FitNews*. They are reprinted with permission on pages: 6-8, 9-10, 40-41, 50-51, 55-57, 59-61, 65-67, 72-74, 75-76, 102-103, 108-111, 118-119, 123-124, 152-157, 164-165, 169-172, 173-174, 239-241, 242-244, 245-246, 247-250, 262-264, 265-266, 271-273, 287-289.

Library of Congress Cataloging-in-Publication Data

Conquering athletic injuries.

  Bibliography: p.
  Includes index.
  1. Sports—Accidents and injuries. 2. Overuse injuries. 3. Physical fitness. I. Taylor, Paul M., 1946-   . II. Taylor, Diane K., 1946-   .
  RD97.C66 1988   617'.1027   87-33905
  ISBN 0-88011-305-7

Developmental Editor: Judy Patterson Wright, PhD
Production Director: Ernie Noa
Projects Manager: Lezli Harris
Copy Editor: Peter Nelson
Assistant Editors: Kathy Kane, Julie Anderson, JoAnne Cline
Proofreader: Laurie McGee
Typesetter: Sandra Meier
Text Design: Keith Blomberg
Text Layout: Denise Mueller
Cover Design: Jack Davis
Cover Photos: Kirk Schlea and Melanie Carr/Focus West
Illustrations By: Patrice Moerman
Interior Photographs By: Greg Merhar
Printed By: Versa Press

ISBN 0-88011-305-7

Printed in the United States of America

10 9 8 7 6 5 4 3

Leisure Press
A Division of Human Kinetics Publishers, Inc.
Box 5076, Champaign, IL 61825-5076
1-800-747-4457

UK Office:
Human Kinetics Publishers (UK) Ltd.
P.O. Box 18
Rawdon, Leeds LS19 6TG
England
(0532) 504211

Dedication

Conquering Athletic Injuries is dedicated to the members of the American Running and Fitness Association. It is through the support of its members that the association is able to continue to serve the public as a source of information on health and fitness. In turn, the members have gained motivation to continue their fit lifestyles and to share this objective with their families and friends.

Members continually challenge the medical advisory board with questions about health and fitness. In responding to these questions, valuable information has gradually been accumulated; this material is the basis for *Conquering Athletic Injuries*. Thus, it was the challenge and questions from the membership that provided the initiative for creating this book.

Thank you, members of the American Running and Fitness Association.

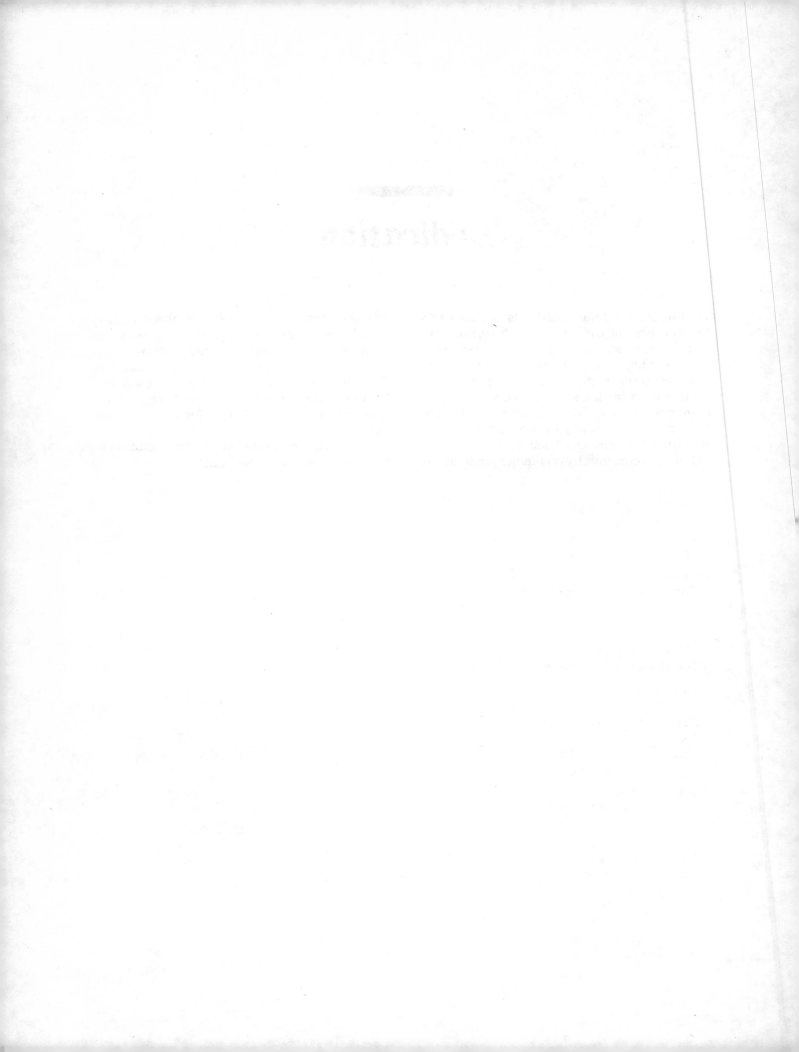

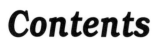

Contents

Chapter 5
Ankle Injuries

Chapter 6
Leg Injuries

Chapter 7
Knee Injuries

A History of the American Running and Fitness Association

Dr. Richard Bohannon

Since 1968, the year I founded the American Running and Fitness Association (originally known as the National Jogging Association), the pursuit of physical fitness has become a national pastime. People in every age group are participating in—and benefiting from—aerobic exercise. What's more important, this wave of interest in fitness continues to grow and is far from cresting. The possibility now exists that the United States may become the healthiest it has ever been.

This possibility makes me proud of the part that AR&FA has played in educating the American people about the benefits of regular exercise and good nutrition. When I suggested that a national association for joggers be founded, I had no idea that it would be in the forefront of the fitness movement only 20 years later.

Back in 1968, American running trails, bike trails, and lap lanes in swimming pools were not very crowded. In that year, participating in a jogging path dedication at Haines Point, Washington, DC, just before retiring as Surgeon General of the United States Air Force, I suggested that a national jogging association be founded to help educate the American public about the benefits of aerobic exercise. Because I had some time on my hands, I began to follow up on this suggestion. Soon, on September 21, 1968, in the company of a number of notables from around the country, the NJA was launched from the steps of the Lincoln Memorial with a symbolic jog around the reflecting pool.

The word *aerobic* was not generally known at the time. My good friend, Kenneth H. Cooper, M.D., had already begun to change that, though. Through his research in Dallas,

Ken was documenting the essentialness of aerobic exercise to the building of good physical condition. In an article in *Reader's Digest* (March, 1968) and through the release of his best-selling book *Aerobics* the following month, Ken introduced an exercise program that awarded points based on the aerobic benefits derived from certain activities. Running was pointed out as the most efficient, inexpensive, and convenient exercise by which to gain aerobic benefits. With this information, the help of Ken, and that of Ron Lawrence, M.D., I knew the NJA would be successful in efforts to improve the level of fitness in America.

During the 1970s, NJA's membership grew steadily; as the NJA grew, so did its programs. We published *Guidelines for Successful Jogging*, which became a basic text for beginning joggers. We initiated National Jogging Day—now Running and Fitness Day—which annually involves millions of Americans. We have published the most consistently informative health newsletter on the market. Moreover, during the seventies, statistics began to indicate a significant decline in mortality from heart disease. I can't help but think that we played a part in this improvement.

As the National Jogging Association entered the 1980s, it became clear that its name did not nearly encompass the wide range of aerobic activities in which Americans were participating. I had founded NJA to encourage jogging, believing—as I still do—that this is the best exercise for most persons. However, people have a variety of favorite fitness ideas; soon, swimmers, bikers, and aerobic dancers were everywhere.

Joggers certainly helped to introduce the

nation to the cardiovascular and pulmonary benefits of aerobic exercise. One- to two-mile jogs became 5K and 10K runs; 5K and 10K runs led to marathons, and marathons led to triathlons. Yet, because NJA's primary goal was to educate and motivate our fellow Americans to participate in aerobic exercise, it was logical to expand the association's focus to include *everyone* in the fitness movement. Thus, the NJA was transformed into the American Running and Fitness Association. Today, AR&FA's 30,000 members include not only persons who run, but also persons who cross-country ski, walk, bike, swim, and aerobically dance their way to good health.

Conquering Athletic Injuries is the next step in AR&FA's continuing educational efforts. It makes me proud that an idea I had has led to the publication of a book presenting contributions from so many experts in the sports-medicine field. This book represents what the association was meant to be—a cooperative effort to bring correct fitness information to as wide an audience as possible.

My special thanks go to Paul and Diane Taylor for their efforts in compiling *Conquering Athletic Injuries*. It is people like them who will make my dream a part of the twenty-first century. For additional information about AR&FA write: American Running and Fitness Association, 9310 Old Georgetown Road, Bethesda, MD 20814.

Preface

The running boom of the 1970s helped create a much greater awareness of health and fitness. The initial enthusiasm for running as a way of developing fitness soon spread to many other aerobic activities. Participation in many sports—aerobic dance, swimming, biking, tennis, triathlons, basketball, racquetball, handball, walking, and other activities that help develop fitness—have shown a continuous increase.

Unfortunately, along with the benefits of fitness programs there has also been an increase in injuries—particularly overuse injuries. This increased activity and the subsequent injuries have generated an increased demand for knowledge of how our bodies respond to this added stress. The athlete has progressed to a point where he or she not only needs to know about the benefits of exercise but also needs to understand the injuries that do occur and the best way to treat—or prevent—these injuries. The contributors to *Conquering Athletic Injuries* have recognized this need for more information; through the efforts of the American Running and Fitness Association, this text has been prepared.

Anyone who participates in an exercise program—whether it be running, aerobic dance, tennis, basketball, or any other sport—recognizes the benefits of activity. However, he or she must also recognize that there is a high potential for injuries that may interfere with activity. Few athletes like to accept the fact that injuries occur that may stop their participation in sports. However, accepting this and being able to treat injuries appropriately is an important part of an exercise program.

There are two basic types of injuries that can occur in sports. The acute trauma, such as a fracture or dislocation, is obvious and requires immediate attention. The overuse injury is more subtle and may not be recognized initially. The overuse injury results from minimal stress applied to a particular part of the body repeatedly over a period of time. The overuse injury may be caused by overtraining, improper training techniques, biomechanical imbalance, or structural abnormalities within the body, or by external forces within the environment.

These nagging overuse injuries develop slowly, can interfere with training, and can be very slow in improving. It is primarily examples of this type of injury that are discussed in *Conquering Athletic Injuries*. This book provides understanding about most of the common sports overuse injuries. For completeness, some of the acute injuries that may occasionally be self-treated, such as ankle sprains, are also included.

This text should be valuable not only to the fitness runner, but to anyone involved in sports. This includes coaches and trainers, who frequently initially treat injuries, and aerobic dance instructors, who are also in a position to recognize and treat minor injuries.

Aerobic dance is showing tremendous growth, similar to that of running when it first became popular. Unfortunately, the number of injuries is also increasing rapidly. The aerobic dancer, especially the instructor, can use *Conquering Athletic Injuries* to better understand the injuries that can occur. These include some of the most common overuse injuries, such as sesamoiditis, shin splints, Achilles tendinitis, heel pain, and Morton's neuroma.

Walking for exercise is also rapidly increasing in popularity. Since walking places less stress on the body, people feel that the increase of injuries may be reduced. However, as in all other forms of exercise, the overuse injuries are occurring. It is just as important for people who walk for exercise to be aware of the potential for overuse injuries.

It is hoped that this text will be found to supply valuable information to any person interested in sports-related injuries. It can be used as a basic sportsmedicine book. For athletes who require more than basic information about the various injuries that they may sustain, this book provides an extensive reading list for obtaining additional information.

Acknowledgments

Staff members of the American Running and Fitness Association have made many contributions to the development of this book. Three persons deserve special recognition for their efforts on behalf of AR&FA.

Ms. Liz Elliot, Executive Director of AR&FA from 1978 to 1986, who also served as editor of *Running and FitNews*, suggested many ideas for articles that were incorporated into this book. The development of *Conquering Athletic Injuries* is a continuation of her commitment to providing information on health, fitness, and injury prevention to AR&FA members.

Two other staff members, Susan Kalish and Julie Widdifield-Wisor, are the heart of this association. It is through their hard work, professional expertise, and belief in the goals of AR&FA that it has been possible to accumulate the information presented in this book.

Our thanks also go to Karen Lips and Michael Schlossman, who were the models for the stretch and strength exercise illustrations.

Contributors

David L. Berman, D.P.M. Clinical associate professor, Department of Community Health, Pennsylvania College of Podiatric Medicine; Professor, Department of Orthopaedic Surgery, Temple University School of Medicine.

David A. Bernstein, D.P.M. American Academy of Podiatric Sports Medicine; Sports consultant to Haverford College and Villanova University.

Katherine A. Braun, R.P.T., A.T.C. Physical therapist; Medical advisor to the Board of Directors, Washington Squash and Nautilus Club; Health consultant to the Board of Directors, YWCA, Washington, DC; Department of Physical Education, George Washington University Team Athletes.

Vincent G. Desiderio, Jr., M.D. Clinical instructor, Division of Orthopaedics, Georgetown University.

Mark D. Dollard, D.P.M. Clinical instructor, Division of Orthopaedics, Georgetown University Hospital; National secretary, Sportsmedicine Committee, Amateur Athletic Union; Vice-chairman, Team Aerobics Dance Committee, AAU.

Jeri Fink Freelance writer, Bellmore, NY.

Ayne F. Furman, D.P.M. Sportsmedicine Committee, Road Runners Club of America; Private practitioner of podiatric sportsmedicine, Alexandria, VA.

Harold B. Glickman, D.P.M. American Academy of Podiatric Sports Medicine, American Academy of Hospital Podiatrists; Clinical professor of orthopaedic surgery, George Washington University Medical Center; President, District of Columbia Podiatric Medical Association.

Denis R. Harris, M.D. Assistant professor of surgery, Department of Orthopaedics, Georgetown University Hospital.

Karen Lenz Jones, B.A. Freelance writer, Washington, DC.

Richard L. Jones, M.D. Director, Sports Medicine Program, Adolescent/Youth Services, Department of Pediatrics, Georgetown University Children's Medical Center.

Mark E. Julsrud, D.P.M. American College of Sports Medicine, American Academy of Podiatric Sports Medicine; Private practitioner of podiatric sportsmedicine, La Crosse, WI.

Susan Kalish Director, American Running and Fitness Association; Editor, *Running and FitNews*.

Mark Landry, D.P.M. American Board of Podiatric Surgery, American Academy of Sports Medicine; Consultant, Mid-America Track and Field Association; Clinical professor, School of Podiatric Medicine, Des Moines, IA; Clinical instructor, Truman Medical Center, University of Missouri; Director, Podiatric Education, Kansas City Residency Program.

Wayne B. Leadbetter, M.D. Attending orthopaedic surgeon, Shady Grove Adventist Hospital; Medical director, Shady Grove Center for Sports Medicine and Rehabilitation, Rockville, MD.

Greg Merhar Freelance photographer, Washington, DC.

Gabe Mirkin, M.D. Syndicated columnist, *New York Times*; Fitness broadcaster, CBS Radio; Professor, Georgetown University School of Medicine; Medical editor, *Running Times*.

Patrice Moerman Freelance illustrator, Washington, DC.

Terry L. Nelson, M.D. Director, Southwestern Michigan Sportsmedicine Clinic.

Lloyd Nesbitt, D.P.M. President, Canadian Podiatric Sportsmedicine Academy; President, Ontario Podiatric Medical Association.

Raymond J. Olkin, D.P.M. Private practitioner of podiatric sportsmedicine, Fairfax, VA.

Michael O'Shea Contributor, *Running and FitNews*.

Charles M. Peterson Contributor, *Running and FitNews*.

Rebecca Riales, Ph.D. Clinical nutritionist, Parkersburg, WV.

Alan Rogol, M.D., Ph.D. Professor, Department of Pediatrics, University of Virginia School of Medicine, Charlottesville.

James R. Snyder, M.D. Founder and director, Washington Cardiovascular Evaluation Center; Founding member, Youth Sports in Northern Virginia.

Diane K. Taylor, B.A. Editorial consultant, *Running and FitNews*; Freelance author and editor.

Paul M. Taylor, D.P.M. Clinical instructor, Division of Orthopaedics, Georgetown University Hospital; President-elect, American Academy of Podiatric Sports Medicine; President, American Running and Fitness Association; Podiatry consultant, Washington Bullets.

Walter R. Thompson, Ph.D. Director of applied physiology, Department of Physical Education, University of Southern Mississippi.

Debra S. Wehman, D.P.M. Attending staff, Westview Hospital, Indianapolis; Consultant, Women's Athletics, Ball State University.

Anthony H. Woodward, M.D. Orthopaedic surgeon, Westminster, MD.

Robert F. Weiss, D.P.M. American Academy of Podiatric Sports Medicine; Medical Advisory Committee, 1984 U.S. Olympic Marathon Trials; Connecticut State Police Surgeon.

Jeffery L. Young Exercise physiologist, New York, NY.

How to Use This Book

Conquering Athletic Injuries is organized so that the injured (or just plain interested) athlete can find discussion of a particular injury according to either the name of the condition (diagnosis) or the location of the injury (pain).

Part I, Recognition of Overuse Injuries, deals with the initial recognition of an injury. This recognition includes being able not only to identify the physical aspects of an injury but also to accept and deal with the psychological problems associated with being injured (chapter 1).

Chapter 2 can be used to identify an injury according to the part of the body involved. For example, you may be having intermittent pain on the outside of a knee. It's understandable that you may not want to visit a doctor with this and every other minor injury; if safe to do so, you'd like to help yourself get better. So, you can turn to *Conquering Athletic Injuries* for answers. If you do not know where in *Conquering Athletic Injuries* to look, refer to the illustrations in chapter 2 to see which common problems may be causing your knee pain. Then refer to part II for specific injury information.

However, caution is necessary here because there may be multiple causes of pain in a particular area. If this is the case, you should refer to all the possible relevant discussions to determine what is most likely causing your pain. Because the basic treatments for different injuries are often similar, treatment may be started without a specific diagnosis. However, if pain persists, professional treatment should be sought.

Referred pain may cause some confusion here, also. This phenomenon occurs when pain is felt in one part of the body but is caused by a problem somewhere else. This can be difficult to identify and may require professional help to diagnose. When an area of pain does not respond to local treatment, additional help is needed.

Chapter 3 deals with the principles of self-care and the self-treatment of injuries. It provides guidelines for dealing with an injury, information on how the body responds to injury, principles related to the use of physical therapy modalities (such as ice or heat), advice on self-medication, and a three-step plan that provides the basis for the treatment of most overuse injuries.

Chapters 4 through 11 deal with specific injuries. Because most sports-related injuries happen to the lower extremities, the list starts with the most distal injuries (toenails) and proceeds to the top of the head. The outlines of every injury chapter follow a common pattern. A definition of an injury is provided, followed by a description of how the injury occurs. Then a recommendation for self-treatment is provided, with an explanation of professional care that may be necessary if self-care is not adequate. Finally, methods of preventing the injury or its recurrence are suggested.

Confusion often arises from the variety of terms used for a particular condition, as there is generally a common term and a medical term. Wherever possible, all terminology relating to a particular condition is mentioned. The table of contents, index, and glossary help here. *Conquering Athletic Injuries* should provide you with rapid access to information about most overuse injuries due to the extensive cross-referencing system used.

For example, you may be told that your problem involves tendinitis. Because this general term refers to inflammation of any tendon, the first thing to do is to identify the specific tendon injured. This can be done either by looking in the table of contents or index under the joint involved (e.g., knee or hip) for "tendinitis" or by referring to chapter 2,

"Injury Identification by Anatomic Location." Once the specific injury has been identified as, for example, patellar tendinitis, reference can be made to chapter 7 for details (see Table 1).

Chapter 12 demonstrates stretching and strengthening exercises that are recommended within the specific injury articles. Because a particular exercise is used in treating a number of injuries, all exercises are presented in chapter 12, rather than being repeated throughout the book. Some of these exercises are specific for certain injuries and should be done only as recommended in the "Injuries" chapters. For the athlete involved in a particular aerobic sport, "Sport-Specific Exercises" are recommended. When the athlete participates primarily in one sport, certain muscle groups become stronger, whereas opposing groups do not develop as well. This imbalance increases the potential for overuse injuries, but any imbalance can be prevented by a proper stretching and strengthening program.

The best solution to overuse injuries is prevention (part III). Chapter 13 offers a number of suggestions on how to avoid injuries. These include various tips and techniques you can use to control abnormal biomechanical stresses, maintain fitness while injured, and protect yourself from environmental forces. Nutritional factors that affect exercise, bone and joint factors involved with exercise, and considerations for exercise for children are discussed in chapters 14, 15, and 16, respectively. Lastly, chapter 17 covers immediate first aid and common skin problems.

The reading list can be used for additional references. At the end of many articles, there is a list of suggested readings. You may want to refer to these references for more information. Many of these references are from medical texts and journals not commonly available in most public libraries; however, your library may be able to obtain copies for you or refer you to a nearby medical school or hospital library.

If you need a definition of commonly used terms, see the glossary. If you need a reference to the human skeleton or specific body plane and movement terms, see Appendices A and B.

It is hoped that *Conquering Athletic Injuries* can serve runners, coaches, trainers, instructors, and athletes of every sport as a source of information for better understanding the injuries and problems that occur during sports and fitness-related activities.

Table 1 How to Locate Information About Injuries in *Conquering Athletic Injuries*

Problem	Answer
You know the medical or common name of the injury. Example: patellar tendinitis (medical name) jumper's knee (common name)	Refer to the table of contents or index.
You don't know the injury's name, but only where it hurts.	Refer to chapter 2, "Injury Identification by Anatomic Location."
You know a general term for an injury, but not its specific name. Example: tendinitis	Refer to the table of contents and to part II to try to identify the specific injury. Example: patellar tendinitis (chapter 7, "Knee Injuries")

PART I

Recognition of Overuse Injuries

There are two types of injuries that the athlete may sustain: the acute trauma and the overuse syndrome. The acute trauma is a sudden, violent injury, such as lacerations, torn ligaments, or broken bones caused by a fall. Acute injuries usually require immediate professional help. The type of problem most frequently encountered by the athlete, however, is the overuse syndrome. This develops from mild or low-grade abnormal force being applied repeatedly for a long period of time. This type of injury frequently responds well to self-treatment.

Understanding these injuries and recognizing how the body responds to them allows you, the athlete, to be more effective in overcoming their damage. Also, by being in tune with your body, you can learn what to do to prevent injuries, how to recognize when an injury may be developing, how to treat it, and when to seek professional help.

CHAPTER 1

———

Understanding and Accepting Overuse Injuries

The first consideration in the prevention of injuries is accepting the fact that we are not indestructible. The human body is an amazing composite of delicate structures that can withstand tremendous stress; however, there are limits. Once you have been injured, you must first accept your injury (see the article entitled "Runner's Withdrawal"). Then you need to work with your injury (see "Rest—A Critical Factor in Training and Improvement").

With the frequency and variety of injuries that can beset the athlete, the dilemma of whether to seek medical help often occurs. It is impossible to offer any universally applicable solutions for this problem; however, a few guidelines can be helpful (see "Self-Care Versus Professional Care"). In some cases, the decision may be obvious. A small blister on the foot, for instance, can almost always be self-treated. If this blister becomes infected, causing a red, painful, swollen foot, the decision to seek professional help is easy. With common sense and basic understanding of the mechanisms of injury and of the body's healing response, you can make educated decisions as to whether medical care is necessary.

Runner's Withdrawal

Jeri Fink

Bill was running 30 miles a week when he tripped and twisted his ankle. His doctor diagnosed the injury as a mild sprain; Bill would be back to running in 3 weeks. Yet, a few days later, Bill became cranky and irritable, impatient with everyone around him. No one understood why—after all, he would be running again in a few weeks. Even Bill himself didn't know why he was so down. His mood got worse, until he eventually fell into a depression that hung on until he was able to resume running.

Runner's withdrawal—it happens when we're injured or sick, when we have to stop running for reasons beyond our control. One out of every three runners will be injured seriously enough this year to force them to stop running, and they may suffer the pain of withdrawal—a very real, yet seldom discussed, problem.

Negative Versus Positive Addiction

Withdrawal occurs when we give up something that has become an important habit in our lives. Most of us associate withdrawal with negative habits or addictions. A negative addiction controls one's life, taking precedence over other needs and responsibilities. The only way to be freed is to go through an often painful withdrawal. We're all familiar with what happens to alcohol- or drug-dependent persons who can't get a "fix" or to cigarette smokers going "cold turkey." They must undergo physical and psychological ordeals to break their dependencies.

There is also positive addiction, where some constructive habit is an important, but not a controlling, part of life. "Positive addictions, such as running and meditation, are thought to provide psychological strength and increase the satisfaction derived from life" (p. 117) explains Michael L. Sachs, Ph.D. (1981).

The basic difference between positive and negative addictions is in how much each controls your life. For example, a drug-dependent person, negatively addicted, is consumed by the need to obtain a fix; this need takes precedence over family, friends, and work. On the other hand, an habitual runner, a positively addicted person, loves the sport and feels a need to run, but is able to skip a day or rearrange his or her schedule, if necessary. Both kinds of habits *are* addictions, however, and need to be renewed on a regular basis. If any addiction is not renewed, withdrawal begins.

How Addiction Starts

How do people become positively addicted? Most of us start running, for example, for such physical reasons as weight control, cardiovascular conditioning, or fitness improvement. As we become more involved, we discover that there are other, more subtle, side effects. "Running makes you feel good," explains John Papalia, a registered physical therapist and the director of a prominent Long Island, New York, sportsmedicine group. "When you reach the appropriate fitness level, you experience the nice, smooth, liquid feel of the joy of running."

Running has been credited with numerous psychological benefits: increasing a feeling of well-being, improving self-esteem, alleviating depression, relieving tension and anxiety, and boosting assertiveness. The new runner discovers these feelings and finds himself or herself sleeping better, eating better, feeling less tension, and even looking better. These feelings reinforce the pattern of exercise. The new runner begins to schedule runs on a regular basis; eventually, after 4 to 6 months, running becomes a part of the daily routine. To maintain the positive effects and to renew the "high," the runner must continue running. Running has become a habit, a method to maintain a positive sense of well-being. "I feel there is something missing when I don't run for a day or two," explains one habitual runner. "It's part of my life, part of my daily itinerary, and I'm just not comfortable without it."

Withdrawal Symptoms

The positive addiction seems to work very smoothly—until something breaks down, until something happens that forces the runner to stop. Maybe this something is an injury, sickness, or family or business demands. Whatever the reason, when an addicted runner has to stop, the chances are pretty strong that he or she will start to suffer withdrawal symptoms about 24 to 36 hours after missing the first scheduled run.

In a study at Hofstra University, Bruce Serkin concluded that some 75 percent of runners become addicted. Another study, at Georgia State University, has shown that even slight variations in the running schedules of habitual runners can have negative effects, causing an unpleasant mood, or a "down." When an habitual runner misses a day or two, he or she might feel guilt or tension, both of which are emotions that are readily relieved by a new run.

However, what happens when you can't run for an extended period of time? "When an addicted runner stops," notes Dr. Sachs, "he or she will experience withdrawal symptoms like irritability, tension, anxiety, depression, and guilt, and physiological sensations like a bloated feeling, muscle twitching, sluggishness, and lethargy."

Why does all this happen? Many experts feel that, actually, when habitual runners stop running, they simply return to their prefitness emotional states. "You just go back to feeling like you did when you didn't run," suggests Ray Fowler, Ph.D., founder of Running Psychologists, a division of the American Psychological Association. "You don't feel any worse; you just drift back to the way you felt before you started running."

Extent of Withdrawal

The extent of withdrawal can be influenced by the reasons you run. Many people use running as a coping mechanism to deal with stress, anxiety, or even depression. As long as they run, it works. If they're injured and have to stop, though, they may have no other way to cope, and everything comes flooding back—in the form of withdrawal. Others use running for daily reinforcement of their positive self-esteem. Without running, there may be no other reinforcement, and their self-image suffers. Not running can represent a very real psychological deprivation.

On the other hand, those people who use running as an escape or as a way to avoid stress are less likely to have as severe a withdrawal. Their running serves as an outlet, an emotional release, rather than as a defense mechanism. Removing it doesn't affect the amount of stress or how they cope, but only how they escape from the rigors of daily life.

"Most of the people I see going through withdrawal are those who have become athletes in their 30s or 40s," remarks Papalia. "They deny their aging with a fanatical devotion to running. They feel running will enhance life . . . make them live longer. Not to run is to go back to their old lifestyle, their fears of ineffectiveness, aging, and physical decline."

Physiological Effects

There are also critical physical components to runner's withdrawal. "I had a stress fracture and couldn't run," relates one habitual runner. "I would get up in the middle of the night, my muscles all cramped up and in pain. The only way I could alleviate it was to do some long, slow stretches."

The facts are not pleasant. Physical fitness deteriorates rapidly. You can be inactive for only a short amount of time before your level of conditioning starts to decline. An athlete in peak condition loses 10 percent of his or her level of fitness per week for the first 4 to 6 weeks of inactivity, with a more gradual loss of conditioning thereafter.

"Fitness is not like money," explains Papalia. "You can't just put it in a bag and have it whenever you want. You can't expect to stop and then go back 2 or 3 weeks later and pick up where you left off. Fitness is something that has to be earned every day."

All of this further compounds the injured runner's distress: Not only are there psychological withdrawal symptoms, but there also is a steady physical decline. Anxiety, depression, and irritability commonly are exacerbated by such physical sensations as bloatedness, cramping, and lethargy. A runner might come to fear other effects of not running such as gaining weight, losing self-esteem, and aging. Some experts speculate that many injured runners continue just to avoid the unpleasant sensations of withdrawal.

How to Avoid Withdrawal Feelings

How can a runner cope? One obvious way is to stick to your schedule as closely as you can. However, if you're injured or if your family, business, or other responsibilities make it impossible to continue running for a while, your first goal should be to maintain your level of fitness as much as possible. This may mean temporarily going to another sport or exercise. "I give my patients alternatives," states Papalia. "If someone gets an injury in the lower extremities, I'll keep him or her active on the upper extremities, maintaining cardiovascular fitness, so he or she doesn't go through withdrawal. I'll have them do stationary rowing, cycling, swimming—alternative activities that can satiate them during the down time."

Actively maintaining your fitness level throughout recuperation helps lessen your psychological as well as physical discomfort. The alternative activities might not be as enjoyable to you as running, but they can temporarily serve as substitutes.

Another way to prevent or alleviate withdrawal is to try to enjoy more activities than only running in the first place. If you swim or cycle as well as run, then you can more easily switch gears until you're able to resume your normal routine. Total dependence on running for physical activity and psychological well-being makes you more vulnerable to withdrawal if the running ceases.

Finally, understand what is happening both physically and psychologically. Remember that it is only a temporary situation. You can use alternatives to maintain your fitness. Assure yourself that you will never return to your old lifestyle; you won't regain weight, lose your assertiveness, or become depressed if you take control of the situation. It might mean forcing yourself to do things you don't already enjoy, such as swimming or working out on machines, but this is only a means to an end—getting you out and running again.

Rest—A Critical Factor in Training and Improvement

Terry L. Nelson, M.D.

In the past, medical prescription for injuries was very simple: stop exercising. Then the pendulum swung the other way. The old definition of rest being a cessation of activity for months was ignored by athletes continuing to train despite debilitating ailments. Adamant athletes rejected rest as an unacceptable solution for treatment of injuries. Many believed time off from exercising would be cruel and unusual punishment, something prescribed only by insensitive physicians who knew nothing about the athlete's psyche. A sportsmedicine physician's reputation—among athletes, at least—could be directly related to how rapidly the athlete was returned to activity.

However, most sportsmedicine physicians who treat athletes realize that rest is an integral part of every successful program. This is true when the athlete has not been injured, and it is *essential* once an injury has occurred.

Rest, though, does not have to mean complete inactivity. Often, in fact, it means controlled activity. The awareness of this may be the key difference between sportsmedicine doctors and general physicians.

To the athlete, controlled activity simply means cutting back on speed, duration, and frequency of activity. A substitution of another aerobic exercise might be the answer to the question of how to rest an injury. If your injury is too serious for weight-bearing activity, running in water while wearing a flotation jacket can replace the regular workout. The water's buoyancy protects recuperating feet, knees, and hips from weight and pressure while the muscles, heart, and lungs are being exercised.

Each exercise session puts stress on the body. The higher the intensity and the longer the duration, the greater is the stress. Daily high-intensity training does not allow the body adequate time to adjust and recover. In general, for every hard training day, you need one easy day afterward. Most athletes get hurt because they try to do too much, too fast, too soon, too frequently.

In fact, more than 50 percent of all running injuries are due to training errors involving an imbalance of hard and easy workouts. Insufficient rest during training results in mental and physical fatigue. Mental fatigue may surface as sleep difficulties, mood swings, listlessness, and easy irritability. Physical fatigue may result in colds, flu, sore throats, stiffness or soreness, and a greater susceptibility to injuries. Athletes also get injured more frequently when tired.

As your cardiovascular function improves with regular aerobic exercise, your body can go farther and faster while remaining in an aerobic state. These are effects of conditioning. If you do not allow this gradual conditioning to occur, you run the risk of injury. You are more likely to develop overuse problems when stressing the body without proper rest. Some of us take longer to break down than others, but we all break down eventually if adequate recovery time isn't provided.

When You Need More Rest

How do you know when to rest, or when you're risking an impending injury? Several signs may precede a breakdown:

- Taking your pulse daily just after awakening, while you are still in bed, can be an accurate personal guide to overtraining. First, over the course of a week, establish an average pulse. Thereafter, a rate 10 beats higher than average at waking may indicate overtiredness from the preceding day's training. Take it easy in the day ahead—a hard session may result in injury.
- A feeling of fatigue during normal daily activities signals overtraining. If training has sapped your energy, exercise and work may suffer.
- Nagging aches and pains, especially in the muscles, may indicate overtraining. After exercise, lactic acid accumulates in

muscles. This buildup is felt in the form of muscle aches. This is due to oxygen debt, which must be repaid through balancing your anaerobic and aerobic training sessions.

- Finally, overtraining may cause sleep disturbances. These include difficulty getting to sleep, waking up frequently during the night, and greater difficulty waking up in the morning.

Each of these signs indicates overtraining. Ignoring these warning signals could lead to significant injury.

Rest When Injured

If you suffer an injury, carefully assess your training schedule and begin a treatment program. Rest until acute pain diminishes. Apply ice and take aspirin for its anti-inflammatory effects.

The following injuries require complete rest and evaluation by a physician:

- Back pain that radiates down the legs
- Knee pain with fluid buildup in the joint; also, if the knee locks, catches, or gives out
- Pain, swelling, or a lump in the Achilles tendon
- Pain in any area that persists through daily activities

Rest is an integral part of any successful training program. The body must be allowed adequate time to recover from strenuous exertion. Be sure to watch for signs of overtraining. When an injury does occur, assess its severity. Treat yourself if it's minor; see a sportsmedicine physician if it continues.

Self-Care Versus Professional Care

Paul M. Taylor, D.P.M.

It helps to differentiate two basic types of injuries. The acute injury is a sudden injury, such as an ankle sprain, whose cause is immediately known; there is sudden pain related to the injury. The other basic type of injury is the overuse syndrome. This develops slowly from the low-grade, repeated microstress that occurs in sports. The pain is minimal initially, and it is usually difficult to relate the onset of pain to any particular incident.

With acute injuries, the symptoms that develop soon after the injury determine whether medical help should be sought. If the injury causes immediate pain, swelling, inability to use the injured body part, or severe pain on pressure that does not resolve in 30 to 40 minutes, then help should be sought. If there is any deformity present, immediate help is necessary. Also, with a musculoskeletal injury, if the athlete hears or feels a crack, pop, or tear, and pain persists, help should be sought. In the time between being injured and getting help, first aid should be administered as indicated (see the section on first aid, chapter 17).

With the overuse injury, it is usually more difficult to determine whether professional help is necessary. This type of injury comes on gradually, and the pain is usually not severe. Frequently, the athlete feels that if the pain is ignored, it will go away. The pain often persists, though, and eventually the decision as to whether to seek help has to be made. Although there are no hard-and-fast rules for this decision, several guidelines can be used to determine the necessity of getting help:

- If after the level of the activity is reduced, you continue to have pain with exercise
- If the pain persists for more than 10 to 14 days
- If the pain resolves with rest but recurs on resuming exercise
- If it is necessary to take oral anti-inflammatory medications continually in order to exercise
- If there is any question at all that any chest pain or discomfort may be heart related (for more information, see chapter 10)
- If there is a persistence of any general medical problem, such as continued malaise, fatigue, recurring upper respiratory infections, bloody urine, or any other chronic symptom

The above recommendations are only guidelines; it is necessary to evaluate each problem individually. In a case in which there is any doubt, a call to the family doctor may help determine whether a visit is in fact necessary.

Once the decision to call or visit a doctor is made, the next dilemma arises: whom do you call for help? With today's many medical specialists, you may not be sure who is the most approriate doctor to treat your problem. Generally, if you are unsure about who to see, the initial contact should be with your family doctor. Upon being made aware of what is happening, in many cases the doctor can provide immediate recommendations and treatment. If the family doctor does not decide to treat this problem, though, he or she can recommend an appropriate specialist.

If you have been treated previously by a doctor for a sports-related condition, you could call that doctor's office for advice. Even if this is ultimately not the right person to see about your particular problem, the doctor can suggest someone you should go to see. People who specialize in sportsmedicine usually know other specialists interested in sports. Recommendations of other runners and running clubs also help in finding the right doctor.

All these things may help avoid a situation in which two or three visits are made before finding the best specialist to treat a particular problem. Sportsmedicine covers all health-related fields and includes the family doctor, dentist, orthopedist, podiatrist, physical therapist, internist, chiropractor, nutritionist, cardiologist, exercise physiologist, psychiatrist, and anyone else who is involved in health and fitness.

This menagerie can be very intimidating to the athlete who wants to know why the knee pain does not go away. Fortunately, the medical community has become more aware of the needs of the athlete, and these specialists are becoming more effective in dealing with wellness, as well as with illness. The various specialists are cooperating more in multidisciplinary approaches to treating the injured athlete. This cooperation will lead to more effective treatment for athletes. This will also lead to a more efficient system in which athletes will quickly know whom to see for initial treatment of specific problems. Although almost any health-care specialist may be used to treat sports-related problems, there are certain specialists who are involved more frequently. Understanding who these specialists are and how their educational background has trained them helps in selecting the right person to treat an injury. The following health-care personnel most frequently treat sports-related problems.

Family Practitioner. The family doctor—a medical doctor (M.D.) or, in some geographic areas, a doctor of osteopathy (D.O.)—is usually the athlete's initial contact with the health-care system. The medical doctor is a graduate of a medical college, has completed internship and residency, and is licensed by the state. The doctor of osteopathy has graduated from a college of osteopathy, has also completed an internship and residency, and is also licensed by the state. Both are involved in treating all problems that may arise in a patient, but the doctor of osteopathy has had more emphasis on the musculoskeletal system during his training. Of course, with over 400,000 practitioners, medical doctors are seen much more frequently than doctors of osteopathy, who number only around 20,000.

Orthopedist. The orthopedist is a medical doctor who has completed a 4- or 5-year residency. He or she specializes in the evaluation and treatment of the musculoskeletal system. The orthopedist treats injuries involving any part of the musculoskeletal system. Many orthopedists have developed a special interest in sports-related injuries.

Podiatrist. The podiatrist specializes in the treatment of foot and foot-related problems. A podiatrist is a graduate of a college of podiatric medicine, holds the degree of doctor of podiatric medicine (D.P.M.), has completed a residency, and is licensed by the state. The podiatrist's education emphasizes lower extremity function and biomechanics; because most sports-related injuries affect the lower extremities, the podiatrist is frequently utilized to treat injuries.

Physical Therapist. The physical therapist provides injury treatment through various physical modalities and offers rehabilitation for recovery and to help prevent future injuries. Most therapists have a college degree, and they must be licensed by the state board either as a physical therapist (P.T.) or a registered physical therapist (R.P.T.). The therapist is actively involved in the evaluation, treatment, and prevention of sports injuries. Some therapists are in private practice, but the majority practice in hospitals, clinics, or doctors' offices.

Physiatrist. The physiatrist is a medical doctor who specializes in physical therapy. He or she evaluates patients, provides special testing techniques, prescribes medications, and recommends additional treatment and rehabilitation programs. Most physiatrists are associated with clinics, and physical medicine and rehabilitation centers in hospitals.

Trainer. The team trainer is generally the first provider of care to an injured athlete who is involved with a team sport. The educational background of a team trainer can vary from hands-on training to a college degree. The trainer is actively involved with the team to treat emergencies and to help prevent injuries through taping, recommending better equipment, establishing strengthening and stretching programs, and working with the coach and team physician to help maintain the health of the athletes.

Cardiologist. The cardiologist is a medical doctor who specializes in the evaluation and treatment of heart problems. The family doctor generally evaluates people initially for any heart problem; however, with certain changes peculiar to the athletic heart, a referral to a cardiologist may be necessary.

Dentist. The necessity for proper mouth protection in contact sports is obvious. Dentists involved in sportsmedicine have determined that special mouthpieces that control bite may also have positive effects on strength. Sports dentistry may offer more advantages to the athlete in the future.

These types of specialists treat the majority of sports-related problems. Because of the unique demands of sports on the mind and body of the athlete, though, almost every health-care provider is involved in the care of athletes.

Suggested Reading for "Self-Care Versus Professional Care"

Blackburn (1984)

Block (1982)

Bridges (1984)

Cavanaugh (1980)

Cooney (1984)

Fedo (1983)

Fraser (1985)

Garrett (1983)

Grant & Boileau (1943)

James et al. (1978)

Koplan et al. (1982)

Lehman (1984)

Massimino & Baxter (1983)

Mirkin (1981)

Pagliano & Jackson (1980)

Renstrom & Johnson (1985)

Stanish (1984)

Stover (1980a, b)

Temple (1983)

"Too Many Electrolytes" (1981)

Wassel (1984)

See reading list at the end of the book for a complete source listing.

CHAPTER 2

Injury Identification by Anatomic Location

Paul M. Taylor, D.P.M.

An athlete who has been involved in sports for several years begins to notice a slight ache in his knee after running. It has developed gradually over the past few weeks. The knee pain does not seem serious, but there is concern about it. It does not seem bad enough to warrant a visit to a doctor, but the athlete would like to know what it is and what can be done to correct it. However, without knowing the name of the condition, it is hard to know where to begin looking for an explanation of this problem.

This chapter is intended to help overcome this difficulty. The drawings of body parts showing areas of pain common to athletes can help you identify possible causes of pain in specific areas. For example, our athlete could turn to the pictures of the knee to locate the common causes of knee pain. For pain localized in the front of the knee, the drawing of the front view of the knee illustrates the possible cause. The athlete can then turn to part II, chapter 7, "Knee Injuries," to obtain more specific information about the particular knee condition. It is possible that more than one condition may be causing pain in that part of the knee. By reviewing the different injuries,

the athlete may be able to distinguish his or her particular problem. Once the problem is identified, some of the self-treatment recommendations can be implemented.

It is not always necessary to identify every specific condition, though, because the initial recommendations for self-care may be similar (see chapter 3). If there are serious questions as to the cause of the pain, and if it does not respond to initial attempts at self-treatment, professional help should be obtained. Because there is a significant overlap of symptoms in a number of sports-related conditions, it is difficult at times—even for a doctor who regularly treats these types of problems—to determine a specific diagnosis.

The descriptions of pain areas and the possible causes of pain in this chapter are intended only as guides and cannot possibly cover all the injuries that can occur (see Figures 2.1 through 2.18). Some conditions that may cause pain over a wide area of the body are not listed in this section. An example of this is sciatica, which comes from a pinched nerve and can cause pain and other symptoms from the lower back to the toes.

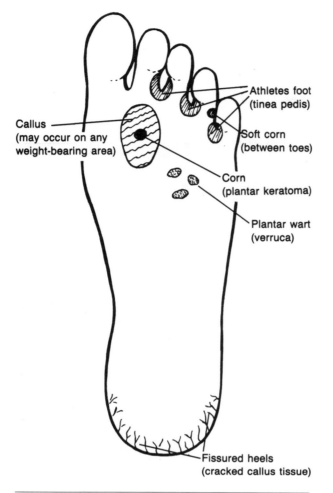

Figure 2.1   Skin changes on the bottom of the foot.

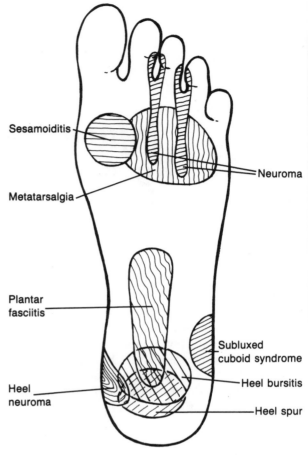

Figure 2.2   Deep pain areas on the bottom of the foot (plantar surface of foot).

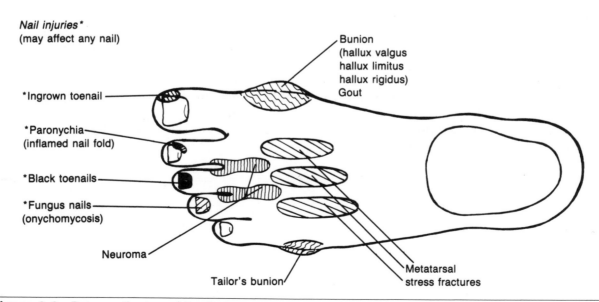

Figure 2.3   Pain on the top of the foot.

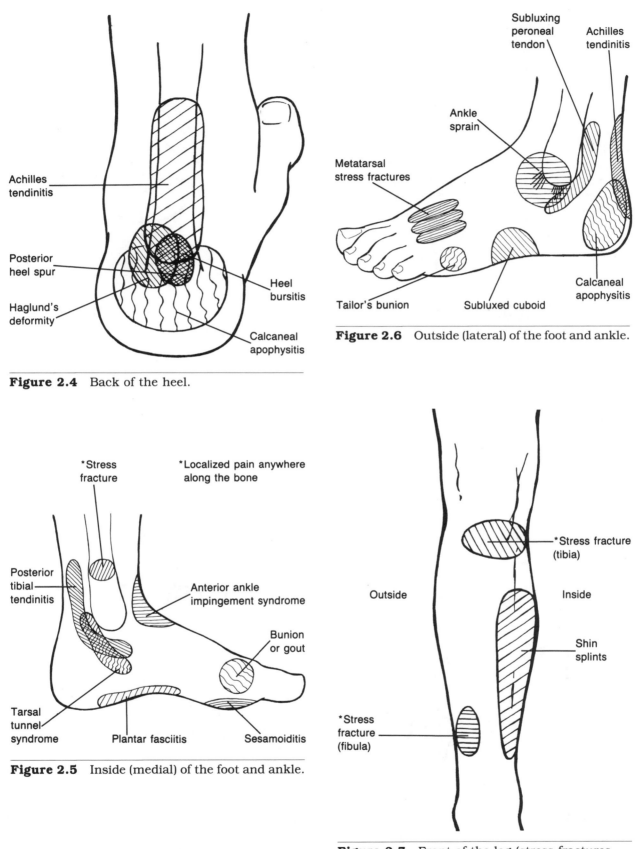

Figure 2.4   Back of the heel.

Figure 2.6   Outside (lateral) of the foot and ankle.

Figure 2.5   Inside (medial) of the foot and ankle.

Figure 2.7   Front of the leg (stress fractures may cause localized pain anywhere along the bone).

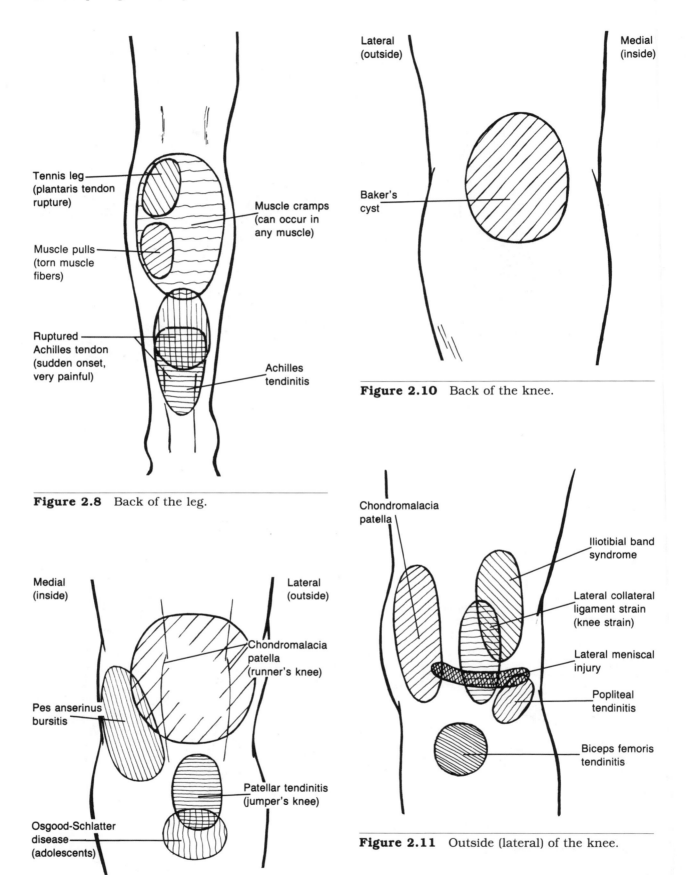

Figure 2.8   Back of the leg.

Tennis leg (plantaris tendon rupture)

Muscle cramps (can occur in any muscle)

Muscle pulls (torn muscle fibers)

Ruptured Achilles tendon (sudden onset, very painful)

Achilles tendinitis

Figure 2.10   Back of the knee.

Lateral (outside)

Medial (inside)

Baker's cyst

Figure 2.9   Front of the knee.

Medial (inside)

Lateral (outside)

Chondromalacia patella (runner's knee)

Pes anserinus bursitis

Patellar tendinitis (jumper's knee)

Osgood-Schlatter disease (adolescents)

Figure 2.11   Outside (lateral) of the knee.

Chondromalacia patella

Iliotibial band syndrome

Lateral collateral ligament strain (knee strain)

Lateral meniscal injury

Popliteal tendinitis

Biceps femoris tendinitis

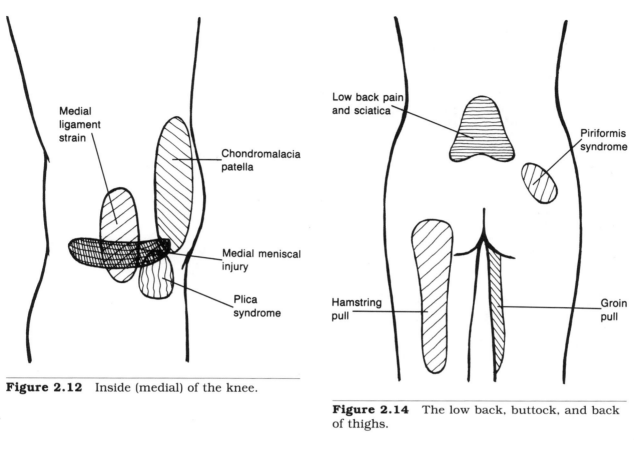

Figure 2.12 Inside (medial) of the knee.

Figure 2.14 The low back, buttock, and back of thighs.

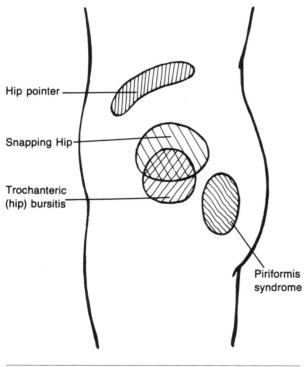

Figure 2.13 Outside of the hip and thigh.

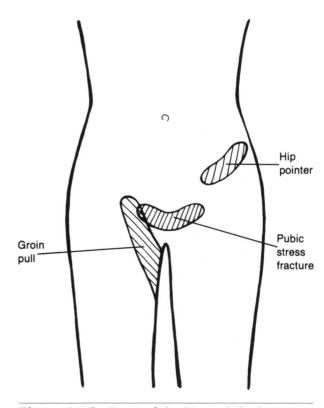

Figure 2.15 Front of the hip and thighs.

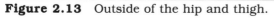

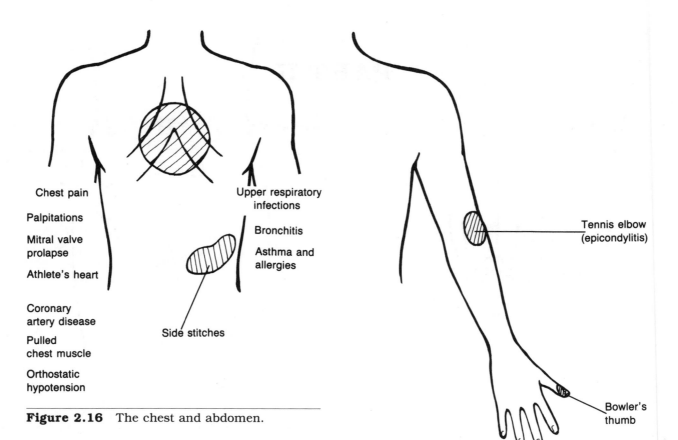

Chest pain

Palpitations

Mitral valve
prolapse

Athlete's heart

Coronary
artery disease

Pulled
chest muscle

Orthostatic
hypotension

Upper respiratory
infections

Bronchitis

Asthma and
allergies

Side stitches

Figure 2.16   The chest and abdomen.

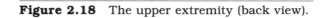

Tennis elbow
(epicondylitis)

Bowler's
thumb

Figure 2.18   The upper extremity (back view).

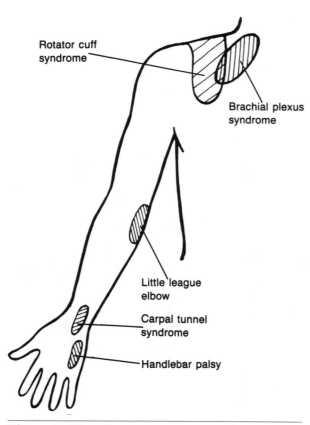

Rotator cuff
syndrome

Brachial plexus
syndrome

Little league
elbow

Carpal tunnel
syndrome

Handlebar palsy

Figure 2.17   The upper extremity (front view).

PART II
Treatment of Overuse Injuries

This part is designed to allow you to develop a self-treatment plan for specific injuries. It first gives a general overview of self-care principles (chapter 3), then details individual injuries (chapters 4 through 11). Before you try to treat a particular injury, you should have a firm understanding of the mechanisms of injuries and the effects of inflammation. Listening to your body and being able to interpret its changes provide you with the ability to recognize the early warning signs of overuse injuries. Exercises for both treating and preventing injuries are recommended in chapter 12.

CHAPTER 3

▬

Establishing a Self-Treatment Plan

Once the effects of inflammation are understood, a basic, three-step treatment plan can be initiated (see "Principles of Self-Care"). This basic plan can be applied to most overuse injuries. In fact, on reviewing the recommended treatments for specific injuries, note the recurrent themes that reflect this basic plan. Also included are methods that can be used at home, such as physical therapy and over-the-counter medications. You should become familiar with the general concepts in chapter 3 before proceeding to the information on specific injuries in chapters 4 to 11.

Principles of Self-Care

Paul M. Taylor, D.P.M.

Recognizing that it is impractical and costly to see a doctor for every minor injury, the athlete frequently finds it necessary to provide self-care. The injury chapters of this book provide information on treatment for specific problems, but it is also necessary to have an understanding of the basic principles that should be considered in self-treatment.

Of the two types of injuries an athlete can sustain, acute trauma and overuse syndrome, by far the most common is the overuse syndrome. The acute trauma usually requires immediate professional attention. By contrast, the overuse syndrome is not of sudden onset, but occurs because of repeated small traumas over a long period of time. This type of injury responds well to self-treatment; therefore, these are the injuries dealt with most in this text.

The athlete must become aware of developing injuries to prevent more serious problems. By listening to your body, treating injuries early, and learning to prevent further injury, you will become adept at self-diagnosis and treatment as well as when to seek professional help.

One aspect of the body's response to injury that must be understood is inflammation. Inflammation results in localized pain, heat, redness, and swelling. When inflammation is severe enough, it may also result in a loss of function. These changes may be minimal in a mild overuse syndrome or extensive in an acute trauma, such as a broken bone.

Recognizing the signs of inflammation is critical in learning how to become aware of developing injuries. Recognizing inflammatory changes early allows early treatment and prevents more serious injuries. Being able to recognize inflammatory changes is the first step in listening to your body. The second step is initiating treatment or preventive measures, as outlined in the "Treatment of Overuse Injuries" part of this book.

One other aspect of inflammation that should be understood is that it is a delayed reaction. It takes time for the body's chemical reactions to initiate the inflammatory changes,

so the signs of inflammation may not be seen until after the injury. This is especially true for overuse syndromes. This is why a runner may not have any pain while running but feels pain a few hours later or even the next morning. The initial tissue damage is occurring during the running, but the changes may not be felt until later. The inflammation may continue to build up for 24 to 48 hours afterward.

Realizing how the body responds to an injury allows determination of how treatment should be initiated. In an acute injury, the severity of the injury usually requires that physical activity be discontinued and immediate treatment rendered. In an obviously severe injury, such as a possible broken bone or a severe laceration, standard first aid should be administered, and immediate medical attention should be obtained (see chapter 17).

For the overuse type of injury, generally, self-care can be attempted. No matter what the overuse injury, a basic treatment plan can be utilized. The three steps in this basic treatment plan are:

1. Reduce or stop the stress causing the injury.
2. Reduce the inflammation and encourage the natural healing process.
3. Correct any factors that can contribute to reinjury.

When pain develops in a part of the body, usually it is caused by inflammation; the inflammation is due to excessive stress or overuse. This is the body's early warning system. The stress may be due to an old injury, to a biomechanical imbalance, or simply to overtraining.

To reduce the stress causing the injury, it may be necessary to reduce or stop activity. The reduction in the level of activity can be done in a number of ways. The level of pain and when it occurs can be used as a guide to determine how much the activity should be reduced. If the pain is severe, occurs at the start of exercise, and remains painful, the activity should be stopped completely. If the pain is present at the beginning of the activity but lessens and does not return until a few hours later, then the level of activity should be reduced by 50 percent until the pain subsides. If the pain does not reduce at this level, the activity should be engaged in only every other day. The reason for this is that inflammation sometimes continues for 24 to 48 hours after an activity; participating every other day gives inflammation time to subside before it is put under stress again. Once the pain has gone away, the level of activity can gradually be increased.

If there is only mild pain at the beginning of activity, and it is present only for a short time afterward, then it may be necessary to reduce the activity by only 15 to 20 percent. In some cases, in order to avoid losing any conditioning, the athlete may elect to substitute other aerobic activities to remove the stress from an injured part. For instance, a runner having knee pain may cut back on running to rest the knee, substituting swimming or biking to avoid any reduction in time spent in training.

In addition to reducing the stress by reducing the level of activity, it is also necessary to initiate step 2 in the basic treatment plan. This requires taking steps to reduce inflammation and encourage healing. This can include the use of ice or heat, whirlpool, and over-the-counter medications. These alternatives are discussed in detail in the "Home Physical Therapy" and medication sections of chapter 3. Suggestions on reducing inflammation are also offered in the individual injury sections.

The third step in the basic treatment plan is to correct any factors that can contribute to reinjury. Because there can be several potential factors involved, the actual trouble points are sometimes difficult to identify. One common problem in sports is the overdevelopment of certain muscle groups. All muscles work in pairs. An example of this is the quadriceps and the hamstrings in the thigh: The quadriceps extend the knee, whereas the hamstrings flex the knee. In many sports there is a greater de-

mand on the hamstrings; as a result, they become stronger and frequently tighter. This causes a relative weakness in the quadriceps and a muscle imbalance, which make the athlete prone to injury. The basic treatment plan should include a program of stretching the tight muscle groups and strengthening the weaker muscle groups.

Another factor that should be considered in evaluating injuries is biomechanical variation. This may include such things as a short leg, bowleg, curvature of the spine, or excessive foot pronation. Any structural malalignment in the body reduces its efficiency and makes it more prone to injury. It is possible to compensate for most of these problems through better shoes, wedges in the shoes, orthotic devices, exercise, or, on rare occasions, surgery.

There are also external biomechanical forces that can contribute to injuries. These can include running on one side of the road, where the surface is always canted in the same direction. This places more stress on one leg than the other. Running in the same direction all the time on a circular track has the same effect. This becomes more noticeable on a shorter track. Shoes that are excessively worn out also create abnormal mechanical forces on the lower extremities. Riding a bike with the seat adjusted improperly or using a bike that is the wrong size results in stress on various parts of the body. Playing basketball on an asphalt surface creates more stress on the feet and knees than playing on a wooden floor. Performing the same high-impact aerobic dance activity on a continual basis places repeated stress on certain parts of the body. If any of these biomechanical imbalances is severe enough, it can cause a recurring injury; it must be corrected.

The three steps in the basic treatment plan must be followed in order for the athlete to effectively self-treat the myriad of overuse syndromes to which he or she may be subjected.

Home Physical Therapy

Paul M. Taylor, D.P.M.

Physical therapy modalities, or treatments, are frequently used for sports-related injuries. Physical therapy utilizes physical agents such as light, heat, ice, diathermy, ultrasound, electrical stimulation, and mechanical techniques to treat injury or disease. For severe or acute injuries, supervision by a registered therapist may be necessary. However, for many overuse injuries, various modalities may be used easily and effectively in self-treatment at home.

Once the mechanism of an injury and the resultant inflammation are understood, many physical therapy modalities can be applied knowledgeably by the athlete. Proper application of these agents helps reduce inflammation, which promotes the healing process.

Generally, when an injury occurs, cold should be applied as soon as possible. Cold compresses reduce bleeding within the tissues and stop the swelling. This applies to both acute injuries and overuse syndromes. With an acute injury, such as an ankle sprain, physical activity should be stopped, and ice should be applied immediately. For an overuse injury, such as mild tendinitis, cold should also be used after the completion of the activity. With an overuse injury, it may not be necessary to discontinue the activity; reducing the length or intensity of the activity may be sufficient. In any injury, after the initial inflammation has subsided with rest and ice, the application of heat helps the body carry more blood to the area to remove injured tissue and to begin repairing the damage.

RICE

One of the primary principles in treating an injury is referred to as *RICE* (rest, ice, compression, and elevation). The immediate objective being the reduction of inflammation, RICE should be started as soon as possible after an injury. *Rest* is necessary to keep from making the injury worse from continual stress. The amount of rest is determined by the degree of the injury. A severe, acute injury requires complete rest, but a mild overuse syndrome may require only a slight reduction in activity.

Ice refers to applying cold to the injured area to reduce the inflammatory reaction. Ice can be used in a number of ways, which are described in conjunction with specific physical therapy modalities in the following pages.

Compression is the application of slight pressure to the injured area to limit swelling. Compression causes a slight constriction of blood vessels, reducing bleeding into the tissues and preventing fluid from building up in the interstitial areas (which would cause more swelling and slower healing). Various types of elastic bandages can be used for compression. When an elastic bandage is applied, it should be snug but not constrictive. The wrapping should start distal to the injured area and wind in a continuous, overlapping fashion to cover the injured site and end proximally (nearer the trunk of the body). This helps force fluids back to the main part of the body, reducing swelling in an injured arm or leg. Compression should not be applied too tightly. If there is any pain, swelling, numbness, or discoloration beyond the compression dressing, it should be loosened or removed. Elastic bandage use should be continued as long as there is swelling. If the swelling is localized to a small area, it may be difficult to obtain even compression; a piece of soft foam can be placed over the area, which is then wrapped with the elastic bandage.

Elevation is also utilized to reduce inflammation, especially its swelling. The injured extremity should be propped up on a couple of pillows so that the injured area is above the heart. When elevating a foot or ankle, pillows should be placed under the legs and knees so that the knee is supported. If pillows are placed under a foot without supporting the knee, the knee is hyperextended; after a while, the back of the knee may become sore.

After an acute injury, rest, ice, compression, and elevation should be continued until the swelling is reduced. RICE is the immediate treatment for any injury to a muscle, tendon, or joint. When an injury results in immediate pain, swelling, and loss of function, RICE should be initiated and medical consultation should be sought. RICE should be used even on minor injuries, for it usually allows a quicker return to activity. There is an old adage that ice is used for the first 24 hours, and then heat treatment is started. However, most medical practitioners now recommend that ice should continue to be used if the region is still swollen, tender, or warm to the touch.

RICE is used initially to stop the inflammatory response. Once this has been accomplished, it is necessary to change to heat treatment. Heat increases circulation to the area and aids in the removal of damaged tissue and the repair of the injury by the body. It also helps reduce some of the local stiffness that occurs after an injury. Heat should be applied for 20 to 30 minutes, three or four times a day. Elevation should be continued during this time.

Cold Therapy

Ice is the simplest, and possibly the best, form of cold therapy. Ice can be placed in an ice bag or plastic bag, which is then wrapped in a towel before application to an injured area. Cold packs, which are reusable, are also satisfactory. Chemical types of cold packs are acceptable when refrigeration is not available, but they are generally not as effective as ice and are much more expensive.

Another effective method for cold therapy is ice massage. A styrofoam cup filled with water is placed in the freezer. When the water is frozen, the top of the cup can be peeled off, leaving a small block of ice with a foam handle. The ice is then rubbed gently over the affected area for 5 to 6 minutes. This works well for the overuse injury; the ice massage can be applied to the injured area immediately after a workout.

Yet another method of cold therapy is effective for body parts that are irregularly shaped and make it difficult to apply ice evenly, such as hands or feet. This method consists of simply placing the hands or feet in a basin filled with cold water. Tap water generally is not cold enough, so it is necessary to add ice to the water. The temperature of the water should be between 55 and 65 degrees Fahrenheit.

Cold therapy should be done as soon as possible after activity. Cold should be applied for only 15 to 20 minutes at a time (unless the athlete is instructed otherwise by a therapist or doctor). When applying ice for this period of time, the region first feels cold, then usually becomes achy and stings slightly, and finally becomes numb.

Heat Therapy

Heat application is generally used after initial inflammation has been stopped with cold therapy. Applying heat causes a vasodilatation, the widening of blood vessels. This allows more blood into an area to help with removing the waste products of an injury and with healing. Heat can be used while you are resting an injury; it can also be applied to a tender area before exercise to aid in the warm-up and to reduce any tightness that may be present from a previous injury.

Application of heat therapy can easily be carried out at home. A heating pad is inexpensive and easy to use. The pad should be wrapped in a towel so that the pad is not in direct contact with the skin. The effect of the heat can be increased by using moist heat. This can be done by placing a moist towel under the heating pad. *CAUTION: This should be done only with heating pads designed to be used with moist heat.* Towels dipped in warm water can also be used to provide moist heat. However, the heat is lost quickly, and the towels must be dipped again every 4 or 5 minutes. For localized heat, warm water can be placed in an ice bag, with a towel wrapped around the bag. Local application of moist heat is effective in relieving muscle spasms and pain and in aiding the body's absorption of inflammatory products. For hands or feet, a basin of warm water can be used.

Chemical packs are also available for heat and are useful when other forms of heat are not available. However, they are more expensive, and not more effective, than heating pads or warm towels. Hydrocollator® packs are bags filled with gel that are heated in water and applied. These are effective, but because they are initially applied with a higher temperature, you should use them only after being given instructions by a therapist.

The greatest benefit from heat therapy comes when the temperature is warm, but not hot. Heating pads should be used on low or medium settings, and hot water should be between 98 and 105 degrees Fahrenheit; this is similar to a warm bath temperature. When heat is being used after an injury to help in healing, it should be applied for 20 to 30 minutes, two to three times a day. When it is being used to help increase mobility and reduce stiffness, it should be used for 5 to 10 minutes before exercising.

Contrast Baths

An alternating application of heat and cold is sometimes effective in relieving an inflammatory reaction. Two large basins or buckets are used, one filled with hot water at 95 to 100 degrees Fahrenheit, and the other with cold water at 55 to 65 degrees Fahrenheit. The injured area is submerged in the hot water for 1 or 2 minutes, and then in the cold water for 1 or 2 minutes. This is repeated several times, ending with an immersion in the cold water for 4 or 5 minutes. This should be done on a daily basis.

Whirlpool

Whirlpool treatment is effective in reducing inflammation because in addition to the benefits of heat, there is also the massage effect generated by the air-formed bubbles in the water. This helps to increase circulation in an injured area. Whirlpools are generally available at spas or health clubs. Someone with a chronic problem can purchase a small, relatively inexpensive unit for home use. Basins with vibrator units are available at even less cost, but true whirlpool or hydrotherapy units are more effective. Whirlpool therapy is used with a water temperature of 98 to 105 degrees Fahrenheit for 20 minutes. It should be done on a daily basis.

Massage

Massage is the manipulation of body tissues with the hands. It has effect on the nervous and muscular systems and on circulation. Massage is of positive value following an injury because it helps reduce adhesions between muscle fibers and assists in removing accumulations of fluid.

The use of massage is an instinctive behavior. When a part of the body, such as a muscle, has been injured, a person naturally rubs the most tender spot. This helps in relaxing the area and provides temporary relief.

This basic form of treatment can be expanded by self-administered massage or by having someone else provide massage. Massage therapy includes many different techniques that are specific for obtaining desired effects. Development of these techniques requires training and practice, but some basic massage can be done at home. Sylvia Klein Olkin (1983), in ''Massage for Runners'' in *Running and Fitness*, recommends the following techniques for self-foot massage and partner massage:

Self-Foot Massage

1. Sitting in a chair, place one of your feet on the opposite thigh. Rub a bit of massage oil—preferably almond or coconut oil—on your hand and apply the oil to the foot.
2. Using your thumbs, apply pressure as you work from the bottom of the arch to the top near the big toe. Repeat five times.
3. Make a fist and use your knuckles to move from the heel area to the toes. Repeat five times.
4. Squeeze the fleshy part of the sole of the foot together by intermeshing your fingers and squeezing the foot between them.
5. Hold all of the toes with one hand and bend them backward. Hold 5 to 10 seconds. Move the toes in the opposite direction. Hold. Repeat this sequence three times.
6. Concentrate on the three useful pressure points on the feet and ankles described below. By working these points, which are usually quite sensitive, you make your legs feel lighter and somewhat tingly.

Pressure point number 1 is located just below the ball, almost in the center, of the foot (Figure 3.1). The area is quite sensitive. It's also slightly hollowed, so your thumb should fit quite well. Massage this section with your thumb to relieve tension and induce relaxation and vitality. Using the pad of your thumb, apply moderate-to-firm pressure for 30 seconds.

Pressure point number 2 is located on the inside of the foot just below the bone of the big

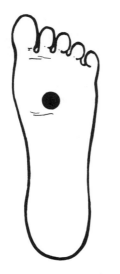

Figure 3.1 Massage pressure point on the ball of the foot.

toe (Figure 3.2). Use the pad of the thumb to massage in a circular motion for 30 seconds.

Pressure point number 3 is located four fingers up from the ankle bone on the calf area of the leg. Place your left hand on your right ankle; using the thumb pad, press in behind your bone and next to where your fingers end (Figure 3.2). Keep massaging until this area feels warm, relaxed, and less sensitive.

These pressure points can be massaged simultaneously for beneficial results.

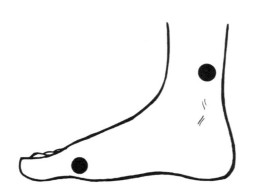

Figure 3.2 Massage pressure points on the side of the foot and ankle.

Partner Massage

Although self-massage is a fine way to learn more about your body and how to make it looser and more comfortable, it pales quickly once you have experienced partner massage.

Following the massage techniques outlined below, you, too, can come to the aid of a fellow athlete and can perhaps teach a friend how to do massage for you.

- Choose a warm, quiet place.
- Massage on a carpeted floor on which you place a blanket, with an old sheet on top in case you spill some oil. If a massage table is available, it is more comfortable for both giver and receiver.
- Massage is most comfortable when the giver uses warmed oil for lubrication. The oil helps the hands apply pressure while they glide over the portion of the body being massaged. Keep an old washcloth handy to eliminate excess oil from hands or body. Never pour oil directly on the body; rub it onto your hands first.
- The person receiving the massage should be nude. Keep a sheet or light blanket handy in case of coolness during the massage.
- Make sure your nails are short, in order to avoid hurting your partner. Be sure he or she removes all jewelry and contact lenses.
- When using different strokes, try to glide from one to another as smoothly as you can. It is best to massage toward the heart.
- Try to mold your hands to your partner's body contours.
- Vary the speed and pressure of your strokes, but do so smoothly.
- The person receiving the massage should be passive and should not try to help during the massage.
- Centering and tuning in to the sensations of being stroked should be the receiver's main concern.
- If massage is done for too long a time, in an irregular pattern, or without lubrication, you could actually make your partner more tense—so, take care.

Athletes are prone to various muscle injuries and general fatigue after activity. Runners frequently develop soreness in the calves and thighs; racquet sports may cause soreness in arms and shoulders; and with football players, almost any muscle group may be stressed or bruised. The use of massage by a partner provides relief of symptoms and assists healing.

When giving massage, you should follow the guidelines described above. When massaging an area, direct the stroking motion toward the heart. Massage should be carried out with smooth, gentle stroking. You should start massage distally, completing the massage for a part of the body, then moving up to the next part of the body. For instance, starting with the foot, you should progress to the leg, and then to the thigh and buttocks. In the larger muscles, if there are any tender areas, the ball of the thumb can be used to apply more localized pressure to loosen up the muscle, but not to the point of causing pain. This same form of thumb pressure can be used in massaging the small muscles on the soles of the feet.

Massage can be applied over the entire body for relaxation and generalized muscle soreness, or it can be applied only to a localized injured area.

Allow your partner to lie still for a few minutes when you finish the massage. Try to be quiet to give him or her time to rouse and slowly get up.

The time and effort you spend giving a massage is well worth the effect: The athlete feels loose, limber, and balanced—and owes you one future therapeutic massage.

Summary

RICE, cold therapy, heat therapy, contrast baths, whirlpool, and massage are all forms of physical therapy that can be provided at home. As an athlete becomes more attuned to his or her body, recognizes some of the early warning signs of injury, and takes early action in treating these injuries, the continued participation in sports is assured, and favorite activities become more enjoyable. Once an athlete understands the mechanisms of an injury and the principles of self-treatment, the treatments recommended in the chapters on individual injuries are much easier to follow. The use of the home physical therapy is frequently recommended in treating many sports-related injuries.

Suggested Reading for "Home Physical Therapy"

Apple (1984)

Basmajian (1984)

Birnbaum (1982)

Block (1982)

Cole (1980)

Gould & Davies (1985)

Kessler & Hertling (1983)

Kiester (1985)

Krusen et al. (1966)

MacLellan & Vyvyan (1981)

Olkin (1983)

Piper & Baxter (1983)

Roberson & Roberson (1984)

Roy & Irvin (1983)

Sheehan (1983)

Southmayd & Hoffman (1981)

Strauss (1984)

Titus (1984)

Wasco (1983)

Wilkerson (1985a, 1985b)

See reading list at the end of the book for a complete source listing.

Over-the-Counter Drugs Commonly Used by Athletes

Richard L. Jones, M.D.

Americans are virtually unaware that only in the last 25 years have over-the-counter (OTC) drugs been required to be both safe and effective. During this quarter century, drug manufacturers have spent billions of dollars developing, marketing, and advertising a bewildering array of OTC medications, with varieties of ingredients that a Federal Drug Administration (FDA) composite report in 1983 concluded contained chemicals only one-third of which are safe and effective. In other words, it took the FDA 21 years (1962–1983) to review OTC drugs and provide some guidelines for their use by the general public. Yet, in the mid-1980s consumers still face the likelihood that in two out of three cases, the OTC drug they buy will not fulfill its prescribed purpose both safely *and* effectively.

Athletes, who are as likely as anyone (or in some cases more likely) to use OTC drugs for self-treatment, should ponder this reality. The potential for *harm* from an OTC drug may be significant, either from the basic action of its ingredients or through a drug interaction.

The 1,249 medically active ingredients used in the over 300,000 brand name OTC products available in the United States have received at least a preliminary review by 1 of the 17 FDA Advisory and Review Panels. The results of these ongoing reviews and evaluations have been published as a catalogue of medically active ingredients in the *Federal Register*, as well as in various books (see reading list). This catalogue has served as the basis for this article's selective review of the OTC drugs that athletes, both weekend and competitive ones, are most likely to use.

Before we discuss some of the OTC drugs athletes may use during illnesses for symptom relief, some guidelines should be remembered (see Table 3.1).

Table 3.1   Guidelines for Taking Over-the-Counter (OTC) Medication

Do	Don't
• Read the label of *any* drug or preparation to be used. Are you allergic to any of its ingredients? Do any of them interact adversely with drugs you already are taking? What are the ingredients' side effects? • Determine whether any ingredient of the drug is contraindicated because of its effect on a congenital, acquired, or chronic illness or disease you have. • Determine whether any ingredient of the drug is banned from use by the NCAA, USOC, or IOC. • Take the OTC in dosages indicated in the directions. Try to use individual, rather than combination, medications. • Contact a sportsmedicine physician whenever symptoms are prolonged or potentially OTC-related side effects occur. • Avoid OTCs that do not list active ingredients.	• Don't exercise vigorously (especially endurance activities) while affected with a presumed viral infection. Such exercise may worsen and/or prolong the illness. • Don't use dosages in excess of those recommended on the packaging. • Don't use multiple medications without checking for drug interactions. • Don't use any medication if you are pregnant or nursing a baby.

Table 3.2   Cough, Cold, Allergy, and Sinus Medications

Drug type and action	Ingredients
Nasal decongestants Reduce nasal and oral mucosal swelling and mucous production. Overuse may produce *rebound worsening* of symptoms when medication is stopped.	*Oral*: (Generally judged safe and effective) Phenylephrine Phenylpropanolamines Pseudoephedrines *Topical*: Ephedrines Naphazoline *Inhaled*: Propylhexedrine (Vitamin C has not been proven effective.)
Expectorants Reduce the thickness of nasal and bronchial secretions. Soothing action *may* help reduce coughing; are *not* cough suppressants, however.	(*None are judged both safe and effective.* They are generally safe, but of uncertain effectiveness.) *Oral*: Guaifenesin Terpin hydrate Ipecac syrup, creosote, potassium guaiiacol-sulfonate, menthol, ammonium chloride, pine tar, and benzoin products *Inhalants*: Turpentine oil Camphor
Antihistamines Reduce stuffiness, sneezing, itchy eyes associated with an allergy.	*Oral*: Brompheniramine Chlorpheniramine Pheniramine Pyrilamine and thonzygamine Diphenhydramine and doxylamine Phenindamine
Cough suppressants Suppress impulse to cough by affecting the cough center in the brain.	*Oral*: Dextromethorphan Diphenhydramine Codeine (prescription) (*All other* oral and inhaled cough suppressants are either unsafe and/or ineffective.)
Anticholenergics **Catropine/belladonna** **Alkaloids** Reduce eye, nasal, and oral secretions associated with colds and allergies.	None considered safe at effective dosages.
Aspirin/acetaminophen Relief of headache and/or malaise.	Combination products may be safe in general. Use of aspirin with some viral diseases may increase the risk of Reye's syndrome.
Caffeine Included in allergy and cold remedies to counteract sedation antihistamines may cause. Safe, but of questionable value.	
Alcohol Used as a solvent. Concentration varies from 1–42%. May interact, or produce sedation when used, with sedatives, hypnotics, antidepressants.	

Medications for Allergies, Asthma, Colds, Coughs, and Sinusitis

The athlete is *more* susceptible to viral diseases of *all* sorts, compared to the nonathlete. In fact, the more "tuned," or conditioned, the athlete is, the more vulnerable he or she may be to viral agents that can infect the respiratory or gastrointestinal tracts, for example.

Differentiating colds from allergy-induced diseases is crucial because OTC drugs containing antihistamines do not reduce viral-induced nasal congestion, whereas the allergically swollen congested nose doesn't respond to a simple decongestant.

Table 3.2 lists the common safe and effective OTC ingredients by their drug action. All OTC cough, cold, and allergy preparations contain some (or all) of these types of drugs. Listed dosages of most of these compounds are standard. Over 200 individual or combination ingredient products are presently available.

In general, viral-induced colds/bronchitis last 3 to 10 days. Recurrent nasal and respiratory symptoms—especially if associated with itchy eyes, sinus congestion, or wheezing (with or without cough)—may more likely be allergic in origin. The athlete with allergies and/or asthma should be careful in the choice and dosage of antihistamines, because asthma (e.g., reactive airway disease) may be worsened by such treatment.

Medications for Fever; Pain; and Joint, Muscle, Nerve, and Soft Tissue Inflammation

OTC drugs marketed for the relief of pain, inflammation (of various types), and fever fall into three categories: aspirin and other salicylates; acetaminophen and related compounds; and nonsteroidal anti-inflammatory agents (NSAIAs), most of which are presently prescription drugs (see Table 3.3).

Salicylates and NSAIAs produce their effects by suppressing the actions of prostaglandins, a group of naturally occurring hormones that

Table 3.3   Analgesic, Anti-Inflammatory, and Antipuretic Medications

Drug type and action	Side effects and drug interactions
Aspirin and other salicylates Suppress production of hormones called prostaglandins, resulting in analgesia in soft tissues, muscles, nerves, bursae, and joints. Also reduce fever by increasing heat loss from body. Reduce joint, muscle, and bursa inflammation.	• 1 in 20 users gets gastric irritation (worsened by alcohol). • Salicylate sensitivity is an allergy seen in 1% of the general population and 20% of asthmatics. • May cause active bleeding (internal), especially if used with anticoagulants. • May cause low blood sugar. • Overdosage can occur. • Associated with risk of Reye's syndrome.
Acetaminophen, Phenacetin Both drugs have analgesic and antipyretic effects similar to aspirin, but by different drug actions. *Neither* has anti-inflammatory effects.	• Both appear less toxic than aspirin in producing gastric irritation, allergic reactions, and bleeding. • Overdoses have occurred. Can produce liver, kidney, and brain damage. Deaths have occurred with massive overdoses. • Phenacetin used regularly has been linked to urinary tract cancers and disorders. Use in OTCs continuing pending final FDA decision.
Nonsteroidal anti-inflammatory agents (NSAIAs), Ibuprofen Have analgesic and anti-inflammatory effects. Mechanism of action similar to salicylates.	• Ibuprofen use has occasionally been associated with abdominal pain, gastritis, nonallergic skin rashes, fluid retention, dizziness, and, rarely, other side effects. • The OTC preparations may be more expensive milligram for milligram than the prescription product.

are involved in many body processes, including the responses to infection and tissue injury. Aspirin, a salicylate, is probably the most used and abused OTC medication. It is a *non*-prescription drug *only* because it was so widely used by so many people before effective regulation of drugs began. Although its uses are many and varied, allergic and asthmatic persons as well as those at risk for gastritis and peptic ulcers clearly should consult their physicians before using salicylates.

For adolescents and adults, total 24-hour doses shouldn't exceed 4 grams divided into 4- to 6-hour intervals, with effective single doses between 325 and 650 milligrams. Salicylate therapy should not be continued for more than 7 to 10 days (5 for children) without a physician's advice being sought.

When fever and/or pain is the symptom the p-aminophenols, acetaminophen and phenacetin (see Table 3.3), are acceptable alternatives to salicylates. Neither has anti-inflammatory activity, however, and is thus not useful in conditions associated with soft tissue, muscle, or joint injury. Side effects are less common, especially in allergic/asthmatic persons, those with stomach or gastrointestinal problems, and persons who drink excessively. However, phenacetin can produce an anemia in individuals with an inherited disease called glucose-6-phosphate-dehydrogenase (G-6-PD) deficiency. This genetic disease is seen in 15 percent of American blacks, who may become severely anemic when exposed to phenacetin or related compounds.

Dosage guidelines for acetaminophen are similar to those for aspirin, with a recommended maximum 24-hour dosage of 3.9 grams divided into 4- to 6-hour intervals, with individual dosages of 325 to 650 milligrams.

Nonsteroidal anti-inflammatory agents (NSAIAs) have only recently become available without prescriptions. This has occurred only because the Upjohn Company's license for ibuprofen, the only NSAIA now available over the counter, expired. The explosion in sports participation among adults of all ages, combined with concern regarding aspirin products, has led to the accelerated marketing of OTC ibuprofen. At present, several OTC ibuprofen products—among them, Advil®, Nuprin®, Medipren®, Ibuprin®, and many generics—compete with Upjohn's prescription Motrin® and generic prescription equivalents.

Dosages vary widely between the OTC and prescription products; the prescription product is sometimes less expensive (not counting the visit to the physician).

In the future, other NSAIAs will doubtless become available without prescription. This group of drugs may become more frequently prescribed and consumed than the salicylates and acetaminophen.

Medications for Motion Sickness and Stomach Upset (Antiemetics)

Motion sickness alone may be treated with OTC drugs. Although antiemetics (see Table 3.4) may curtail nausea and vomiting, these symptoms may indicate serious diseases—such as urinary or digestive tract disorders, brain injury or infection, appendicitis—or reactions to such prescribed drugs as antibiotics and steroids. A physician's advice should be obtained if there is any likelihood of an underlying disease.

Table 3.4   A Selected List of Medications for Motion Sickness

Active ingredient	Adult dosage	Common brand name
Cyclizine hydrochloride	50 mg every 4–6 hr	Marezine®
Meclizine hydrochloride	25–50 mg 30 min before trip	Anti-vert® Bonine® Lamine®
Dimenhydrinate	50–100 mg every 4–6 hr, not to exceed 400 mg in 24 hr	Dramamine® Dimentabs® Dipendrate® Eldodran® Marmine®

Cyclizine, meclizine, and dimenhydrinate have all been recognized as generally safe and effective for the relief of nausea and vomiting. These compounds all can produce sedation (especially if taken with alcohol, sedatives, or tranquilizers), can worsen glaucoma or prostatic enlargement, and are contraindicated with pregnancy.

Antidiarrheal Medications

Athletes, especially competitive ones, are frequently exposed to situations, settings, infectious agents, and foods that may trigger severe, crampy diarrhea of limited duration. Treatment of such diarrheas may be indicated, especially if competition is to occur in the immediate future. Although diarrhea can herald significant infectious, toxic, immunological, metabolic, or surgical conditions, self-treatment may be reasonable if the diarrhea is of sudden onset; is without blood; is associated with variable degrees of cramping pain, nausea, vomiting, and anorexia, but no fever; and if self-treatment is limited to a maximum of 2 or 3 days.

Avoiding solid foods, combined with drinking only clear liquids and soups to compensate for fluid loss, may be all that is necessary. Using OTC medications can moderate the symptoms while the body's own mechanisms correct or eliminate the cause. In treating diarrhea and associated symptoms, remember to avoid tobacco, caffeine, and alcohol.

Choose an antidiarrheal product containing a maximum of two medically active agents, if narcotic agents like paregoric or lomotil are unavailable (Table 3.5). Antidiarrheals principally contain some combination of adsorbents, anticholinergics, and astringents. Other agents, such as certain antacids (containing calcium carbonate), bulk-forming compounds (carboxymethylcellulose), and the bacteria *Lactobacillus acidophilus* and *bulgaricus*, are thought to have antidiarrheal actions.

Adsorbents are thought (but not proven) to bind or absorb the excess water associated with diarrhea, along with toxins or viruses that cause the diarrhea, thus producing solid stools. Commonly used adsorbents include aluminum magnesium silicate, charcoal, kaolin, and pectin.

Anticholinergics, such as atropine sulfate, homatropine methylbromide, and hyoscyamine sulfate, are generally safe and effective in reducing diarrhea. However, effective doses (0.6 to 1.0 milligram) are *not* available over the counter, but are had only by prescription. Avoiding OTC agents containing anticholinergics is probably best.

Astringents are thought to alleviate diarrhea by protein precipitation in the bowel. Astringents include alumina powder, calcium hy-

Table 3.5   Antidiarrheal Medications

A combination of the following may be used to treat diarrhea

Drug activity	Chemical or generic name
Adsorbents	Aluminum magnesium silicate Charcoal Kaolin Pectin Polycarbophil
Anticholinergics	Atropine sulfate Homatropine methylbromide Hyoscyamine sulfate
Astringents	Alumina powder Calcium hydroxide Zinc phenolsulfonate Bismuth salts
Antacids	Calcium carbonate Carboxymethylcellulose *Lactobacillus acidophilis* *Lactobacillus bulgaricus*
Opiates[a]	Opium powder Tincture of opium Paregoric

[a]Require a prescription in most states; when available OTC, dosage may be too low to be effective.

droxide, zinc phenolsulfonate, and bismuth salts.

Reasonable antidiarrhea combinations include the following: aluminum hydroxysilicate and pectin; kaolin and pectin; carboxymethylcellulose and *L. acidophilus*; and kaolin and hydrated alumina powder.

Medications for Corns, Calluses, and Warts

Corns, calluses, and warts are usually caused by excessive friction, pressure, moisture, or a combination of these, induced by overuse and/or abnormal- (tight-) fitting clothing or shoes. Self-treatment of these various skin problems is warranted if they are not widespread, not associated with any existing systemic disease, are of recent onset, and if self-treatment is limited to a month or less, after which medical help should be sought.

Keratolytic agents, such as salicylic acid, pantothenic acid, zinc chloride, and acetic and lactic acids, destroy tissue, resulting in shedding and peeling. Excessive use or use on normal skin may cause irritation and infection. Other agents may be used as lubricants (castor oil or petrolatum), local anesthetics to reduce pain, or astringents to help in the removal of dead skin (thymol, camphor, and methyl salicylate). For more information, see "Corns, Calluses, and Warts" in chapter 4.

Medication for Athlete's Foot

Athlete's foot, a fungus infection on the feet, is common to athletes, whose feet perspire heavily and are more exposed to contact with the fungus in showers and locker rooms. There are many OTC medications available to treat athlete's foot (Table 3.6). For more information on athlete's foot, see chapter 4.

Table 3.6 Common Medications in Over-the-Counter (OTC) Athlete's Foot Preparations

Chemical or generic name	Brand name
Boric acid, potassium alum, menthol, thymol	BFI Powder®
Iodochlorhydroxyquin 3%	Vioform®
Tolnaftate	Aftate® Tinactin®
Undecylenic acid, zinc undecylenate	Desenex®
Sodium propionate, sodium caprylate	Sopronol®
Triacetin	Enzactin® Fungacetin®
Miconazole	Micatin®

Medications for Sunburn

Athletic activity outdoors can frequently lead to sunburn. Although the best treatment is prevention (see "Sunburn" in chapter 17), when a sunburn does occur, there are various OTC medications that can help. Many sunburn sprays contain a topical anesthetic, such as benzocaine, and may provide temporary relief of the burning sensation. Care should be exercised, though, because some people find that these sprays irritate their skin. Topical steroids (cortisone) can also be used to help reduce the inflammation. Moisturizers are also helpful in preventing the skin from drying excessively. Probably the simplest method of treating sunburn is by taking a cool bath.

Summary

The variety of OTC medications available is enormous. Their selective use is warranted in treating certain medical conditions that can adversely affect athletic performance.

You should keep in mind, however, that self-treatment may be harmful if the symptoms treated reflect a serious disease that goes undiagnosed because the symptoms have been relieved. Remember, too, that OTC medications themselves can be dangerous. Always consider seeking the advice of others, including sportsmedicine personnel, when you use OTC drugs.

Suggested Reading for "Over-the-Counter Drugs Commonly Used by Athletes"

Benowicz (1979)

Graedon & Graedon (1985)

See reading list at the end of the book for a complete source listing.

CHAPTER 4

▬▬

Foot Injuries

In most fitness activities, there is continual shock from the legs propelling the body back and forth over the activity surface, often with sharp cuts from side to side and great leaps and landings. The foot, the usual interface between the earth and the moving body, absorbs much of the impact and other stress from movement; it also plays a crucial role itself in propulsion. However, it is vulnerable to a myriad of injuries to many different tissues and parts, from many causes. This chapter discusses a number of foot problems the athlete may encounter.

Ingrown Toenails

Ayne F. Furman, D.P.M.

An ingrown toenail occurs when the sides or borders of any toenail, usually the big toe, curve into the flesh; when flesh is forced up around a nail; or a combination of both (Figure 4.1). This condition is usually accompanied by sharp pain. For some people the nail is bothered only in snug shoes or when knocked or stepped on; for others it is so painful they cannot let even bedsheets rest on the affected toes. If neglected, an ingrown toenail can cause the toe itself to become infected. Signs of infection generally include extreme pain and redness, and frequently pus is seen seeping out around the edge of the nail. If infection occurs, immediate professional attention is needed.

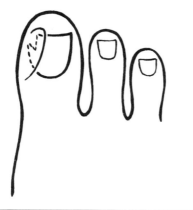

Figure 4.1   Ingrown toenail.

There are several causes of ingrown toenails, among them heredity, foot deformities, trauma, and types of shoes worn. Not only does heredity determine such things as eye color, but it also helps determine the kinds of foot problems persons develop. In the case of toes, some people are simply born with wide nails surrounded by excessive flesh. For such people, shoe wear is a real problem unless they have their wide nails permanently corrected. Foot deformities, such as bunions, can cause the big toe to rotate on its side; this pushes the toe tissue up around the nail, forcing the nail edge into the flesh.

A missed fly ball landing on a toenail, playing kick ball, a stubbed toe, and similar events all can cause trauma to a toenail. Weeks or months after all pain is forgotten from the incident, an ingrown nail may develop. This is due to the earlier trauma that deformed the nail and its matrix (the area beneath the skin behind the cuticle from which the nail grows).

The most easily remedied cause of ingrown toenails is the types of shoes worn. Wearing narrow shoes or shoes that are too small and compress the toe tissue and toenails can cause ingrown nails to develop. To see the amount of compression imposed on the toes, make a foot tracing while standing up. Then place your shoe over the tracing and graphically see how the toes' outline hangs over the edges of the shoe. This is especially evident with fashionable high heels and biking cleats, both traditionally narrow shoes.

When an ingrown nail is neglected and continually insulted by tight shoe wear, an infected toe may develop. The formation of the infection comes from continual pressure of the nail border on the surrounding tissue. This pressure causes a decrease in blood supply to the area under the nail border and encourages tissue breakdown, which is followed by the entry of bacteria.

The worst treatment for ingrown toenails is home surgery, especially when the nail is clipped back as far as possible. This form of treatment tends to create a ledge or spicule along the nail border, which snags the tissue as it grows. Each time the nail border is clipped, the ingrown nail is actually made worse. Another popular home treatment, which is a myth, says that by cutting a "v" in the center of the tip of the nail, pressure will be relieved. This simply does not work, because the nail grows from the matrix out. Self-treatment can be tried, but never by persons who suffer from diabetes or peripheral vascular disease, or who have decreased nerve sensation in the feet. For people with these diseases, self-treatment is dangerous and can lead to ulceration and gangrene very quickly.

Proper self-treatment procedure for mildly ingrown or infected toenails consists of the following steps:

1. Cleanse the toe and nail clippers with 70 percent isopropyl alcohol.
2. Clip off a small portion of the offending nail at the edge of the toe.
3. Soak the foot in epsom salts (2 tablespoons to 1 quart of warm water) for 7 to 10 minutes, twice a day for 3 to 5 days.
4. Apply an antibiotic ointment, such as Bacitracin® or Neosporin®, and wear a Band-Aid®.
5. Wear wide shoes.
6. If pain is not relieved, or if infection develops, seek podiatric care.

Professional treatment is usually geared toward permanent correction via a minor surgical procedure. During this procedure the toe is first numbed with a local anesthetic, usually lidocaine. Lidocaine injection takes place at the base of the toe—not around the nail itself, due to the configuration of the nerves going to the toe. The toe is then usually scrubbed with Betadine®, a type of skin disinfectant, to decrease the risk of infection after the surgery. A small portion of the entire ingrown nail border is then removed back to the matrix. Next, the area is inspected for any signs of infection, which, if present, are then removed.

If the toe was infected, the procedure sometimes stops at this point.

For permanent correction, the nail-producing cells of the matrix must be destroyed. This is done by applying phenol, a strong acid, to the nail matrix. The area is then flushed with alcohol. Some podiatrists use lasers instead of phenol to kill matrix cells. Both methods are completely painless once the toe is numbed, and neither requires stitches. The postoperative site needs to be kept clean via soaks and/or applications of antibiotic ointments or solutions for several weeks.

Pain following a permanent nail correction procedure should be minimal, as long as the foot is elevated after the surgery for several hours. Normally, only aspirin or Tylenol® needs to be taken for the discomfort, if any pain is even felt at all. Usually little or no work has to be missed. Activities such as running and biking can usually be resumed 2 to 5 days after surgery. Wearing pointed shoes or biking cleats, or playing sports (especially soccer, in which the toe easily can be hit) can be uncomfortable for a couple of weeks.

Although prevention is not always possible for some causes of ingrown nails, one can never go wrong cutting toenails straight across, wearing shoes that fit and feel comfortable, and buying the right size of shoes (shoes should be bought at the end of the day, because feet swell during the day and usually measure larger later in the day than in the morning). Always seek professional podiatric care, rather than perform your own surgery.

Black Toenails

Paul M. Taylor, D.P.M.

Black toenails are a common malady among athletes. It is not unusual for a runner to return from a workout, take off the shoes and socks, and find blackened toes—even when no pain was felt during the run. This condition occurs because of pressure on the nail and nail bed, causing a blood blister or blood clot (hematoma) to develop under the nail. There are two types of black toenails.

Acute Black Toenail

The acute form happens suddenly, usually from stubbing the toe or having it stepped on. This can result in bleeding under the nail, with red or blue discoloration and severe pain from the increased pressure. The nail turns black within 12 to 24 hours. If you stub the toe with so much momentum that you tear the nail away, contact your podiatrist immediately.

Chronic Black Toenail

The most common reason runners develop a black toenail is chronic irritation of the nail. Tight socks, short shoes, running downhill, and wearing loose shoes (so that when your foot should stop, inertia keeps it going forward and jams it into the front of your shoe) cause chronic black toenails. This repeated microtrauma causes only a slight amount of bleeding and minimal pressure buildup; thus, minimal or no pain is felt. Occasionally, runners do not realize this is happening until they notice the discolored nail. Yet, if the condition persists, the nail gradually becomes thicker.

Treatment

An acute black toenail should be treated as soon after the injury as possible to prevent loosening or loss of the nail. If the blood is not released spontaneously, it has to be drained. To do this, hold an opened paper clip with a pair of pliers. Heat its end with a match and touch the top of the nail with the heated clip. (This procedure is not painful.) This quickly melts through the nail, releasing the blood. It may be necessary to make two holes to drain the nail completely. You do not need to worry about burning the tender skin under the nail; blood beneath the nail quickly cools the clip. After gently compressing the nail to stimulate drainage, apply an antiseptic and a dry gauze dressing. If this treatment does not give relief, or if the nail is completely torn away from the foot, get professional help. Do not run with a ruptured, untreated toenail.

A chronic black toenail does not need to be drained, because there is no significant accumulation of blood under it. By eliminating the cause of irritation, a new nail gradually forms, pushing out the damaged nail. This requires patience, because it takes 6 to 9 months for a new nail to grow. If the nail becomes thick, file it down.

Prevention

Acute injury to the nail is usually unavoidable, for it occurs by accident. Early treatment, however, can reduce the chances of permanent nail damage.

Chronic black toenails, however, can be prevented. Buy socks that are about ½ inch longer than your longest toe. Avoid tube socks, which generally do not fit well. Never wear socks that restrict the movement of your foot. When buying a running shoe, make sure your fit is perfect. Do not count on the shoes to stretch with wear. Make sure that each shoe bends at the ball of the foot and that you can "pinch" material at the toe. There should be a finger's width of extra space at the toe of the shoe, your toes should be able to wiggle freely, and your heel should fit snugly. Do not be afraid to try on half a dozen or more shoes before deciding which pair to buy. If you have a black toenail, check your running shoes to be sure that there are no seams in front of the shoe that are irritating the toe or nail and, if you have leather uppers, that the leather is not stiff and cracked.

Always keep your nails properly clipped. Cut them to their natural shape—do not round them as you would fingernails. Let your nails extend to the end of your toes. Do not cut them so short as to expose tender skin or let them extend past your toes, which increases the likelihood of injury and irritation to the nail.

Professional Treatment

Acute or chronic black toenails often can be treated at home. However, if a nail is severely torn or off the toe, or if infection or swelling occurs, contact a podiatrist. Also, seek help if you are diabetic, have an unsteady hand, or have circulatory problems. A podiatrist can painlessly treat your nail so you will soon be running again without pain.

Fungus Nails (Onychomycosis)

Paul M. Taylor, D.P.M.

Onychomycosis is a thickening, discoloration, and softness of the nails caused by a fungus infection. The problem fungus is a microscopic organism that invades the nail bed and nail plate and causes a gradual destruction of the nail. The fungus may be of the same type that causes athlete's foot.

In order for onychomycosis to develop, the nail must first be injured, allowing the organism to enter under the nail. There may be no pain associated with this, and the development of the mycotic nail is very gradual. Initially only a small area of discoloration may be noted, which over a period of several months or years can gradually expand to envelop the entire nail. Because the athlete is prone to injure nails and is frequently being exposed to the fungus in showers or gyms, the incidence of this problem in athletes is high.

This condition may appear similar to runner's nails (see "Thick Toe Nails"), which are also thickened, but only from trauma. A nail injured frequently has an increased chance of fungus invasion with development of the onychomycosis. It is the actual presence of the fungal organism that differentiates this condition. It is also the presence of the fungus that makes this a more difficult condition to treat. As the condition progresses, a soft material builds up under the nail, causing increased discoloration, thickening, and an odor from the nail. Mycotic nails are more common on the toenails, but they can develop on the fingernails as well.

Treatment of onychomycosis is most effective if the condition is recognized early. Professional treatment is necessary, because most over-the-counter antifungal medications cannot penetrate the nail plate to reach the organism. Treatment for this condition can still be very difficult. If the nail is not completely involved, treatment can include trimming back the infected portion of the nail, applying an antifungal agent daily, and scrubbing the nails with an antiseptic soap, which may allow a healthy nail to grow. If the major portion of the nail is involved, the nail plate may have to be removed surgically. Then the above topical treatment is carried out. Recently the use of a laser has been recommended to treat the nail bed after the nail plate has been removed. This is an attempt to destroy the fungal elements on the nail bed. The long-term results of laser treatment have not yet been determined.

Oral medication is available to treat the fungus, but it is necessary to take the medication until a new healthy nail grows out completely. For toenails, this could require having to take the oral antifungal medications for 12 to 18 months, and there is no guarantee that this will resolve the problem. Also, being on the medication for such a long period of time requires frequent blood tests to rule out the onset of any adverse side effects. Because of the potential problems with the oral medication, the decision to start this mode of therapy should be discussed in detail with your doctor beforehand.

Because fungus nails are so difficult to treat, preventive measures should be taken. This is especially true for persons who are at high risk, including athletes who have nails that are subject to repeated trauma, who use public showers, or who have chronic athlete's foot problems, their skin being a potential source of infection for the nails. Prevention includes such simple measures as wearing shower slippers; keeping the feet dry; using clean, dry socks; using more than one pair of athletic shoes, so that you never have to wear a pair that has not dried completely; avoiding repeated injury to the nails; trimming the nails frequently, so that they do not get too long and break off; and applying an athlete's foot powder daily.

Onychomycosis can be annoying, and because it is contagious, it can spread to other nails or other people. Thus, preventive measures and early treatment should be initiated as soon as this problem becomes evident.

Paronychia

Harold B. Glickman, D.P.M.

Paronychia is a rather common disorder that affects the toenails and fingernails of athletes of all ages. Defined as an inflammation of the nail fold that may become infected, it is a rather painful and bothersome condition that quite often requires medical attention.

The severity of the condition varies. It may occur as a mild redness and swelling, or may progress with an overabundance of red, pulpy granulation tissue with infection and drainage of pus around the entire nail plate.

Often caused by shoes that are too narrow or tight, paronychia and subsequent infection particularly affect athletes. The chronic rubbing of the skin around the nail irritates and inflames the tissue, sometimes opening the skin to infection. As the inflammation progresses, swelling and an overabundance of skin called granulation tissue occur. Naturally, this is quite painful.

When the paronychia of the toenail becomes painful or infection occurs, it is sometimes necessary to remove that portion of the nail. This should be done by a doctor; otherwise, part of the nail may be left and continue to ingrow. Often if a paronychia becomes chronic due to ingrowing of a nail, part of the matrix, the cells that produce the nail, may need to be removed so that the condition doesn't reoccur.

The distinction between paronychia and an infected ingrown nail may be confusing. Paronychia refers to the inflammation around the nail. This may occur from irritation of the nail without an ingrown nail. An ingrown nail causes paronychia; in such a case, though, the primary problem is the ingrown nail (see section on ingrown toenails).

At the first sign of inflammation, pain, or infection, soaking should begin immediately in warm salt water soaks (2 teaspoons per quart of water) or in Domeboro® or Blueboro® solution. This should be done for 15 minutes, three times a day. Apply a topical antibiotic cream after the soaks. If there is no progress within 24 hours, it is best to see a physician or podiatrist to treat the paronychia and possibly to remove any offending portion of the nail. Paronychia should be treated immediately to prevent the progression of an infection of the nail.

Thick Toenails (Onychauxic Nails; Runner's Nails)

Ayne F. Furman, D.P.M.

Thick toenails are so frequently found among long-distance runners that they have been called *runner's nails*. They appear as thickened toenails with an opaque to pale yellow appearance. The two most common locations for runner's nails to develop are the fifth toe and the longest toe (either the second or big toe).

The cause of thickened nails is trauma to the toenail. This generates a disruption of the arrangement of the nail-forming cells located at the growth plate, or matrix. The trauma can be as direct as dropping a shot-put on the toe, or as subtle as the constant rubbing of the top of the shoe on the nail. Constant rubbing causes microtrauma, which after many miles produces the nail cell disorganization. Once the integrity of the nail cells has been altered, there are most likely permanent changes that take place in the nail.

Thickened nails cause no health problems, unless they become ingrown. Once ingrown, pain is noticed under the nail borders or at the sides of the toe. Do not attempt to do bathroom surgery, because it could cause an infection or make an existing infection worse. If an ingrown toenail occurs, seek podiatric treatment. The offending portion of nail can be removed with very little discomfort and without loss of many training days.

Thick toenails are susceptible to shoe irritation, because they are closer to the top of shoes. Therefore, certain self-treatment measures should be performed to prevent further thickening and blister formation below the nail. The treatment consists of (a) filing the thickened nail down with a nail file or fine sandpaper, (b) covering the tips of the affected nails with strips of moleskin, and (c) buying shoes with ample toe box depth.

Blisters that develop beneath the nails are usually blood filled, which is why they appear black to purple in color. They are noticed after trauma to the nail and may be painful (see "Black Toenails"). In some cases, trauma to the nail loosens the nail from its bed, and the nail falls off. There are no harmful side effects. The nail grows back within 6 to 8 months.

Not all thick toenails are due to trauma. They can be a side effect of systemic diseases, such as diabetes or psoriasis. Thick toenails may also be caused by a local fungus infection of the nail (see "Fungus Nails").

Suggested Reading for "Thick Toenails (Onychauxic Nails; Runner's Nails)"

Bordelon (1985)

See reading list at the end of the book for a complete source listing.

Athlete's Foot

Harold B. Glickman, D.P.M.

Athlete's foot, known in medicine as *tinea pedis*, is an infection of the skin caused by fungi. These fungi are quite opportunistic and often find ideal conditions existing on the feet, especially between the toes and on the soles, due to the warmth and moisture caused by heavy socks and tennis or jogging shoes. The fungi, which are microscopic organisms, tend to remain in the outer horny surface of the skin. These superficial skin infections can become bothersome and sometimes debilitating. However, if treated early, the fungus can be eradicated quickly.

The means by which fungal infections are acquired and transmitted are not entirely known. Some investigators favor the theory that fungal infections are acquired from fungi in the environment. Fungi have been isolated from shoes, locker room floors, shower stalls, foot baths, and so forth in many studies. However, newer studies conclude that this is all circumstantial and that decreased local resistance of the skin accounts for the activation of infection by fungus.

The inflammation caused by superficial fungi varies from slight scaling and occasional fissuring (cracks) between the toes, to more extensive dry, reddish scaling, to acute bullous or blisterlike sores on the soles of the feet.

There are several methods by which the doctor can make a definitive diagnosis through laboratory studies. The first method is through the use of KOH microscopic examination. The doctor scrapes a superficial portion of the infected area, mixes this with KOH (potassium hydroxide), and examines this under the microscope. The fungi are readily visible, and the diagnosis is confirmed.

Another method of diagnosis involves culturing, or growing in a culture medium the fungus obtained from a skin scraping. Most practitioners who deal with athlete's foot have this method readily available.

Usually the diagnosis of the most common types of fungal infections of the feet can be made almost entirely on clinical grounds. The fungal infection caused by *Trichophyton rubrum* is a chronic infection on the sole of the foot that shows a dull red, low-grade inflammation with moderate, dry scaling. This infection resembles the distribution on the foot of a low-cut moccasin and can remain localized to one foot for years. The other common fungal infection of the foot is caused by *Trichophyton mentagrophytes*. This type of infection usually causes recurrent itching and scaling between the toes, with small blisters and scaling on the soles of the feet. This infection is subject to acute flare-ups, particularly during warm weather and when occlusive footgear is worn.

All types of fungal infections have a tendency to be more severe under conditions of poor hygiene, heat, and humidity. It is therefore highly recommended that proper foot bathing and drying are essential to help control *tinea pedis*.

Treatment of fungal infections has advanced markedly over the past 20 years. There are now many products available over-the-counter that are highly successful, including topical products that contain undecylenic acid and tolnafate. At times a prescription medication is in order, and your physician or podiatrist will have to be contacted. There are several oral antifungal medications containing griseofulvin, or ketoconazole. These medications should be administered only by your doctor and monitored very carefully. Like any drug, these may produce unwarranted reactions, such as skin rashes, gastrointestinal upsets, and headaches. They are usually used only in severe cases of tinea pedis. There are also available by prescription stronger topical medications, which may be tried before proceeding to the oral medications.

Tinea pedis can be a rather bothersome superficial skin infection of the feet. Proper hygiene is essential, and successful self-treatment can usually be obtained with topical over-the-counter medications. In more severe cases, do not hesitate to call on your physician or podiatrist for definitive diagnosis and treatment.

Soft Corns (Heloma Molle)

Paul M. Taylor, D.P.M.

Soft corns are a thickening of the outer layer of the skin between the toes, occurring because of pressure and irritation to the toes. These corns remain "soft" due to the moisture that is usually present interdigitally. As the buildup of the skin continues, these soft corns can become painful, due to pressure on the deeper layers of tissues containing the nerves and blood vessels.

The cause of soft corns is pressure from an enlargement or malposition of bones in the adjacent toes (Figure 4.2). Shoes and stretch

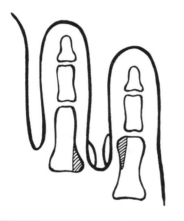

Figure 4.2 A bony prominence on adjacent toes causes repeated pressure on the skin and the development of soft corns.

socks also increase the pressure that contributes to the formation of corns. Dress shoes usually impose more pressure than do athletic shoes. The thickening of the outer layer of skin is a normal response by the body to protect itself from excessive pressure and irritation. However, if the irritation persists, the buildup of the skin becomes excessive, and a soft corn

develops. In late stages of this condition, an abscess or ulcer can develop under the corn, which may become very painful and infected.

Self-treatment for soft corns requires avoiding tight shoes and socks and applying a lubricant between the toes to stop the irritation. Noxzema® or Desitin® are effective for this. Placing a small, soft pad between the toes also helps relieve the pressure. Using an adhesive aperture pad also relieves the excessive pressure. The use of medicated corn pads or corn medications should be avoided, because these contain acids that can irritate the normal skin in the area.

Prevention of soft corns requires attention to shoes and socks. Tight shoes, due to either improper fit or a narrow toe box, should be avoided. Any socks or hose that stretch can increase pressure on the toes, especially the smallest toe, and aggravate a soft corn.

If a soft corn persists, professional podiatric care may be necessary. For temporary relief, the podiatrist can debride (remove) the corn and apply protective padding and medication. Also, x-ray studies can determine the extent of the bony involvement. If the corn remains symptomatic and does not respond to conservative treatment, surgical correction should be considered. Surgical correction requires removing the portions of the toe bone that cause the soft corn to develop. These procedures can be done as an outpatient, office procedure under local anesthesia. The patient is ambulatory immediately; however, strenuous activity may have to be avoided for 2 to 3 weeks.

Soft corns can be a chronic source of irritation. However, they can usually be self-treated successfully. If they do not resolve, the problem can be corrected surgically.

Morton's Syndrome and Morton's Neuroma: Two Different, but Often Confused, Problems

David A. Bernstein, D.P.M.

There are many reasons for the development of forefoot pain in athletes. Morton's syndrome and Morton's neuroma are frequently mistaken as being the same condition.

Morton's Syndrome

In 1935 Dr. D.J. Morton initially described a heredity-related syndrome that involved a shortened first metatarsal, a posterior displacement of the sesamoids (two small bones located under the first metatarsal head), and hypertrophy of the second metatarsal (Figure 4.3). The external appearance of this foot type includes a first toe that is abnormally short when compared to the second toe. It may present plantar calluses under the second and possibly the third metatarsal heads and a mild to moderate bunion deformity of the big toe joint.

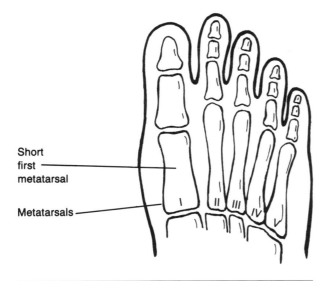

Figure 4.3 Morton's syndrome has a short first metatarsal.

Pain in the forefoot is the most frequent complaint; however, a burning sensation is usually reported after activity, due to the abnormal, excessive weight-bearing stress placed under the lesser metatarsal heads. The shortened first metatarsal is not able to provide the support that is required for normal function. Arch fatigue and discomfort throughout the foot are common complaints, because excessive pronation almost always accompanies this problem.

Treatment of Morton's Syndrome

Treatment of Morton's syndrome depends on the severity and progression of the deformities and symptoms. Early detection in children can be treated with prescription foot orthoses, which significantly help prevent the associated degenerative changes from occurring. In adults, orthoses allow for better function and less discomfort, but do nothing to help correct imbalances.

For the athlete who still relates painful foot problems after receiving orthoses, surgery can help return the foot to a more normal weight-bearing alignment. A great deal of surgical expertise, with careful preoperative clinical and x-ray evaluation as well as postoperative orthoses, is essential. The athlete can expect a minimum recovery period of 6 to 8 weeks before returning to exercise. In most cases, swimming and cycling can be resumed earlier, in 3 to 4 weeks.

Morton's Neuroma

Morton's neuroma (neuralgia) was first described by T.G. Morton in 1876. It presents as a benign nerve tumor that produces an assortment of painful symptoms involving the third intermetatarsal space and the adjacent third and fourth toes (Figure 4.4). Patients have described tingling, numbness, cramping, burning, and even an electrical-like shooting sensation to the end of these toes. Neuromas are less frequently found in other intermeta-

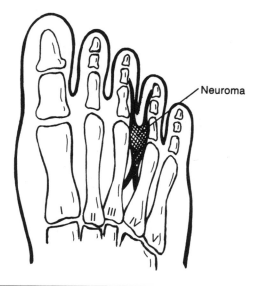

Figure 4.4 Morton's neuroma has a thickening of the nerve between the metatarsals.

tarsal spaces, the outer side of the first metatarsalphalangeal joint, and the inside portion of the heel. Women are affected more often than men, possibly due to tighter fitting and higher heeled shoes. A neuroma can develop anywhere that a normal nerve is subjected to constant trauma. The third intermetatarsal space is the most common location for this lesion, because two nerve branches combine to form a nerve larger than usual between the third and fourth metatarsal heads. Over an extended period of abuse, this nerve enlarges and can become entrapped in the surrounding scar and inflamed tissue.

Treatment of Morton's Neuroma

The most important concept in treating a neuroma is to begin as soon as any symptoms are observed. Early attention may allow the nerve to return to normal function and prevent permanent damage.

Initial treatment includes the disposal of all foot gear that is symptomatic (both athletic and street shoes). The appearance of neuromas has lessened over the past 20 years, due to the attention given to better fitting shoes. Running and other sports shoes have become quite specialized to accommodate many different types of feet; however, athletes are still plagued with painful neuromas. A shoe that

seems to fit well in the store may be injurious during activity. The human foot absorbs an enormous amount of stress and undergoes certain changes that must be allowed by the shoe. As the foot pronates and the arch lowers, the overall length of the foot increases, and it moves forward in the shoe. The foot also slightly enlarges with increasing intensity of activity, lateness in the day, and increasing temperature and humidity. All of these factors can produce a poor-fitting shoe that compresses the metatarsal heads together, traumatizing the nerve. It is recommended that there should be at least ½ to ¾ of an inch of additional room between the tip of the longest toe and the end of the shoe for the athlete bothered by neuroma. This space may vary, depending on the nature of the involved sport.

Other treatments to reduce neuroma discomfort have to do with altering the biomechanics of the foot. Prescription foot orthoses are helpful, due to their controlling excessive pronation. Also, the placement of a felt pad between the third and fourth metatarsal heads is helpful. Other shoe modifications include skipping the lower eyelets when lacing the shoe and even removing the sock liner to provide additional room.

Local injections of cortisone mixed with an anesthetic, such as Xylocaine®, may reduce inflammation and pain if there has not been any permanent damage to the nerve. In cases that are unresponsive after two or three injections, surgical removal is indicated. This can be done in a properly equipped office under local anesthesia, or in a hospital. The excision of the damaged portion of the nerve produces only minimal loss of sensation between the third and fourth toes, without any decrease in muscle strength or function. Patients are ambulatory the same day, but 5 to 6 weeks of healing are required before attempting to return to full activity. However, swimming and cycling can be started in 3 weeks.

Conclusion

There has been confusion in the past in regard to these two problems that cause forefoot pain. They are two different problems, described by two different persons with the same last name. Dr. D.J. Morton's syndrome is a heredity condition that results in a short first metatarsal and an apparently long second toe. Dr. T.G. Morton's neuroma is of functional and traumatic origin, causing nerve inflammation and pain, usually in the third and fourth toes. Still, either condition adversely affects an athlete, but early and appropriate treatment usually provides complete relief of symptoms.

Sesamoiditis

Deborah S. Wehman, D.P.M.

Some athletes, especially those with high-arched feet, suffer from pain under the ball of the foot. This condition, called sesamoiditis, is an inflammation of the sesamoid bones (shaped like sesame seeds) under the head of the big toe (see Figure 4.5).

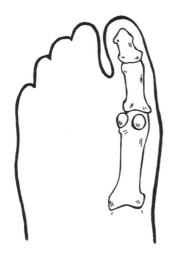

Figure 4.5 The sesamoids are located under the first metatarsal.

Sesamoid bones, found inside tendons, help distribute weight-bearing pressure. The best-known sesamoid bone, the patella, or kneecap, is in the quadriceps tendon. *Sesamoiditis*, however, refers only to the sesamoids of the foot.

The two sesamoid bones located in the foot are the medial and the lateral, located in the tendon of the flexor hallucis brevis muscle. Their function is to increase the mechanical advantage of the muscle by acting as a fulcrum.

Causes

Causes of sesamoiditis vary, but it is most commonly found in runners, and other athletes, with high-arched (cavus) feet. The athlete with a cavus foot exerts more weight on the balls of his or her feet. The force is accentuated by sports that involve pounding or jumping, such as sprinting, basketball, volleyball, or gymnastics. The trauma can lead to an irritation of the sesamoids and the surrounding tissue; if the pounding is great enough, it could lead to a fracture.

A stress or traumatic fracture of the sesamoid bones also causes sesamoiditis. Stress fractures can result from continuous landing on the ball of a foot that does not absorb shock well, such as a foot with a high arch.

Bipartite sesamoids—when more than two sesamoid bones are present or when one of them is split—commonly cause pain under the ball of the foot (see Figure 4.6). Some experts

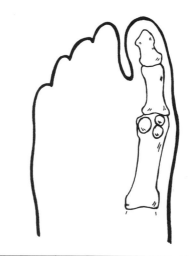

Figure 4.6 A sesamoid bone may develop in two or more segments.

theorize that bipartite sesamoids—usually three sesamoid bones, although four have been seen—actually were fractured at a younger age but didn't hurt because there was not enough stress on them at the time of the fracture. Bipartite sesamoids can lead to pain because they may not be properly positioned beneath the toe and could be pushing against a nerve, bone, or other structure.

Symptoms

You can evaluate your condition by pressing on the ball of your foot. There should be a specific spot that hurts the most. If this same spot hurts when you pull back on your big toe to stretch the tendon of the muscle the sesamoids are in, this may also indicate sesamoiditis. This pain is greater during activity and subsides with prolonged periods of rest.

You can treat sesamoiditis at home by doing the following:

1. Apply an ice cup to the painful area for 10 to 15 minutes after you exercise.
2. Take aspirin (the usual recommended dosage is two aspirin four times a day, as long as there is no stomach upset).
3. Pad around the painful area to relieve pressure (see Figure 4.7). Insoles can increase the cushioning under the sesamoids, decreasing the force on those bones.

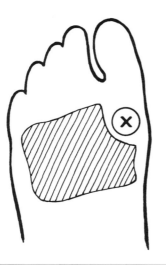

Figure 4.7 Protective padding should be applied around the painful area.

4. Exercise on softer surfaces.
5. Finally, decrease your activity or stop altogether for a time to decrease the pain and inflammation and give the sesamoids a chance to heal.

Last Resort

If this self-treatment doesn't relieve the problem, consult a sportsmedicine podiatrist. Your podiatrist should suggest the above treatments first. However, if these have not already eliminated the pain, x-rays should be taken to determine whether there is a fracture. If no fracture is found, a steroid injection may be given along with padding to relieve the pressure below the big toe. Anti-inflammatory medication may be prescribed to reduce pain and swelling. The podiatrist may also suggest orthotic devices to help relieve the pressure.

If these relatively conservative treatments do not work, or if the pain continues to return after long periods of rest, surgical removal of the painful sesamoid should be considered.

If there is a fracture, a cast may be applied for 4 to 6 weeks. Often, though, even immobilizing the area with a cast does not relieve the pain. If this is the case, surgery may be required to remove the fractured sesamoid. Although not the treatment of choice, surgery sometimes is the only method that eliminates the pain.

Conclusion

Sesamoiditis may be a debilitating condition for runners, jumpers, or other athletes. Initial treatment of ice, padding, and rest may relieve the condition. Changing to a softer running surface and adding insoles to the shoes may also be helpful. If the above self-treatments do not resolve the condition, consult a sportsmedicine podiatrist.

Suggested Reading for "Sesamoiditis"

Scranton (1981)

Van-Hal et al. (1982)

See reading list at the end of the book for a complete source listing.

Metatarsalgia

Paul M. Taylor, D.P.M.

Metatarsalgia is a symptom in which there is pain on the bottom of the foot, just behind the toes. This condition is given this name because the bones in this part of the foot that carry the body's weight are the metatarsals, and the suffix *-algia* denotes pain. Metatarsalgia is not an injury, but only a symptom of pain in that particular part of the body. Because this part of the foot supports all the body weight in walking, running, or playing sports, it is an area that frequently is injured. Some undesired conditions in this area include Morton's neuroma, stress fractures, bursitis, tendinitis, and arthritis.

When pain first develops in the metatarsals, it is possible to treat the symptoms without knowing the exact cause of the pain. Most of these symptoms are due to inflammation within the tissues. Treatment involves measures that should always be used to stop inflammation. These include rest, ice, compression, elevation, and the use of aspirin or other anti-inflammatory medication (see chapter 3). A metatarsal pad can also be placed behind the painful area, in order to keep weight off the area (see chapter 13, "Shoe Modifications," Figures 13.11 and 13.12).

If the above measures do not resolve the metatarsalgia symptoms in 10 to 14 days, it is necessary to identify the cause of the pain in order to treat it appropriately. This may require professional evaluation in order to determine the exact cause of the pain. Such an evaluation includes an examination, x-rays, and possibly other diagnostic tests. Once a diagnosis is made, more aggressive therapy can be initiated, possibly including strapping and padding, physical therapy, injections, orthotic devices, or surgery.

Metatarsalgia is a common symptom that occurs in sports. It usually resolves spontaneously if given enough rest and appropriate initial self-treatment. Professional help is indicated when the pain does not resolve or continues to recur.

Blisters

Paul M. Taylor, D.P.M.

Blisters are one of the most common injuries sustained by the athlete. The blister is a collection of fluid between the outer layers of the skin. It is caused by friction, pressure, and heat. A combination of these types of physical microtrauma results in a separation between the layers of the skin (dermis and epidermis) and a resultant inflammatory infiltration of fluid that distends the outer layer of skin. This results in the fluid-filled blister, with the outer layer of skin forming the roof of the blister. As the microtrauma continues, deeper layers of skin are involved; small blood vessels may rupture, with bleeding into the blister. This is usually more painful, with an initial reddish discoloration of the blister that gradually develops a blue discoloration.

Blisters often occur when the athlete begins a new activity or increases his or her level of activity. New shoes are also a frequent cause of blisters. Changes in court surfaces may also cause new blisters. Environmental conditions such as moisture or heat also contribute to the formation of blisters. Some persons, particularly those with fair skin, are more prone to blister formation.

Blisters are common, and they usually respond well to self-treatment. When the athlete develops a blister, immediate treatment usually results in relief of symptoms and a rapid healing, without any loss of time from activity. Once the fluid has built up under the skin, forming the blister, the blister needs to be drained. Cleanse the area with an antiseptic, such as alcohol, and, using a needle that also has been disinfected, place two or three puncture holes in the roof of the blister, allowing the fluid to drain out.

The roof of the blister should not be removed at this time, because it provides the best protection available to the sensitive skin underneath. An antibiotic ointment or antiseptic should be applied to the area, and a sterile gauze pad should be taped over the blister. The tape should not be applied directly to the blister, because, when the tape is removed, the skin that was the blister's roof would be pulled off with the tape.

The gauze dressing should be applied for 2 or 3 days; by this time the blister should be dry and not showing any signs of redness. If the roof of the blister has reattached to the underlying skin, it should be left on. If the skin is very loose, it should be carefully trimmed off. This initial first aid and self-treatment should resolve most blisters.

If the athlete suffers from repeated blisters, measures should be taken to try to prevent their development. In order to prevent the formation of blisters, it is necessary to try to eliminate any factor that contributes to their development. If starting a new activity or increasing the level of activity causes blisters, a more gradual increase may be necessary. Because blisters are caused by pressure, friction, and heat, a change in shoe wear, an additional pair of socks, or thicker socks may be needed. For the runner in a hot climate in which the temperature of streets may result in blisters, it may be necessary to run at a time of day when the roads have cooled down. Wearing shoes that are damp from rain or from perspiration from a previous activity contributes to blister formation. A second, dry pair of shoes should be available. New shoes should always be broken in gradually. Careful attention should be given to proper fit (see "Shoe Selection for Prevention of Injuries" in chapter 13).

For chronic areas of irritation, blisters may be prevented by applying petroleum jelly or lotions. Many products are available to help prevent blisters. These include special socks, various insole replacements, and soft tissue supplements such as moleskin, foam padding, and Second Skin®. One method to try to toughen up the skin is to paint a problem area with tincture of benzoin, allow it to dry, and then powder the area before putting on socks. By using preventive techniques and by properly treating any blister that does develop, problems with blisters should be avoided.

If blisters persist, or if any complications develop, medical help may be necessary. Professional help may be needed for blisters if they continue to recur, if they do not respond to self-care and interfere with activities, or if any suspected infection develops. An infection is evident, with increasing pain, swelling, and redness. The clear drainage from the blister changes to a thicker, yellow material, although drainage from an infection can sometimes be other colors as well. Small red streaks may also be seen around the area. If any of these signs of infection are evident, professional help should be sought as soon as possible.

Blisters are a common problem for athletes. In most cases, they can be adequately self-treated and will be only a temporary nuisance.

Corns, Calluses, and Warts

Raymond J. Olkin, D.P.M.

Corns, calluses, and warts are common foot problems that have afflicted the general population for centuries. Runners and fitness enthusiasts who are active on their feet often have to limit their activities because of pain from these ailments. Simple self-treatment or professional treatment by a foot specialist usually reduces or eliminates their discomfort.

Corns and Calluses

Corns and calluses are areas of dry, dead skin caused by friction and pressure. Heredity is the most important factor in their formation, because it dictates skin type, biomechanical function, and foot structure. Corns usually appear on the toes, both on the top and on the sides. Calluses normally form on the bottom of the foot—the ball, the end of the large toe, or the heel.

Corns

Most corns are found on the side of the small toe. They also appear on the top of the other lesser toes, but rarely on the large toe.

Corns can form wherever prominent bones rub the shoe, if there is friction and pressure. They usually are caused by a bony deformity of the toe, most often due to heredity. Contracture deformities, which include hammer and mallet toes, are the most common. A hammer toe is bent at the joint close to the ball of the foot, causing the top of the toe to be raised and rub on the shoe, forming a corn. A mallet toe is contracted at the joint nearest the toenail, causing a corn on the bottom or top of the toe.

Contracture deformities resulting in corns may also be due to various types of arthritis, faulty biomechanics, or injury, or they may be congenital. Friction and pressure from shoes contribute to corn formation, but alone usually do not cause it.

Corns that form between the toes are called soft corns. These are usually caused by small bumps on touching areas of two toes. These bony areas rub against each other; the friction results in the development of corns. Tight-fitting or pointed-toe shoes may contribute to soft corns, but heredity, arthritis, trauma, disease, or congenital formation are usually the underlying causes.

Corns are normally circular, localized, yellowish lesions. If left untreated, hard tissue can thicken to the point at which pressure on the underlying healthy skin becomes too great to bear. The skin beneath the corn may break down and ulcerate, making the surrounding skin red, warm, and more painful. Inflammation or red streaks may be evident. These are signs of spreading infection and warrant immediate medical attention.

Calluses

Calluses are usually larger than corns. Foot structure and the manner in which the foot strikes the ground are of primary importance in their formation. High-arched feet can cause metatarsal and heel calluses. Forefoot and rearfoot imbalances can result in calluses beneath certain bones, depending on the imbalance and how the body compensates.

Often a circular area of considerable pain lies beneath a callus. A bony protrusion at the ball of the foot, usually a metatarsal bone of abnormal length or slant, can cause this type of painful skin thickening.

If calluses are left unattended and become thick, then underlying blistering, ulceration, and infection are possible. People with circulatory diseases or diabetes are prone to these complications and should seek regular professional foot care.

Warts

Warts differ from corns and calluses because they result from infection, not friction or pressure. A wart is a benign tumor caused by a virus. It can appear anywhere on the body; on the feet, it can occur at a site of trauma or at a break in the skin.

Warts on the bottom of the foot are called

plantar warts. They lie deeper in the skin than other warts, because of pressure from the body's weight. They usually are covered by hardened tissue and are painful. Warts can multiply quickly and spread to family members or other people in close contact. People whose feet sweat excessively seem to contract warts at a greater frequency than those whose feet do not sweat as much. They frequently appear on children and adolescents.

Warts have a distinctive spongy appearance and usually have tiny pinpoint dark areas within them. Normal skin lines stop at the outer border of a wart. They can appear singly or in a mosaic pattern.

Corn and Callus Care

People who notice corns or calluses on their feet should lubricate them daily. Before running, petroleum jelly should be applied. Regular lubrication with dry-skin lotions, oils, or creams slows their development. Corns can be lubricated and wrapped, or covered with gauze or an adhesive bandage for a few days at a time, to keep them moist; however, they should be left uncovered at intervals to dry. Acid preparations should not be used for calluses or corns, because acid cannot distinguish them from normal, healthy skin; serious ulceration of underlying tissue may result.

The athlete with corns between the toes should place lamb's wool or a nonadhesive foam pad between the affected areas prior to putting on shoes and socks, in order to separate the toes. With hammer toes or mallet toes, loose-fitting shoes with depth in the toe box should be worn. A small, lengthwise slit can be cut in running shoes just above the area of the deformed toe to allow it more room. Runners with more severe toe problems should inquire about open-toed running shoes.

Friction-reducing insoles can be inserted in athletic and street shoes to help minimize callus development. This is especially helpful for the athlete participating in sports requiring quick changes of direction, such as basketball and racquet sports.

Professional care for corns and calluses usually provides instant relief. In many cases, the underlying causes can be treated and the problems permanently resolved. Many problems can be corrected with orthotic shoe inserts.

In some instances, surgical correction of an underlying deformity is advised. Less traumatic surgical procedures than were previously available have been developed for corns and calluses and, when necessary, bring quick results. Hammer toes, mallet toes, bone spurs, and deviated metatarsals can all be surgically corrected, with accompanying corns and calluses therefore permanently resolved.

Sometimes periodic trimming by a professional of dead tissue from the corn or callus is necessary to maintain comfort. This does not correct the situation but does allow pain-free activity.

Wart Care and Treatment

Treatment of warts differs from that of corns and calluses. Here, over-the-counter acid preparations can be used by the patient (if there is no underlying diabetes or vascular disease) because the acids are specific for wart tissue. (Persons with diabetes or vascular disease should check with their physician at the first sign of warts, corns, or calluses.)

There is no medicine available that kills a virus. At home, the patient can apply over-the-counter acid preparations regularly. The usually whitened destroyed tissue should be removed between applications. Vitamin E oil or castor oil applications can also be tried. Children seem to respond well if the treatment used is presented very positively. If children believe the treatment will be successful, it normally is. Plantar warts usually require professional care, because they lie so deep within the tissue.

Because there is no specific treatment for viral infections, foot specialists can destroy warts by various methods. Those available include surgical excision, burning with different acids, electrodesiccation, injection technique, laser beams, oral vitamin A therapy, freezing, and many others. No one technique is better than another. Each specialist develops his or her favored treatments. Most are relatively painless and have a success rate of 70 to 80 percent.

Proper Care First

Corns, calluses, and warts are relatively small, benign problems, but the pain they can cause often leads to a loss of fitness, due to a diminishment of physical activity. A sore foot can make even the natural, uncomplicated act of walking difficult. Properly fitted shoes are the best prevention. Simple self-treatment relieves most minor irritations. If problems linger, however, medical care usually corrects the underlying causes.

Tailor's Bunion (Bunionette)

Paul M. Taylor, D.P.M.

A tailor's bunion is an enlargement along the outer side of the foot, just behind the little toe. The bump is due to a malposition or abnormal enlargement of the fifth metatarsal (Figure 4.8). These changes may be secondary to an old injury, a congenital anomaly, or chronic irritation from shoes. It was originally termed a "tailor's" bunion because tailors at one time would sit on the floor cross-legged; the constant pressure on the outside of the foot would cause this bump.

The tailor's bunion is currently a problem most frequently caused by aggravation from women's dress shoes. However, at times it can also be a source of irritation to the athlete. Bursitis (inflammation of a fluid-filled sac) may develop between the skin and bone, with increasing redness, swelling, and pain in the area.

If a problem appears to be developing in this area, initial treatment should consist of trying wider shoes or shoes with a softer upper. A protective aperture pad of self-adhesive felt or foam can be cut to fit around the area (Figure 4.9). In most cases, this relieves the problem. However, if the bony changes are very prominent and subject to repeated irritation, the pain may persist. If this happens, a surgical procedure may be necessary to remove the enlarged portion of bone.

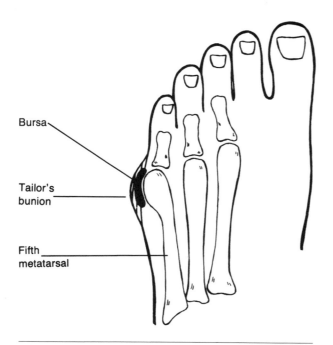

Figure 4.8 The tailor's bunion is composed of the head of the fifth metatarsal and an overlying bursa.

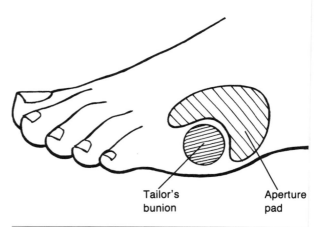

Figure 4.9 The tailor's bunion can be protected with an aperture pad.

Bunions (Hallux Valgus Deformity)

Robert F. Weiss, D.P.M.

The term *bunion* is used to denote a painful swelling of the soft tissue, and bone enlargement occurring over the inner aspect of the ball, of the great toe. The appearance of the bunion varies with its stage of development. In the initial, developmental phase, a bunion consists of a partial dislocation outward of the great toe (hallux valgus), which renders the head of the metatarsal bone unduly prominent (compare Figure 4.10 and Figure 4.11).

Causes

There are many causes of bunion deformities. One of the most common is hereditary tendencies. This contributes to biomechanical imbalances, which may be both functional and structural. These biomechanical imbalances along with other hereditary tendencies can lead to the development of the bunion deformity. Metabolic conditions such as arthritis, gouty arthritis, and rheumatoid arthritis may be predisposing factors to the deformity. Injuries, which may include traumatic arthritis, may also lead to bunion manifestation.

Mechanics

A biomechanical evaluation and gait analysis demonstrate mechanical causes very easily. One of the most common mechanical deviations is pronation of the foot, which appears as a flat-footed gait. It is evident while standing, because of the lowering of the arch and the tilting inward of the ankle. During walking or running, the excessive pronation continues throughout the midstance and propulsive phases of the gait cycle. This places excessive

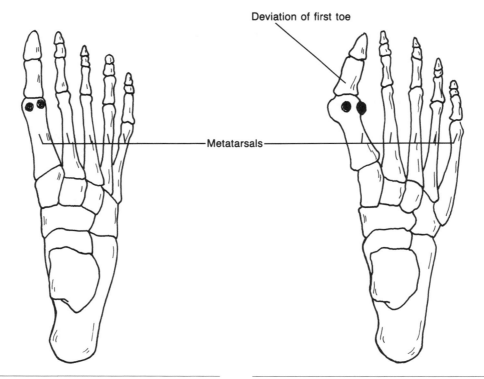

Figure 4.10 Normal alignment of the first toe.

Figure 4.11 The abnormal alignment of the first metatarsal and toe that occurs with a bunion (hallux valgus).

stress on the inside of the big toe during the propulsive phase of the gait, forcing it in a lateral direction toward the smaller toes. It is the combination of abnormal biomechanical forces and hereditary factors that leads to the development of the bunion deformity. (For additional information, see "Pronation" and "Supination" in this chapter.)

Symptoms

As the bunion develops, the head of the metatarsal bone enlarges from shoe irritation. The bunion sufferer begins to experience pain and discomfort in the area of the ball of the great toe, especially after exercise. As the case continues to advance, a bursa (sac of fluid) forms over the inner or top aspect of the bony prominence. The pain then becomes more intense, owing to an acute attack of inflammation in the bursa and possibly also in the neighboring joint. Very often, the great toe is angled toward the smaller toes and may overlap or underlap the second toe. Therefore, the mechanical imbalances and the development of the bunion can create deformities of all the lesser toes.

Self-Treatment

The first choice in the treatment of bunion deformities is a conservative, mechanical approach. Without changing the functional causes of the deformity, even the most sophisticated surgical procedure will not be the answer.

There are many different devices to help in the self-treatment of bunion deformities, including toe posts, springs, and levers. The simplest home treatment is to place a toe separator (a piece of ¼-inch thick foam or polyurethane foam) between the first and second toes. You may then place a small piece of tape around the separator from the inside of the base of the great toe to around the outside of the great toe.

Another form of home treatment is to create a bunion shield by cutting a hole in a ⅛- or ¼-inch felt pad and placing it over the enlarged bump on the metatarsal head. You may then hold the toe in a straight position by using 3-by-3-inch adhesive tape. Hold the toe in this position by anchoring the tape around the

base of the great toe, then extending it behind and over the bump (over the pad). Follow with one or two pieces of tape transversely to lock it in place.

Home treatment should also involve checking shoes for fit and style. Shoes that are too short or narrow or have a narrow or pointed toe box aggravate the bunion deformity.

If home therapy fails, seek the advice of a sportsmedicine podiatrist, who can evaluate the problem from a radiologic standpoint as well as consider the biomechanical, functional, and structural deviations. X-ray evaluation is essential in determining the joint status, viewing changes in the joint space, and assessing the possibility of cartilaginous changes that may lead to arthritic changes.

Again, the first choice in the treatment of bunions is the conservative approach, here using a biomechanical functional orthotic device. This is made following an examination and casting of the lower extremities, using engineering equipment and a gait analysis. If the orthotic therapy does not give successful relief of the symptoms, the patient must be evaluated from a surgical standpoint. However, the patient must continue to wear the orthotic devices postoperatively for better control of the original biomechanical imbalances.

Surgical Intervention

If the bunion deformity is of a simple nature, with enlargement of the metatarsal head, a simple bunionectomy (removal of the bump) can be performed to reduce the enlarged bone. However, when the great toe is also deviated into a valgus position toward the lesser toes, this deformity must be reduced by a surgical osteotomy (fracturing of bone) of the great toe to place it in proper anatomical position relative to the metatarsal head.

In cases of severe deformity, there may be a need to reduce the intermetatarsal angle, in addition to the bunionectomy and great toe osteotomy (see Figure 4.11). This is performed by a surgical osteotomy at the inside base of the first metatarsal for the bone to regain better anatomical position and function. For the person whose x-ray shows a narrowing of the joint space and a limited range of motion, due to arthritic changes, the procedure of choice would either be to create a joint space between the base of the great toe and the metatarsal head, or to form a new joint by placing a medical grade plastic joint, or spacer, in the base of the great toe to articulate properly with the metatarsal head.

Prevention

Most athletes want to know what needs to be done to get back on the road. Often a successful treatment regimen is based on the athlete's understanding of the problem and its cause. Most overuse injuries can be related to a triad of critical factors, which are (a) conditioning and training, (b) lower extremity structure and function, and (c) shoe gear. If all these areas were examined by the physician and patient together, the etiology, diagnosis, and treatment of most overuse injuries could often be simple and successful.

Suggested Reading for "Bunions (Hallux Valgus Deformity)"

Lillich & Baxter (1986)

_____

See reading list at the end of the book for a complete source listing.

Stiff Toe (Hallux Rigidus; Hallux Limitus)

Paul M. Taylor, D.P.M.

Hallux rigidus and hallux limitus are conditions in which motion in the first toe is gradually lost, usually due to arthritic changes. This loss of motion occurs at the joint formed by the first metatarsal of the foot and the phalangeal bone of the first toe. This joint is called the metatarsal phalangeal joint (Figure 4.12). The terms *hallux rigidus* and *hallux limitus* are derived from "hallux," which refers to the first toe; "limitus," having a limited motion in the joint; and "rigidus," meaning rigid or motionless.

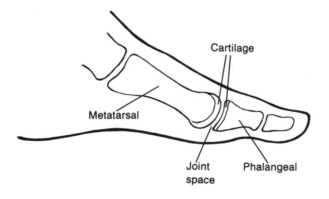

Figure 4.12 Normal first metatarsal phalangeal joint.

Loss of motion begins to occur usually after an injury. This may be either a sudden, severe injury—such as dropping a heavy object on the toe—or it may be due to repeated, minor injuries—such as catching the toe in the grass while playing soccer. Generally the problem starts with hallux limitus and progresses to hallux rigidus.

The initial injury causes damage to the articular cartilage lining the joint as well as a resultant inflammatory change. The articular cartilage is the smooth lining of the joint, which allows the joint to glide smoothly and freely. When the cartilage is damaged by an injury or becomes rough due to chronic inflammation, motion is gradually lost and hallux limitus results. If the damage continues, with inflammation and swelling within the

joint, this causes a pulling on the bone by the capsule that surrounds the joint; the body responds by forming new bone. This new bone forms a lipping or spurring around the joint, which impinges on free motion of the joint and results in hallux rigidus (Figure 4.13).

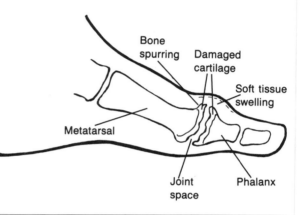

Figure 4.13 Abnormal changes in first metatarsal phalangeal joint that result in a stiff toe (hallux limitus or hallux rigidus).

During the development of hallux limitus or rigidus, there are all the signs of inflammation within the joint, including pain, redness, and swelling—as well as the gradual loss of motion. These signs, even if they appear to be minor, should not be ignored, because this problem tends to become progressively worse.

Early treatment for hallux limitus or rigidus begins by trying to identify any factors that are irritating the joint. If it is an improperly fitted shoe, a shoe change is necessary. If a certain sport seems to be the primary cause, it may be best to consider an alternative sport. Frequently, a hallux limitus indicates that there may be a biomechanical imbalance within the foot or lower extremity. Therefore, when this problem occurs, an early evaluation by a podiatrist may be indicated. If there is a biomechanical problem, it may be controlled by an orthotic device; this may stop the progression of the hallux limitus.

If the hallux limitus was caused by a sudden injury, there may be a small bone fragment in the joint from a small fracture, or a piece of the cartilage may have broken off and it may be floating in the joint. Either of these conditions causes a chronic inflammation in the joint and increasing bony proliferation around the joint, with a decreasing range of motion. An x-ray usually identifies these problems. When they occur, surgery is generally necessary to remove the fragment, or there will be continued damage to the joint.

Occasionally, due to work or other commitments, it is not possible for the athlete to have surgery on this joint initially. If the joint is painful after activity, it should first be treated with rest, ice, compression, and elevation. A shoe modification or orthotic device should be fabricated. Physical therapy helps resolve the symptoms; when temporary relief is needed, cortisone injections can be considered. Cortisone should not be used to treat this problem repeatedly, because it increases the potential for more damage to the joint.

A hallux limitus or rigidus can cause limitation of activity in an athlete. The damage that can occur to the joint can be limited by early recognition and treatment of this condition.

Gout

Paul M. Taylor, D.P.M.

Gout is a metabolic condition in which there is an increase of uric acid levels in the blood (hyperuricemia). This can result in deposition of crystals of uric acid in body tissues, most commonly in the joints and subcutaneous tissues. In later stages, other organs may also become affected. Gout is much more common in men than women.

The exact mechanism for hyperuricemia is unknown. In some persons with gout, the increase is due to an excessive rate of production of uric acid, whereas in others it is due to faulty renal excretion of uric acid. The initial attack of gout may be precipitated by sudden changes in diet, such as fasting, or by excessive alcohol intake, sudden stress on the joints, or certain medications, such as diuretics. In many cases, a particular cause cannot be identified.

The initial attack of gout is fairly sudden and very painful. It usually begins at night. The big toe joint is most commonly affected, but other joints, including the heel, ankle, or knee, may be involved. The joint becomes red, swollen, hot, and intensely painful.

Treatment includes rest, warm compresses, and elevation. Medical treatment should be obtained as soon as possible, in order to confirm the diagnosis and to begin immediate treatment. Blood tests, x-rays, and joint fluid aspiration may be needed to confirm the diagnosis. This confirmation is necessary because other problems, such as injury or infection, can cause similar symptoms. Treatment then includes medication that is specific for gout. Colchicine relieves the symptoms within several hours but usually also causes nausea or diarrhea. Other potent anti-inflammatories can also be used to relieve the acute attack.

The acute attack may subside within several days, but the metabolic problem will still be present. Continued medical evaluation and treatment is necessary to control the hyperuricemia and to prevent repeated attacks and later damage to the body. Gout persisting over a period of time can lead to repeated acute attacks, chronic gouty arthritis, kidney damage (gouty nephritis), subcutaneous deposits of uric acid (tophi), deposits in bursa (olecranon bursa), and vascular changes. The potential for these problems can be greatly reduced through medical care. If symptoms recur, or the blood levels of uric acid remain high, medication such as allopurinal, probenecid, or sulfinpyrazone can be used to treat chronic gouty problems.

Gout, both in its acute and chronic stages, can adversely affect the athlete. However, with proper medical care, these adverse effects can be well controlled.

Stress Fractures

Harold B. Glickman, D.P.M.

Stress fractures are one of the most misdiagnosed injuries suffered by athletes. Also called "march fractures," because they frequently strike military personnel, stress fractures are incomplete breaks or cracks in normal bone caused by repeated trauma or pounding. When the bone can take no more stress, the crack occurs. The injury can happen after a short period of stress, as little as several hours, but usually follows a longer period of cumulative trauma.

Stress fractures are understandable in a military population, whose training includes long, hard marches. A young, out-of-shape recruit who suddenly marches or hikes 10 miles in one day is a prime candidate for a stress fracture. Reasons for stress or march fractures in the general population, particularly among athletes, are not completely agreed on by medical experts. Yet today more athletes than ever before are developing the problem and seeking professional help to remedy it.

Causes

Athletes with stress fractures have no apparent systemic conditions predisposing them to the injury. Most who incur such fractures, particularly in the foot, are in good physical condition. A high level of fitness and lack of previous systemic ailments cause stress fractures to be frequently misdiagnosed as problems of the ligaments or muscles.

A change in your normal fitness routine can result in a stress fracture. Switching to a harder surface or increasing your distance or speed too rapidly (e.g., going from 5K to 10K racing without proper conditioning or training) may lead to a cracked bone. Returning to activity after a layoff and trying to exercise at the same intensity as before may cause a stress fracture.

Shoes also play an important role. If you normally exercise in rigid, thick-soled shoes and suddenly change to light, flexible footwear, you should protect yourself by working at an easy pace until you adapt to the new shoe. Because a high-arched foot doesn't absorb shock as well as a foot that hits the ground on a flatter plane, this shock is transmitted to the bone and may cause a stress fracture. Well-cushioned shoes or orthoses can help prevent such injuries in athletes with exceptionally high arches. Athletes with hypermobile flat feet (characterized by excessive mobility in a foot that fails to land squarely on the ground and that doesn't become stable at toe-off) can also suffer stress fractures due to the way their feet strike the ground.

Symptoms

The first symptom of a stress fracture is the gradual onset of pain, whether the fracture is located in the lower leg (tibial stress fracture), foot (metatarsal stress fracture), or heel. The pain commonly occurs during athletic activity and may be very mild at first, so the athlete may ignore the discomfort and continue to exercise through the pain. This can be very dangerous, because if you don't heed warning signs of a stress fracture, you risk much more serious damage. If you continue to exercise on hard surfaces or return to activity too soon after suffering a stress fracture, a complete fracture (with a separation of the bone) can occur.

Pain may cease when the activity ends and the athlete rests, but the pain will return when normal or athletic activity resumes. The pain becomes increasingly intense, more constant, and deeper during exercise. Downhill running and deceleration may be particularly painful. Local swelling and tenderness may occur.

In diagnosing stress fractures, one of the physician's best approaches is to press or manipulate the injured site. A stress fracture hurts when pushed on with a finger, both from above and below. Touching the skin over a simple muscle strain or overuse syndrome injury does not produce nearly the extent of tenderness or pain of a stress fracture; an injured tendon or ligament hurts only when pressure is applied on one side.

Pain and swelling, then, are the hallmarks of stress fractures. Without an overt injury or physical trauma to the area, the athlete becomes concerned when the pain and swelling do not subside after a few days of self-enforced rest and the use of ice and elevation. Athletic and some normal activities become difficult, and professional help is needed.

Treatment

Once the athlete is in the doctor's office, x-rays of the injured site often are taken. However, x-ray results may be negative for stress fractures for the first 5 to 10 days after the injury. Osseous, or bony, changes and the healing process usually do not show up on x-rays until a week or more have passed, until the stress fracture has begun to heal as new bone forms to fill in the tiny crack. Repeat x-rays during the first week of active professional treatment, therefore, are needless if a stress fracture truly is present.

The cornerstone of treatment for a stress fracture is to discontinue the injurious activity immediately. However, the athlete should remain in the best physical condition possible. If you are recovering from a stress fracture, you should continue the basic stretching exercises you have always used to prepare for exercising. Just be sure to take it easy. Swimming and bicycling can help you maintain cardiovascular fitness while placing less stress on feet and lower legs. In general, other daily activities should continue as normally as possible.

Very infrequently, a plaster of paris cast is applied, most often in tibial (lower leg) stress fractures. In many cases, walking with crutches—without a cast—is sufficient to relieve pressure and weight from the leg.

A fractured heel can be treated by wearing a heel cup or special protective padding. Metatarsal stress fractures may require casting for 4 to 6 weeks because these bones move a lot and need stronger measures to immobilize them. (For your information, you have five metatarsal bones in each foot. The big toe is designated *number one*; the little toe, *number five*. The big toe is so strong that it rarely sustains a fracture. Metatarsal stress fractures occur most frequently in numbers two, three, and four—the bones enduring the greatest shock when your foot strikes the ground.)

Oral nonsteroidal anti-inflammatory medications can be used to alleviate pain and swelling.

A fractured bone heals as new bone forms a bony callus around the fracture site. This normal healing growth often can be felt beneath the skin the fourth or fifth week after the injury and eventually subsides.

One of the discouraging aspects in treating stress fractures is the usual need to delay returning to athletic activity. Pain subsides by the second week of treatment, so the athlete wishes to return to running or other sports endeavors when he or she is asymptomatic. However, as stated above, returning to normal vigorous exercise too soon only delays healing and can cause permanent damage. There is no set time for resuming activity, but a good rule is to wait as long as possible—from 4 to 8 weeks, depending on the location and severity of the injury.

Prevention

Once the injury heals, prevention of further stress fracturing should be of uppermost concern to both doctor and patient. Discuss the causes of your injury with your doctor (training methods, shoes, biomechanical limitations), so you can avoid reinjury.

Stress fractures in the metatarsal region can be prevented by wearing properly cushioned shoes or orthoses and by adhering to proper training guidelines (e.g., avoiding hard surfaces and foregoing rapid increases in speed and distance). When the athlete realizes what has caused the stress fracture, further injuries can be prevented. Proper biomechanical evaluation by your sportsmedicine physician can help you learn how to alleviate your own particular stresses on legs and feet.

Stress fractures among the civilian population are more prevalent than ever before. With proper diagnosis, treatment, and elimination of the causative factors, the athlete may gradually resume normal activity and consciously work to make sure future stress fractures do not occur.

Suggested Reading for "Stress Fractures"

Pavlov et al. (1983)

Shangold (1983)

Sullivan et al. (1984)

Van-Hal et al. (1982)

———————

See reading list at the end of the book for a complete source listing.

Plantar Fasciitis

Harold B. Glickman, D.P.M.

Persistent pain located on the plantar, or bottom, aspect of the heel and closest to the inside, or medial, aspect of the foot can be a challenging problem to both the athlete and the medical practitioner. This plantar fasciitis is most noticeable in the morning upon waking up and taking those first few steps. It subsides as walking becomes more prolonged. However, after the sufferer sits for long periods of time, especially at work, those first few steps can once again produce discomfort and irritation. During athletic activity, discomfort may come early and then subside. There are few injuries to the athlete that can be more persistent and aggravating than plantar fasciitis.

A careful look at the anatomy and biomechanics of the area can go a long way toward understanding, and therefore alleviating, the symptoms of plantar fasciitis. Anatomically, the plantar fascia is a fibrous, tendonlike structure that runs the entire length of the bottom of the foot. It originates on the calcaneus, or heel bone, and extends to the base of the toes (Figures 4.14 and 4.15). The plan-

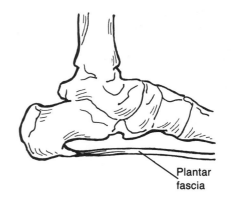

Figure 4.15 The plantar fascia inserts into the heel, as viewed from the side of the foot.

tar fascia helps support the plantar aspect of the foot. During the excessive stress of activity, the plantar fascia can become irritated, inflamed, or even torn if enough repetitive stress occurs at the area.

The main difference between running and walking, other than in speed, is that both feet can be off the ground at the same time in running, whereas this does not happen in normal walking. The heel serves as a shock absorber for the body. During the gait cycle, heel contact occurs first in the supinated, or "up and in," position of the foot, just before full heel contact. As full heel contact occurs, the foot begins to roll the opposite way, or pronates, and goes "down and out."

This repetitive stress usually occurs at a specific area on the bottom of the heel. Known in medical terms as the medial-plantar aspect of the heel, it is at the junction where the plantar fascia is attached to the heel bone. In the athlete, the continued stress can produce scarring, fibrosis, degeneration, and quite often a heel spur or calcium deposit located on the bottom of the heel bone. X-rays are needed to confirm the diagnosis of heel spur. In the absence of undue stress on the plantar fascia the heel spur can be asymptomatic. However, in athletes who do have plantar fasciitis and damage to the plantar fascia, a heel spur may be present. The area can become so inflamed that swelling is present and the area is quite painful to the touch. In this instance, an acute

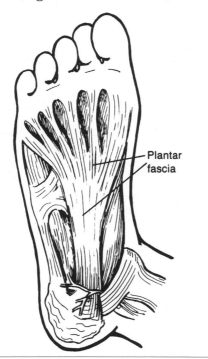

Figure 4.14 The plantar fascia forms a wide band extending from the heel into the toes, viewed from the bottom of the foot.

condition is present and treatment should be instituted immediately.

Causes of Plantar Fasciitis

Biomechanically, the athlete who has the high-arch, rigid type of foot, or the flat, pronated type of foot, is more susceptible to plantar fasciitis than others. Because the high-arch foot has a tight bandlike plantar fascia, it is unable to move during the gait cycle. Repetitive stress and pulling occurs, then inflammation and pain. In the flat or pronated type of foot, excessive motion is the culprit. Here the plantar fascia is working overtime. As the foot pronates past neutral or normal position at the midstance of the gait cycle, the excessive pulling causes undue stress and strain at the origin of the plantar fascia at the heel bone.

Improper shoe wear is also implicated as a causative factor in plantar fasciitis. A person who has a flattened longitudinal arch or a pronated foot and wears a light, flexible shoe only accentuates the stress and strain of the plantar fascia. Shoes that have been worn excessively also allow the foot to roll or pronate beyond normal, thereby causing stress on the plantar fascia.

Improper training methods are often found to be the most common cause of plantar fasciitis. The athlete who suddenly increases activity either on a daily or weekly basis is putting undue strain on the plantar fascia. This does not mean that the athlete should not increase activity but, rather, that it should be done at a gradual rate.

Treatment

Often, if plantar fasciitis is not caught early, its treatment can be slow and lengthy. Hot or cold packs, strapping, massage, functional or biomechanical orthoses, cortisone injections, stretching, and oral anti-inflammatory medications are some of the modalities used.

In deciding the best form of treatment, it is imperative that the athlete and medical practitioner first eliminate all causative factors. A complete history and pedal examination, including gait analysis, is warranted. X-rays are recommended not only to check for a heel spur but also to check for structural or positional osseous changes.

Once the causative factors, such as improper training methods, are eliminated and gait analysis performed, relief of discomfort can be instituted. Ice application and strapping are two of the most common forms of early treatment. Rest, either through reduced activity or complete rest, is usually necessary. Physical therapy involving whirlpool and ultrasound application has been found to be very successful. Anti-inflammatory medication is also quite successful in alleviating severe discomfort in acute cases.

The importance of correcting biomechanical problems and alleviating stress and strain on the plantar fascia cannot be ignored. For long-term therapy and control, functional orthotic devices are the most widely accepted form of treatment in cases that are persistent. It is imperative that pronatory forces exerted on the plantar fascia be halted. A neutral position cast of the foot should be obtained to allow the foot to function in its proper fashion. A full weight-bearing cast is not recommended, for this does not prevent the foot from pronating past neutral. Materials for orthoses range from sponge to plastic. In general, the more rigid, high-arch foot should have an orthosis made from softer materials for shock absorption. The hypermobile, flexible, flattened-arch foot, though, should make use of a more rigid orthosis to control pronation and excessive stress and strain on the plantar fascia. Such materials for rigid orthoses include a flexible plastic or semirigid leather material.

Cortisone injections are often used. The painful area is injected during the acute phase and as a temporary measure to alleviate pain. More often than not, the pain usually returns unless the causative factors are found and corrected. Plantar fascia and calf muscle stretching exercises help prevent recurrence once the acute pain has subsided (see chapter 12, Stretch Exercises 1, 2, and 3).

Most patients respond to these forms of treatment. In a small percentage of patients, though, surgery is indicated. However, this should be discussed in full detail with the doctor, and it is recommended that all conservative forms of treatment be instituted first.

Summary

Most athletes with plantar fasciitis respond to conservative forms of treatment. Once the causative factors are found, treatment can be instituted. Improper shoes, training methods, and biomechanical reasons are all implicated in causing plantar fasciitis. Too much stress and strain, causing wear and tear with inflammation and fibrosis, leads to pain and discomfort. With appropriate initial treatment and a functional biomechanical orthotic device, the athlete can resume normal routines without difficulty.

Suggested Reading for "Plantar Fasciitis"

Baxter & Thigpen (1984)

Goulet (1984)

Herrick & Herrick (1983)

Snider et al. (1983)

See reading list at the end of the book for a complete source listing.

Subluxed Cuboid Syndrome

Mark D. Dollard, D.P.M.

The outside, or lateral, aspect of the foot is a key stabilizer of the foot. The calcaneocuboid joint is a vital link in lateral foot stability. The calcaneocuboid joint is formed by the calcaneus and cuboid bones (Figure 4.16). This joint is susceptible to sudden injury or chronic strain in certain foot types, which can cause this joint to mildly dislocate, or sublux.

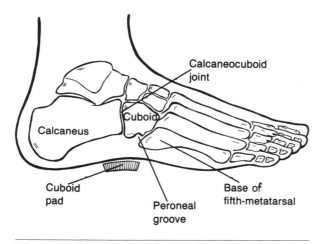

Figure 4.16 Subluxed cuboid syndrome.

When the cuboid subluxes downward, the athlete may experience a dull ache along the central portion of the lateral border of the foot. The long calcaneocuboid ligament, extending from the heel to the cuboid, may become strained, mimicking heel spur pain along the bottom of the heel. Direct pressure at the calcaneocuboid joint often elicits the primary pain symptoms. On stance, the athlete experiences discomfort when attempting to stand on his or her toes or when rolling the arches toward the outside border of the foot.

Because this joint is involved with locking the foot for strength during various stages of the gait cycle, any instability or dysfunction around the cuboid inhibits functional stability in the foot during the propulsive phase of gait. The athlete shies away from forcefully pushing off with the foot. Lateral, side-to-side sports, such as tennis or racquetball, place the greatest strain at this joint. Stair climbing and lateral cutting movements aggravate the condition. Tight heel cords, causing an early heel lift, disturb the normal weight transfer through the lateral column and initiate the syndrome. Anatomically, the cuboid aids the function of the peroneal tendons by stabilizing the tendons as they pass under the foot. The subluxed cuboid may disturb normal peroneal function, with ensuing tendinitis and referred pain to either the lateral ankle or the plantar aspect of the forefoot.

Treatment for a subluxed cuboid syndrome consists of a series of manipulations of the joint and secure strappings to reduce the subluxation. The manipulation needs to be done by a professional; however, applying a cuboid pad sometimes provides relief. This can be done by trimming a ¼-inch thick felt pad approximately 1 inch square and taping it under the cuboid. This is the area under the outer border of the foot, just behind the bump (which is the base of the metatarsal) at about the middle of the foot. If this padding causes increasing pain, it should be discontinued. Anti-inflammatory medication and physical therapy help ease any discomfort. After care with orthotic control, use calf-stretching exercises to guard against reinjury.

Subluxed cuboid syndrome is an uncommon problem but, once recognized, responds well to appropriate treatment.

Pronation

Mark Landry, D.P.M.

The term *pronation* signifies the flattening of the arch during weightbearing, causing the kneecap and foot to roll inward during running and walking.

Some pronation is natural, desirable, and necessary to allow the foot to adapt to various surfaces and absorb shock. However, in some persons this inward rotation of the knee and flattening of the arch is excessive, putting too much strain on the muscles, tendons, and ligaments of the hip, thigh, leg, knee, and foot. The extra force of hyperpronation can cause stress fractures or shin splints in the lower leg. It also can lead to arch strain and fatigue, heel spur syndrome, plantar fasciitis (an inflammation of the pressure-absorbing fibrous sheet covering the muscles on the bottom of the foot), Achilles tendinitis, bunions, and stress fractures of the foot.

Pronation is a three-dimensional motion involving several joints of the foot and ankle. As your heel strikes the ground your leg twists inward, your ankle bulges inward, and the knee flexes to help absorb the impact, while your forefoot and heel rotate outward. This compromise motion of the forefoot and heel going one way while the ankle and leg go another occurs because the joint axes of the rearfoot and midfoot bones move with a lot of horizontal motion, increasing total pronation. Both the degree and level of pronation at the midfoot, rearfoot, or ankle most often are assessed by a physician through x-rays taken of the standing patient.

Identifying Pronation

Experienced athletes often can identify an overly pronating athlete when they observe the other's ankles bulging inward during walking or running. Eventual telltale signs of excessive pronation are more compression of the inside of the heel, compared to the outside of the heel. A hyperpronator's shoe heels always wear down first because, in compensating for excessive pronation, he or she lands too far back on the heels. When the shoes are re-

moved and looked at from the rear, they are seen to slant inward.

Whereas excessive pronation can be observed by standing behind another and observing the ankles turning in, there are other, less obvious, structural foot changes that occur that can be viewed from the side (seen as a sagging of the longitudinal arch) (Figure 4.17). Therefore, pronation has an effect on both the foot and the leg in all three dimensions and can be observed and measured from behind, above, and the side.

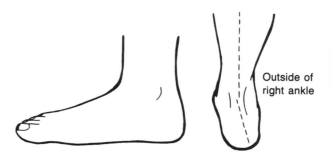
Outside of right ankle

Figure 4.17   Pronation of the foot causes a positional change in which the arch rolls in and the heel rolls out, giving a flattened appearance to the arch.

Pronation during walking is normally observed when the foot is on the ground (stance phase). Supination (ankle and foot rolling outward) provides leverage during the propulsive phase of the walker's gait. In running, the foot markedly pronates on impact with the ground and remains relatively pronated for a longer period of time—about 70 percent of the stance phase—when compared to walking. Persons who hyperpronate do so throughout the stance phase when walking, and even more so when running. This foot action contributes to many of the overuse injuries seen in athletes.

Though people who hyperpronate tend to develop injuries in distance running, they do quite well in other sports, such as basketball and sprinting. The repetitive and similar foot-strike activity in distance running magnifies what otherwise might be a minor degree of pronation.

With foot strike, gravity thrusts the foot (and leg) into pronation. Muscles and tendons work to rotate the leg externally and supinate the foot for pushing off. When the bony structure is hyperpronated, muscles and tendons strain as they fail to align the leg and foot. Undue stress from the force of the body's weight and from stretching of the muscles and tendons ultimately is absorbed by bones and joints. Muscle cramps and tendon strain appear initially. If this condition is left untreated, more serious joint damage and stress fractures may occur.

Anatomical Causes

Pronation seldom is caused by problems in joints of the rear- or midfoot. Occasionally an athlete born with an irregular joint surface may develop hyperpronation, but this is rare. Pronation more often occurs to compensate for some other anatomical aberration. Among such irregularities within the foot are the following:

- Morton's syndrome, in which the long bone (metatarsal) behind the big toe may be too elevated or too short, making the big toe shorter than the next toe and causing the foot to rock inward and pronate
- Loose joints or double-jointedness
- Abnormal leg anatomy (for example, a bowlegged person brings the foot fully to the ground by pronating)
- Tight calf muscles, which may mean a normal- to high-arched foot when not weightbearing, but marked pronation on weightbearing; a severely tight calf pulls the heel upward and outward while the midfoot laterally collapses to allow the foot to flatten on the ground

Genetic background plays a role in most anatomical predispositions toward hyperpronation. Heredity patterns of foot, knee, and leg structures are not difficult to see. Those who hyperpronate with a knocked knee can compare, if possible, their individual structure with that of their parents or grandparents. Older family members with a similar genetic makeup may well have vague arthritic complaints involving the knee or foot.

Athletic shoe designers have countered hyperpronation by tilting the shoe with a varus wedge inserted in the sole to tilt the foot toward the midline of the body, adding reinforcing pegs to the sole, reinforcing the heel counter, and using a multitude of other components, such as flared heels and arch supports, to stabilize the foot and keep it from turning inward excessively as it strikes the ground and then pushes off. Though some current shoe devices may be somewhat trendy, shoe companies should be credited for an overall improvement in the quality of footwear now available for athletes.

Functional Causes

The exercise surface is the most important nonanatomical cause for excessive pronation. Soft, dry sand causes your foot to hyperpronate because of the lack of ground resistance. Muscles easily strain in an attempt to stabilize an overpronated foot with internal leg rotation. As your foot strikes sand, it often remains pronated throughout stance phase and does not exert leverage. Abnormal force is exerted on the joint ligaments and capsules within the foot and leg. Exercising on dry sand is not recommended. Also, sloped surfaces pronate the high-sided leg and foot more; consequently, you should use a level surface.

A faulty shoe often can cause hyperpronation. Inspect the heels of a new pair of shoes from behind. Are they vertical? Make sure one shoe does not lean or bulge toward the other.

The athlete's style of movement may also contribute to functional hyperpronation. The bounce gait sometimes seen in the novice runner requires more knee flexion and foot pronation at ground impact. Good running style involves less up-and-down swinging of the body's center of gravity than walking. Overstriding, however, increases the need for knees and ankles to absorb excessive shock. The impact from overstriding overwhelms what the knee and foot normally can do and often results in injury.

Just as the ballet dancer who "wings" the foot for style in a pronated attitude prior to landing may develop ankle and knee injuries, so may the athlete whose foot is allowed to flare or flop outward during the swing phase of gait. This causes the foot to land in an overpronated position. Also, the tired athlete may lean forward more, allowing the foot to land in an excessively dorsiflexed (upward) and pronated position.

Controlling Hyperpronation

Exercise style and all of the shoes you wear regularly—athletic and nonathletic—should be checked to determine functional causes for excessive pronation. Exercise on level, firm surfaces. After all functional causes are ruled out, a thorough anatomical evaluation should be done by a sports podiatrist.

Once the physician has ascertained which joint is causing your problem and has determined the magnitude and possible anatomical causes for your hyperpronation, a customized orthotic device can be made to control the hyperpronation. If one of your legs is longer than the other and pronates, a lift can be incorporated in the shoe worn on the shorter leg. If pronation occurs primarily in midfoot and within the horizontal plane, the orthotic device may need to be made with more side-to-side control.

Conclusion

Many shoe companies, running stores, and salespersons have recently improved and expanded their lines of shoes as well as footwear advice for the athlete. The diagnosis of hyperpronation and related injuries also has expanded in scope during the last decade. The precise nature of an injury must be diagnosed, followed by conservative measures to determine what role, if any, hyperpronation plays in the injury. Functional hyperpronation from shoes, terrain, or faulty style should either be ruled out or corrected. If anatomical hyperpronation coexists with an injury, the rear- and midfoot can be evaluated to determine the precise joints involved and how an orthotic device should be constructed to control the excessive pronation.

Suggested Reading for "Pronation"

Brody (1980)

See reading list at the end of the book for a complete source listing.

Supination (Pes Cavus; High-Arch Feet)

Paul M. Taylor, D.P.M.

Supination is a normal motion that occurs in the foot. Important to proper foot function of the athlete, supination is the reverse of pronation. Both essential movements, supination and pronation become important injury considerations when either is excessive or impaired, or occurs at the wrong time during the gait cycle.

To understand supination, visualize the motion of your foot as taking place on three planes: it turns inward (adduct), flexes downward (plantarflex), and rotates inward (invert), all at the same time. This three-plane motion, possible because of the complex configuration of the foot joints, allows the foot to function differently during each of the three motions.

While the foot is pronated, the arch flattens, making it more flexible, so it can adapt to changes in surfaces. When the foot is supinated, it is more rigid and can act as a lever to propel the body forward while moving. For optimum function of these unique features of the foot, there must be a normal sequence to pronation and supination while the foot contacts the ground.

As the heel hits the ground at the beginning of the stance (or ground) phase of the gait cycle, the foot is in a slightly supinated position. As the entire foot contacts the ground, it becomes more pronated, to adapt to any unequal surface. Then, as the body weight shifts over the foot, it again supinates, to become the rigid lever needed to propel the body forward.

Excessive pronation results in a hypermobile (moving excessively) and unstable foot, causing a myriad of foot and leg problems commonly recognized by many athletes (e.g., muscle, tendon, and ligament strains; stress fractures; runner's knee; tendinitis; etc.). Although it does not occur as frequently as pronation, excessive supination also can lead to a number of injuries.

Potential Injuries

Injuries that occur in the supinated foot are due to positional changes in the foot structure.

The supinated foot appears to have a high arch. A footprint may show contact only at the heel and the ball, without any arch area contact. The heel appears inverted (turned inward) when viewed from behind. The toes may be contracted, and usually there is a tight heel cord. These changes contribute to injuries in this foot type (Figure 4.18).

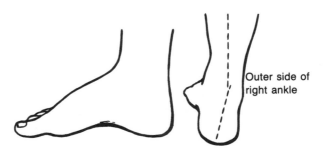

Outer side of right ankle

Figure 4.18 Supination of the foot causes a positional change in which the height of the arch is increased and the heel rolls inward, as viewed from behind.

Athletes with supinated feet frequently complain of heel problems. Achilles tendinitis can develop on the back of the heel, due to the tight heel cord. Pain and swelling can develop on the back portion of the heel from the tilt of the heel bone (calcaneus). This causes a rubbing by the shoe that irritates the area. If this goes on too long, bursitis (inflammation of the friction-reducing sac of fluid protecting the heel) may result.

Several sites on the bottom of the heel can cause pain. Plantar fasciitis (an inflammation of the protective fibrous tissue covering the muscles on the bottom of the foot) may develop due to the traction on this thick fibrous band connecting the heel to the front of the foot and helping support the arch. This structure is more prone to injury in the high-arch foot.

Because the heel contacts the surface more to the outside when the foot supinates, a small nerve on the outer border of the heel can become traumatized and may develop into a heel neuroma, a very painful thickening of the nerve. If stress on the plantar fascia where it inserts into the calcaneus, or heel bone, persists long enough, a heel spur, or outgrowth on the heel bone, can result.

Supination causes more weight to be shifted to the outer border of the foot. This can lead to an irritation to the joint at the base of the little toe. When this continues, an enlargement called a *tailor's bunion* can develop at this joint.

A muscle imbalance is also frequently present in the supinated foot, accounting for the contraction of the toes that may occur. This, in conjunction with the more prominent bones in the balls of the feet due to the high arch, causes increased pain and formation of a callus on the bottom of the foot.

Prevention

If the athlete has a supinated foot, there are several ways to prevent the injuries described or to self-treat some of these problems when they begin to occur.

Selection of proper shoes should be the first step. Though the clerk at your local athletic shoe store should be able to help in choosing the best shoes, be sure to look for high shock-absorbing capability, a sturdy heel counter, a contoured innersole for heel protection, and, most important, a good fit. Things to avoid if you have a supinated foot include shoes with a varus wedge (an insert in the shoe that tilts your foot slightly toward the midline of your body) and other shoes designed to control pronation. In some cases, due to the supination and other leg and ankle positions, it is necessary to obtain a shoe that does control pronation. Although this seems a contradiction, it sometimes does happen. To determine if this is necessary, you will probably require a thorough biomechanical evaluation by a sportsmedicine physician.

Another preventive technique is to increase shock absorption by placing an additional innersole in the shoe or using heel pads. Also important for athletes who supinate is stretching, particularly of the calf and hamstring. Refer to chapter 12 for recommended strengthening and stretching exercises. Strengthening exercises emphasizing the muscles in the front of the leg (anterior tibialis) (Strength Exercise

25) and the thigh (quadriceps) (Strength Exercises 18a and b) should be done. Stretching exercises should include the wall push-up (Stretch Exercises 2 and 3) and toe touches (Stretch Exercise 12).

Treatment

If problems develop despite preventive measures, localized self-treatment should include rest, ice after activity, and aspirin. Occasionally, resting an injury for 5 to 7 days allows it to heal. If you continue activity, ice should be applied to the injured area for 5 to 10 minutes afterward to prevent inflammation. If you have stopped activity, heat should be applied for 15 to 20 minutes two to three times per day to help the local healing.

Two aspirin can be taken four times a day to reduce inflammation. Consult your physician if you have had allergic reactions to aspirin or if you have any stomach problems or bleeding tendencies, because aspirin can be hard on the stomach and can interfere with normal blood clotting. In such cases, your physician can prescribe a nonaspirin anti-inflammatory medication.

When problems persist, professional help may be needed. Supination injuries are not as common as pronation injuries, but they can be more difficult to treat. A doctor may suggest some of the things you have already tried (e.g., ice, rest, heat, and aspirin). Be sure to inform the physician of any self-treatment, so he or she can implement more aggressive therapy if needed. This may consist of injections, physical therapy, stronger oral anti-inflammatories, or orthotic devices. Orthotic devices that normally work best for supination problems are soft or semiflexible. Specific corrections or posting can be applied to the device to accommodate your individual foot type. The doctor may also suggest changes in stretching or strengthening techniques.

Supination and pronation are opposite motions. Both can cause foot problems for the athlete. Excessive supination can lead to several specific injuries; an understanding of some of the mechanisms involved in these allows you to appreciate the complexity of your foot, to be patient in recovering from an ailment, and to accept changes that may be necessary.

Heel Spurs

Robert F. Weiss, D.P.M.

Heel spur syndrome is one of the most common, and potentially most devastating, injuries that the athlete can suffer. The heel bone (calcaneus) is a thick, rectangular bone. At the bottom of the calcaneus is a pad to cushion the heel with the ground. There is also a band of connective tissue that runs longitudinally along the arch from the heel to the toes. This is the plantar fascia; it elevates, or supports, the arch. The plantar fascia is a tough, fibrous band composed of three strips. The middle strip is the thickest; the thinner medial and lateral strips are thickest at the heel region, becoming thinner at the metatarsal-toe joints (Figure 4.19).

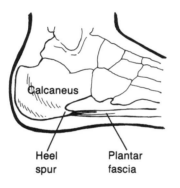

Figure 4.19 The plantar heel spur develops where the plantar fascia inserts into the heel bone (calcaneus).

The spur formation is usually a shelf of bone along the entire width of the heel bone. It is formed by the continual tearing away of the periosteum or lining of the heel bone by the strong plantar fascia, due to abnormal pronation of the foot during the heel contact, midstance, and toe-off phases of gait. As the tearing occurs, a layer of new bone (a calcium deposit) forms. This layer gradually thickens, forming a heel spur located at the insertion of the plantar fascia, at the bottom of the heel bone. This bony prominence penetrates into the surrounding tissue as an irritant and can cause a heel bursitis.

Causes

There are several possible causes of heel spurs. One such possibility is poor training shoes. They may be worn down on the heel area or may lack rearfoot control or cushioning. Another cause may be running on hard surfaces, including concrete roads. Although it has been said that running on dirt or grass is better for you, I have not always found this to be true, due to the uneven terrain. Increase in training, sprinting, track workouts for speed training, and hill running are often contributing causes of heel spurs. However, spurs are primarily due to the abnormal biomechanical changes of the pathological foot mechanics due to excessive foot pronation.

Symptoms

A heel spur manifests itself as a deep tenderness on the bottom of the heel. The pain may radiate into the sole of the foot. Actually, the pain is not from the spur itself, but from the irritated fibrous bursa, the sac that surrounds the spur. In its early stages, the heel spur syndrome has a characteristic pain cycle of greater soreness in the morning or after sitting for a long period of time, becoming less painful after walking or jogging.

Depending on the extent of the deformity, pain may be variable, being present during rest or only after vigorous exercise. There may also be local swelling. The pain is usually tolerable. After a few weeks, a pattern of dull, aching pain occurs with standing, after a period of rest.

Treatment

Therapy for a heel spur includes rest from the event putting stress on your heel; go to an alternate aerobic activity, such as swimming or biking, to stay in good cardiovascular condition. I am a believer in long-distance walking to increase blood flow to the tissues because blood contains the body's own natural healing elements. Start at just a few miles; then walk up to the distance that you were running. One rule of thumb is that if you can walk without pain, you may start back with your activities—in moderation.

Massage the heel with ice for 10 minutes. Follow this with moist heat (a hot washcloth in a plastic bag) for 3 to 5 minutes to increase blood supply to the injured area. This sequence, which should be done two or three times per day, is very helpful.

An extremely important move that is often overlooked is to change into a proper running shoe with good heel and forefoot cushioning. This protects the area from additional trauma.

Heel cushion padding placed directly into the shoe (using sponge rubber or felt cut to the shape of the heel, or shaped like a horseshoe, to take the pressure off the lateral portion of the heel) may be of some value. Also, taping the longitudinal arch holds the plantar fascia in place and retards the pulling during the abnormal pronation.

If symptoms and pain persist or recur after a few days of self-treatment and rest, seek the help of a sports-oriented physician. In my professional experience with the less severe cases of heel spur syndrome, various physical therapy modalities, including ultrasound with electrical muscle stimulation and exercise, have been very helpful in treatment when used along with the home physical therapy methods already mentioned.

In more severe cases, anti-inflammatory medications can be used successfully. Another form of treatment is the utilization of a local injection of steroid preparations with lidocaine (a local anesthetic). For patients who do not like the idea of steroids (although this is a very safe and effective treatment) vitamin B-12 may be injected in place of it. This vitamin works as a therapeutic nerve block above the inner aspect of the heel to create vasodilation, or increased blood supply, to the area of the heel spur.

A biomechanical evaluation—including a gait analysis, preferably on a treadmill—should be instituted. Engineering instruments should be utilized to measure any degree of abnormal foot imbalances that may result in extra stress on the foot structures. A temporary, soft orthosis with heel lifts and wedging for forefoot and rearfoot balancing can be used until the proper functional sport orthotic devices can be fabricated to correct any lower extremity or foot deformity.

In the most severe cases, a surgical procedure may be warranted when all conservative and biomechanical therapy efforts have been unsuccessful and there is extreme pain on motion.

It is also wise to remember that perhaps the best treatment for the athlete is rest.

Prevention

The symptoms of a heel spur can be painful in acute stages and, if not dealt with early, can become chronic—creating problems for years to come.

The athletic culture is beginning to understand the enormous stress fitness activities put on the feet and legs. Therefore, it comes as no surprise that the athlete looks for the best shoes available. In order to best protect the foot, you need a running shoe with a thick sole, a thicker heel, and a semiflexible forefoot.

In addition to careful selection of shoes in preventing heel spurs, stretching exercises are also important. If the calf muscles and fascia are tight, this will increase the traction effect by the fascia on the heel spur—resulting in pain. Refer to chapter 12, Stretch Exercises 1, 2, and 3.

Suggested Reading for "Heel Spurs"

Baxter & Thigpen (1984)

See reading list at the end of the book for a complete source listing.

Heel Neuroma

Paul M. Taylor, D.P.M.

A heel neuroma is a painful thickening of a sensory nerve along the inside border of the heel. When a nerve is subjected to repeated trauma, it develops a fibrous thickening around it. As this fibrous tissue increases, it places increasing pressure on the nerve fibers. This increased pressure causes pain on the nerve, and pain can also be felt in the area that is supplied with that nerve.

The nerve along the inside plantar aspect of the heel is subject to irritation as the heel strikes the ground during running. This is more prevalent in persons who pronate excessively, because they place more pressure on the inside of the heel. The early symptoms of a heel neuroma are initially more evident after exercise. There may be a mild pain that may be felt only as a burning or tingling along the inner border of the heel. This may gradually increase, with radiating pain farther under the heel or back up toward the ankle. If the irritation on the nerve continues long enough, the nerve becomes increasingly thickened and painful. In the later stages of this condition, the enlarged nerve can be identified under the skin by rolling the thumb over the painful area; a small, movable nodule or bump can be felt.

The heel neuroma can be treated initially by the sufferer using a shoe with better rearfoot stability and adding a heel cup, which can be obtained at most athletic shoe stores or sporting goods stores. An ice massage should be applied over the area for 5 minutes after activity.

If the pain does not respond to this initial self-treatment, professional help may be necessary. This could include additional shoe modifications, physical therapy such as ultrasound, orthotic devices to control any abnormal foot function, cortisone injections, and, ultimately, surgical excision of the neuroma if other treatments do not resolve the pain.

The more radical treatments, such as surgery, can be avoided if early treatment is initiated when the first symptoms of a heel neuroma are observed.

Heel Bruise (Stone Bruise)

Paul M. Taylor, D.P.M.

A heel bruise can occur during running by striking the heel against an object, such as a stone, or during jumping by landing hard on the heel. The bottom of the heel is normally well protected. The skin on the bottom of the heel is the thickest of any part of the body. A thick layer of dense fat, supported by strong fibrous tissue, protects and cushions the heel bone. Despite this, a sharp blow to the bottom of the heel can damage these tissues, cause rupture of blood vessels, and damage the periosteum, or covering, of the heel bone (calcaneus). When this occurs, the bleeding causes a bruise of the fat layer; if the periosteum is damaged, pain can develop that may last for several weeks. The periosteum (tissue which surrounds all bone) is very sensitive, and an injury to this tissue can be very painful.

When the athlete sustains a heel bruise, he or she can usually recall the incident that caused the pain. When this happens, the activity should be discontinued, ice applied to the heel, and the foot elevated. Returning to full activity should be avoided until it is comfortable to walk on the heel. Thick, soft foam pads should be worn in all shoes. On resuming activity, the athlete should wear a shoe with high shock absorption in the heel and should continue to use the soft pads. Ice applications should be continued after activity until there is no longer any tenderness in the heel.

There are also many other causes of plantar heel pain; if there is no recollection of a specific episode when the heel was injured, and it does not improve in 2 to 3 weeks, then it is possible that the heel pain may not be due to a simple stone bruise. If other causes for the heel pain cannot be identified, medical attention should be sought. It is a common error to refer to any painful heel condition as a stone bruise. Actually, most heel pain is due to other causes. Therefore, careful attention should be paid to accurately identifying the cause of heel pain.

Fissured Heels

Paul M. Taylor, D.P.M.

Fissured heels is a condition in which the skin around the heels becomes very dry and callused, and the skin begins to split, causing painful cracks or fissures in the skin. This cracking of the heels is more common in persons who are generally prone to dry skin problems. It becomes worse during winter months, when humidity is reduced by the heating of homes and offices.

The fissures develop because the dry, thickened, callused skin does not stretch like normal skin. Fissures can split the full thickness of skin and become very painful. They are very slow to heal because the callus holds the skin apart.

People who are prone to dry skin should try to prevent fissures from developing. This can be done by applying hand cream or lotion to the heels daily. For more severe cases, heavier ointment such as petroleum jelly should be applied. If this is too greasy, the ointment can be applied at night; a pair of cotton socks is worn over it to bed. It also helps to keep the humidity higher in the house by running a humidifier. If there is thick callus around the heels, this should be smoothed with a pumice stone or callus file two or three times a week.

If the above preventive measures do not work, and the fissures still develop, more aggressive treatment is needed. An antibiotic ointment should be applied to the open fissure, which is covered with a Band-Aid® applied crosswise in order to hold the margins of the fissure together so it can heal. A heel cup should be obtained to wear in the shoes in order to limit the amount of stretching of the heel pad, so as to reduce the number of fissures. The preventive measures described above should be continued as well.

Most cases of heel fissures can be self-treated. However, if pain persists or redness, swelling, or drainage from the fissures develops, professional podiatric care should be sought.

Calcaneal Apophysitis

Ayne F. Furman, D.P.M.

One of the most commonly overlooked causes of heel pain in children is calcaneal apophysitis, a condition in which the epiphysis (growth plate) of the calcaneus (heel bone) becomes irritated and inflamed (Figure 4.20).

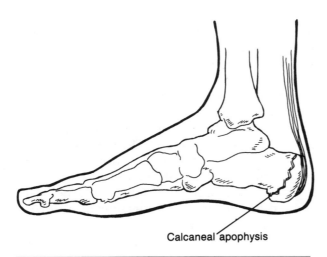

Calcaneal apophysis

Figure 4.20   Calcaneal apophysitis develops at the growth plate of the heel bone (calcaneus).

Calcaneal apophysitis occurs most often in children between the ages of 10 and 14, at a time when the bones of the feet are still ossifying and becoming mature. The child who is affected by this ailment complains of a dull, achy pain in one or both heels. The pain is most intense during and after physical activity—especially activity that involves continual pounding of the feet—but subsides with rest. Many times the pain is so severe it causes the child to limp. The heel may appear swollen, warm, and tender to the touch.

Several years ago it was thought that calcaneal apophysitis was rare in females, but with the increased participation of young girls in sports, the condition is found equally among boys and girls.

Causes

The epiphyseal plate of the calcaneus is the weakest point of the developing heel and is much softer than the mature bone at either end. The heel is placed under considerable stress with walking, but the amount of stress at this point increases up to six times during activities such as basketball, soccer, and running. It is the result of repeated small amounts of stress, or microtrauma, that is believed to cause inflammation at the epiphysis.

A number of factors have been shown to be associated with calcaneal apophysitis, including two- or three-cleated heels on soccer shoes, faulty foot biomechanics, a tight gastrocnemius soleus (calf) muscle complex, excessive training, poorly constructed shoes, and repeated jumping.

Treatment

Elimination or modification of one or more of the aggravating factors mentioned above may cure the symptoms of calcaneal apophysitis. Some simple changes:

1. Avoid soccer shoes with only two or three cleats at the heel. Shoes should have four-cleated heels to distribute the impact of foot strike more evenly.
2. Faulty foot biomechanics, such as a pronated (flat) or cavus (high-arch) foot structure, may lead to increased stress at the epiphysis. A prescription orthotic device from a sportsmedicine podiatrist often solves the problem.
3. The gastrocnemius soleus muscle complex blends together to form the Achilles tendon, which attaches to the rear fragment of mature bone. If the muscle complex is contracted or too tight, it causes increased pull on the rear fragment of bone in a direction away from the epiphysis. This problem sometimes can be corrected through the addition of a ¼-inch heel lift in each shoe or by stretching the calf muscles. An effective stretch for the calf can be done by standing facing a wall, 2 to 3 feet away, feet pointing straight ahead. Place your hands on the wall

and gradually lean forward, keeping knees straight and feet flat on the ground. Lean forward until tightness in calves and lower leg can be felt. Hold this position for 30 seconds. Straighten up. Repeat four times.

4. The amount of exercise any child can tolerate is individually determined, just as for adults. For one child, running 10 miles a week and playing soccer may be excessive and could induce enough heel trauma to cause calcaneal apophysitis, whereas another child may have no problem. Limiting the training schedule or play level is a good, safe way to initiate home treatment.

5. Due to the high cost of athletic footwear and the child's rapidly changing shoe size, shoes often are worn too long, or less expensive, poor-quality shoes are purchased. Particularly with running, poor footwear can add stress to the epiphysis because the shoes frequently do not offer enough protection or allow the foot to function optimally.

6. The kind of jumping done in basketball games is highly associated with the incidence of calcaneal apophysitis. Many times it is advisable for a child to sit out a season because the pounding aggravates the symptoms. An alternative activity such as swimming can be substituted to make the rest from basketball more acceptable to the child.

Once calcaneal apophysitis develops, the amount of activity must be reduced significantly until the pain diminishes. Only then should a slow increase back to the previous level of activity be attempted. Sometimes complete rest is necessary to relieve chronic inflammation of the epiphysis.

Severe Pain

If the heel pain is severe enough to cause the child to limp, or if swelling is evident, investigation by a trained medical person is necessary. At the time of the exam, x-rays normally are taken of the heel area. This is done not so much to diagnose calcaneal apophysitis (because it often does not show up well on standard x-rays), as to rule out other possible causes of the pain, such as a bone tumor or infection. Once a diagnosis is made, the doctor's treatment is one or a combination of the above-mentioned therapies. If the heel pain is so severe that the child has difficulty walking, a last resort is to place a plaster cast from below the knee to the end of the foot for 3 to 4 weeks. After the cast is removed, activities should be resumed slowly.

Effects of Continued Activity

Unlike some other conditions, calcaneal apophysitis resolves itself by the age of 14 or 15, after the growth plate has ossified. In this age of increased athletic activities for children, however, telling a child to stop all athletics for several seasons normally is not well received and should be done only when all indicated therapies have been attempted.

A common question concerns whether continued activity in a child with calcaneal apophysitis is harmful. Unfortunately, little long-term research and documentation have been done on this condition. It is always best to be conservative. Whenever a child complains of pain, or limps for an unknown reason, the cause should be investigated. See chapter 16, "Developmental Factors Affecting Children's Exercise" for additional information.

Posterior Heel Spur

Paul M. Taylor, D.P.M.

A posterior heel spur is an enlargement of bone that develops on the back of the heel bone (calcaneus). The spur develops at the insertion of the Achilles tendon (Figure 4.21). The mechanism for the formation of the spur is a traction force from the Achilles tendon pulling on the periosteum, or lining, of the heel bone. This occurs on a microscopic level; when the periosteum is separated from the bone, the body attempts to repair the injury by laying down new bone. This is a very slow process that continues over a long period of time.

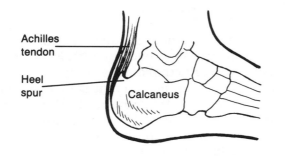

Figure 4.21 The posterior heel spur develops on the heel bone (calcaneus) at the insertion of the Achilles tendon.

As the sequence of traction, separation of periosteum, and new bone formation continues, a bony projection or spur can develop on the back of the heel. Sometimes this process continues on such a low-grade level that no pain is felt during this time. However, as the traction increases and the process speeds up, pain may be felt on the back of the heel, which can be isolated by pressing on that area. Frequently, inflammation and pain extend up along the Achilles tendon. Because of this, the posterior heel spur may be mistaken as an Achilles tendinitis.

Initial treatment for a developing posterior heel spur is to reduce the level of activity to stop the traction on the heel. Ice should be applied to reduce the inflammation. A ¼-inch heel raise helps take some of the tension off the Achilles tendon. If there is excessive motion in the heel because of a foot imbalance, an orthotic device can help. Gentle stretching exercises for the calf muscles should be done after the inflammation subsides. Trying to stretch the calf while the area is still tender may aggravate it, because this places more tension on the developing spur.

Usually a heel spur is most painful during the developmental stage. If local treatment keeps the heel comfortable during this time, which may take several months, the pain eventually resolves—even though the spur may still be evident on x-ray. Because of this, it is not generally necessary to consider surgical removal for the spur. Conservative treatment provides relief during the development of the spur; surgery is necessary only if pain is severe and persistent. Cortisone injections should be avoided for this problem, because they do nothing to dissolve the spur and may weaken the tendon, especially with repeated injections.

The posterior spur is caused by the traction of the Achilles tendon on the calcaneus and usually is self-limiting and responsive to conservative treatment if the level of activity is reduced.

Haglund's Deformity (Pump Bump)

Paul M. Taylor, D.P.M.

A Haglund's deformity is an enlargement of the back of the heel (calcaneus) that causes irritation and pain due to rubbing from shoes. The bony prominence, the enlargement, is usually a developmental variance in the shape of the bone; it is sometimes due to a change in the position of the foot in which there is inversion of the heel. The enlargement on the back of the heel, usually toward the outer side of the foot, is very easily irritated by the stiff, reinforced heel counter of shoes. This especially happens with the pump type of shoe, thus the term *pump bump.*

The rubbing initially causes irritation and blisters on the skin. As the pressure continues, though, inflammation of the deeper tissues develops, with increasing pain and swelling. Eventually a knot of inflamed tissue develops in this area. This is formed by a combination of the enlarged bone, the thickened, irritated skin, the swelling of deeper tissues, and possibly a bursitis between the bone and the skin. As the irritation from the shoe continues, the knot becomes larger and more painful.

Self-treatment of the pump bump involves avoiding shoes that irritate the heel area and applying protective padding to prevent irritation. Foam or felt padding can be placed around the bump and then covered with moleskin to protect the area. A heel cup may also help keep pressure off the area. It may also help to change styles of shoes so that the heel pressure is off the area. The contact point of the heel counter against the bump can also be changed by placing a heel pad in the shoe to slightly raise the heel.

If relief cannot be obtained with the above self-treatment then professional help may be needed. Professional treatment may involve several approaches. Initially, shoe modifications and a different type of padding may be tried. If the area is very swollen and tender, a course of physical therapy may be indicated. A cortisone injection to obtain quicker relief may be considered. In cases in which a particular foot type (such as a high arch) places the heel in an abnormal position, an orthotic device can help to alleviate the pressure by changing the position of the heel.

When conservative measures fail to provide relief, surgical excision of the enlarged portion of the heel bone should be considered. This procedure can be done safely on an outpatient basis under local anesthesia. Recovery time varies with the extent of bone which must be removed; therefore, the expected results, recovery, and options should be discussed with the surgeon.

Prevention of a recurrence of the pump bump requires proper shoe selection, avoiding a heel counter that irritates the area, and, in cases in which a certain foot type contributes to the problem, using an orthotic device.

The Haglund's deformity or pump bump can develop into a very painful problem for the athlete. Fortunately, most of these respond to conservative treatment; for the persistent cases, surgical correction is available.

Tarsal Tunnel Syndrome

Paul M. Taylor, D.P.M.

Tarsal tunnel syndrome is an uncommon injury that is due to compression of the posterior tibial nerve. The posterior tibial nerve becomes entrapped on the inside of the ankle, just below the ankle bone (Figure 4.22). This syndrome can cause multiple symptoms in this area, including pain and swelling on the inside of the ankle, pain radiating up the inside of the leg or down into the foot (sometimes into the toes), pain on the bottom of the heel, or numbness on the bottom of the foot.

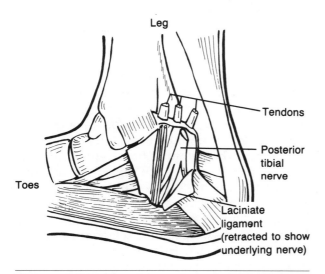

Figure 4.22   Tarsal tunnel syndrome occurs when surrounding structures cause impingement on the posterior tibial nerve.

There are multiple causes for the compression of this nerve. They all occur because the nerve passes through a tunnel formed by the laciniate ligament just below the ankle. This ligament supports the posterior tibial nerve, blood vessels, and tendons in this area. There is only a limited amount of room in this area; anything that causes increased swelling or crowding of the tissues may create the entrapment and compression of the nerve.

Tarsal tunnel syndrome has been attributed to congenital tightness or to thickening of the laciniate ligament itself. A bony enlargement, such as an exostosis, may compress the nerve.

Varicose veins in this area may expand enough to cause the symptoms. Trauma, such as an ankle fracture or severe ankle sprain, causes swelling and possibly adhesions around the nerve. Tarsal tunnel syndrome from an injury may not be evident until late in the recovery stage. Overuse injuries, such as posterior tibial tendinitis, may initiate this syndrome. Excessive pronation of the foot may cause or contribute to tarsal tunnel syndrome by stretching the nerve under the ligament as the foot rolls out and the ankle rolls in.

Because tarsal tunnel syndrome can have multiple symptoms and causes, the initial diagnosis of this condition is difficult. In many cases, patients were treated for other problems before the proper diagnosis of tarsal tunnel syndrome was made. It is easy to misdiagnose this problem, especially when it develops following an injury. The diagnosis can be made based on the symptoms described above, an accurate history, and a positive Tinel sign (pain or tingling into the foot when the nerve is tapped). Once there is a suspicion that tarsal tunnel syndrome exists, it can be confirmed by special tests, including electromyographic and nerve conduction studies.

Treatment requires identifying and correcting the cause. If pronation is present, an orthotic device can help. If there has been an injury with persistent swelling, then rest, heat, compression, and elevation should be used to reduce the swelling. With injuries or tendinitis, the use of oral anti-inflammatories or cortisone injections may be indicated.

Unfortunately, with tarsal tunnel syndrome, especially in cases that are diagnosed late, conservative treatment is not always successful. When this occurs, surgical correction, which includes freeing the nerve from under the laciniate ligament, is necessary.

Prevention of tarsal tunnel syndrome includes early and appropriate treatment of ankle injuries, controlling pronation, and obtaining early treatment when the symptoms of this syndrome are first noticed.

Suggested Reading for "Tarsal Tunnel Syndrome"

Murphy & Baxter (1985)

Ricciardi-Polline et al. (1985)

See reading list at the end of the book for a complete source listing.

CHAPTER 5

Ankle Injuries

The ankle is made up of only three bones, the tibia and the fibula at the leg and the talus of the foot. All are bound together by numerous ligaments, tendons, and bands of connective fibers for support. The ankle joint itself is a hinge joint that only allows movement within the sagittal plane. The ankle can bend in either an upward direction of the foot toward the anterior surface of the leg (dorsiflexion), or in a downward direction of the foot away from the anterior surface of the leg (plantar flexion).

Because of the ankle, the foot can be planted firmly on slanted and irregular surfaces without much loss of balance or speed to the athlete. Often, though, the forces of propulsion push the ankle beyond its limits of flexibility and/or stabilizing support. Then, sudden, acute trauma or gradual overuse injury can result. This chapter looks at a few of the ankle conditions most likely to afflict the athlete. For additional information on terminology used in this chapter, see Appendix A, "The Human Skeleton," and Appendix B, "Body Plane and Movement Terms."

Achilles Tendon Injuries (Tendinitis; Tenosynovitis; Tendinosis; Tendon Rupture)

Mark D. Dollard, D.P.M.

Achilles tendon injuries rank among the most common overuse injuries in athletes, and among the most difficult to treat. These injuries can range from simple tendinitis to severe rupture. The key to diagnosis of the stages of Achilles injuries is recognizing their signs and symptoms.

Anatomy

Comprised of the two conjoined tendons of the soleus and gastrocnemius muscles, the Achilles tendon inserts into the rear part of the heel bone (Figure 5.1). The bulk of the soleus fibers insert into the inside aspect of the heel bone. Surrounding both tendons is an extremely important vascular sheath, the peri-

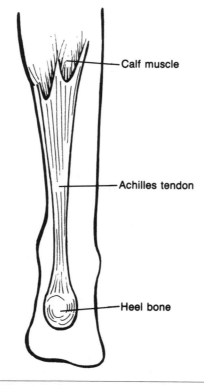

Figure 5.1 The Achilles tendon arises from the calf muscles (gastrocnemius and soleus) and inserts into the heel bone (calcaneus).

tenon, which nourishes the tendon fibers with its blood supply. Because of the specific insertion of these individual tendon fibers, athletes with a tendency to pronate (e.g., become flat-footed) repeatedly stretch the soleus tendon, increasing the likelihood of its injury. Athletes with high-arched, supinated foot types constantly stretch the gastrocnemius fibers, causing injuries higher up in the Achilles complex.

Injury Definitions

Tendinitis is a catchall term for a variety of inflammatory conditions that affect the Achilles tendon. Accurately diagnosing the structural level of an injury to the tendon is important in starting treatment. Usually, the first set of symptoms involves inflammation of the vascular sheath surrounding the tendon; a tenosynovitis of the peritenon. This pain is described as a mild burning or prickly heat sensation about 1 to 3 inches in the Achilles tendon above the heel bone. This area of the tendon has the poorest blood supply and is susceptible to injury even from simple shoe counter irritation.

The second stage of injury causes inflammation and degeneration of the actual tendon fibers: a tendinosis. Second stage pain is described as a shooting, stabbing sensation during physical activity, especially after a sudden change in direction or while running uphill. The athlete may actually feel a crackling sensation while rubbing a hand over the tendon; this is due to inflammatory fluid collecting under the peritenon sheath.

Stage three involves extensive weakening of collagen protein fibers, leading to partial or complete rupture. The athlete may feel a sudden snap or a pop when the tendon ruptures. It may not even be painful; however, a great deal of swelling develops. The torn Achilles provides little strength to allow the athlete to stand on his toes or push off with his foot. To test the integrity of the Achilles, the athlete should lie on his or her stomach. Another person should squeeze the bulky belly of the calf muscle. This normally causes the foot to jerk downward; the ruptured side fails to move the foot in this test.

Mechanism of Injury

When the peritenon is irritated by the back of the shoe rubbing against the tendon, this is easily corrected. In other instances, the sheath may have been damaged by repetitive overstretching during running. Blood vessels are damaged and oxygen supply is lost. Running "cold"—without the proper warm-up necessary to increase the viscosity of the lubricating oils between the sheath and the tendon—allows friction to wear away at the peritenon sheath.

Tendinosis develops in two ways: (a) chronic loss of blood supply from the peritenon, or (b) degeneration in the collagen protein makeup of tendon fibers from the mechanical trauma of repetitive overstretching of the tendon. The primary cause of tendon damage is now known to be due to sudden overstretching of tendon fibers (eccentric stretch) and not from strong contractions (concentric contracture). If the Achilles tendon has not been properly preconditioned with sound flexibility and strength programs, it loses its ability to comply with sudden stretches and to withstand the strain of body weight with each bouncing step. Tendon fibers cannot stretch beyond a certain maximum point. Hill running, stair climbing, and bouncing activities are not handled well by unconditioned tendon fibers.

With normal athletic activities, this physical limitation shows itself when the heel strikes the ground. At this point, as the Achilles becomes fully outstretched with leg extension and ankle flexion, the athlete feels the majority of his or her discomfort. Injured athletes often relate that they experienced the greatest pain when they landed on a curb, ran up stairs, or suddenly changed running directions. If a chronic tendinosis condition is allowed to continue, any sudden stretch may violently snap or rupture weakened tendon fibers. Much as occurs with bony stress fracture repair, the tenocytes—cells that repair tendon—work slowly and cannot overcome daily damage done by the overenthused athlete. The athlete may also be in double jeopardy if his or her foot type is also contributing to strain on the Achilles complex.

Self-Treatment

Prevention with a solid preconditioning program is the best treatment. A flexibility program concentrating on both the soleus and gastrocnemius muscles is advised (see "Stretching Exercises" section for calf stretches). After developing increased flexibility and compliance to stretching, the athlete may adopt certain plyometric drills in order to further coordinate his or her muscle reflexes to counter sudden stretches. These exercises are a series of bouncing drills that should be done only after trained instruction and supervision.

If symptoms do appear, simple self-treatment includes (a) stretching, (b) ice treatment after running, (c) heel lifts, (d) avoidance of hilly courses, (e) avoidance of irritating shoes, (f) use of orthotic devices, and (g) use of aspirin. If symptoms do not resolve after 2 weeks, professional care is recommended.

Professional Care

Don't hesitate to seek professional care in persistent cases. Chronic conditions deteriorate tendon fiber integrity fast. A sports-oriented physician, after examination, can classify your injury as acute—less than 2 weeks duration; subacute—2 to 6 weeks duration; or chronic—greater than 6 weeks duration.

In chronic forms of Achilles injury, degenerative changes and irregularities in the tendon fibers occur. Chronic tendinosis may produce nodular and palpable deformities in the tendon itself. The acute stage is treated with 10 days rest, physical therapy using contrast cold/heat treatment, and oral anti-inflammatory medication. The subacute stage is treated as above, with the addition of heel lifts, orthotic devices, mild compression wraps, or mild restrictive strappings. Some physicians may elect to carefully and judiciously place steroid medication along the outside of the tendon sheath. Direct injections into the tendon is absolutely contraindicated. Direct steroid injection can cause greater deterioration to the tendon material. The chronic stage requires at least 4 to 6 weeks of absolute immobilization.

If conservative treatments prove ineffective, surgery is sometimes warranted to remove nodular irregularities and surgically induce channels for vascular ingrowth into the central core of the tendon. In complete ruptures, emergency surgical repair of the tendon is necessary. This then requires several weeks of immobilization, followed by several months of rehabilitation.

Summary

The key to recovery from Achilles tendon injury is for the athlete to understand both the level and stage of the injury. The athlete must effect appropriate changes in his or her physical activity program or seek professional care in time to avoid serious Achilles tendon damage.

Suggested Reading for "Achilles Tendon Injuries (Tendinitis; Tenosynovitis; Tendinosis; Tendon Rupture)"

Chechick et al. (1982)

Clement & Padmore (1984)

Derscheid & Brown (1985)

Leach et al. (1981)

MacLellan & Vyvyan (1981)

Scheller et al. (1980)

Smart et al. (1980)

See reading list at the end of the book for a complete source listing.

Posterior Tibial Tendinitis

Paul M. Taylor, D.P.M.

Posterior tibial tendinitis is an inflammation of the tendon of the posterior tibial muscle. The muscle attaches in the leg behind the tibia and fibula. The tendon begins in the lower one third of the leg and passes behind the inside of the ankle to attach in the midpart of the foot (Figure 5.2). The tendinitis usually develops from overuse and is more common in people who pronate excessively. Other factors that frequently cause overuse injuries may also contribute to this tendinitis, such as a rapid increase in activity; always running on the same side of the road, with the slope in the same direction; running with worn shoes; or inadequate warm-up or stretching.

Symptoms include pain, swelling, and sometimes crepitus or a feeling of roughness over the tendon. The pain is on the inside of the ankle, usually just behind and below the ankle bone, but it may extend up into the leg. During the condition's early stages, its pain is present at the start of activity, gradually subsides, and then recurs after the activity is completed. If untreated, it can progress to increasing pain and swelling over the area. When the pain involves the tendon higher in the leg, the tendinitis may be mistaken for shin splints or a stress fracture.

Treatment for posterior tibial tendinitis initially should include the basic treatment for inflammation due to overuse: RICE—rest, ice, compression, and elevation. In addition, anti-inflammatories help reduce swelling; and any biomechanical imbalances should be controlled. For more chronic cases, a regimen of ice after activity and heat applied at bedtime may be effective. Professional treatment for resistant cases may include orthotic devices, physical therapy, and stronger oral anti-inflammatories. Cortisone injections should be used only for the most resistant cases and should be followed by 2 weeks of inactivity.

To prevent recurrence, the causative factors of the tendinitis—such as training techniques, worn shoes, biomechanical problems, and training environment—should be controlled. Posterior tibial tendinitis is a common problem that can interfere with sports participation. It should be treated as soon as any symptoms develop.

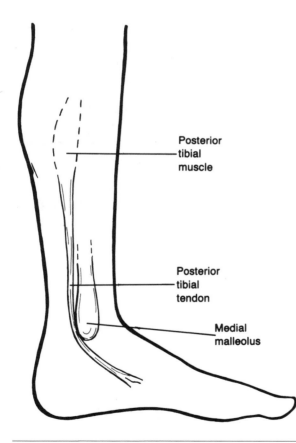

Figure 5.2 Posterior tibial tendinitis can develop anywhere along the course of the tendon on the inside of the ankle.

Suggested Reading for "Posterior Tibial Tendinitis"

Scheller et al. (1980)

See reading list at the end of the book for a complete source listing.

Anterior Ankle Impingement Syndrome

Mark D. Dollard, D.P.M.

Among the many ankle problems affecting athletic performance is a condition of a bony growth on the top of the ankle bone. This bony spur limits the full range of motion available at the ankle joint, greatly reducing the foot's ability to dorsiflex, or bend upward at the ankle. This spur may arise along the entire neck of the talus (ankle bone) to a size large enough to impinge against the front of the tibia (leg bone) (Figure 5.3). The ankle joint capsule attaches in this area. The capsule is the structure that surrounds the joint, maintaining the fluid within the joint.

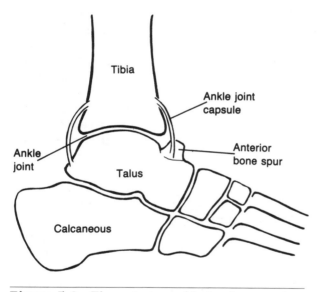

Figure 5.3 The anterior ankle impingement syndrome develops from a bone spur in the front of the ankle joint.

Proper ankle mechanics requires approximately 15 to 20 degrees of ankle dorsiflexion for the leg to roll over the planted foot during normal walking or running. Without this motion being available, the foot is held in a relatively plantarflexed position. There is not enough motion available in the ankle for the foot to function properly during gait, and various problems may develop.

A variety of symptoms can develop either from direct irritation of the ankle capsule and joint structures or from strain at other foot and leg structures associated with the compensated position of the foot. The capsule often becomes entrapped between the spur and the tibia, creating chronic capsular swelling, inflammation, and sharp pain with each movement. Tenderness along the anterior ankle and a gritty puffiness may be felt over this area. Prolonged inflammation of the capsule may lead to fibrotic scarring, thickening, and invagination of the ankle capsule, creating a pathologic fold of tissue into the joint. In this instance, a movable, clicking structure may be sensed by the athlete as the defect snaps in and out of the joint. During examination, both the presence of limited ankle motion and the above symptoms should warrant x-ray evaluation to determine the presence of the spur.

Bony growths at the ankle can result from congenital formation, acquired changes in certain foot types, or consistent trauma in specific sports. Congenital bone formation is present at birth; however, it often remains undetected until immature bone sufficiently ossifies for x-ray detection. Certain flexible, high-arched foot types cause the rearfoot to violently rock backward into the ankle joint as the forefoot contacts the ground. The ankle bone jams against the front of the tibia, and a bony spur eventually forms, with ankle dorsiflexion becoming progressively limited. Trauma in specific sports increases the chance of acquiring the spur. Certain athletes (e.g., basketball players, volleyball players, baseball catchers, football linemen, and competitive weight-lifters) are often affected by this problem. Ankle bone damage resulting from either repetitive bouncing or strain from a low squat position is unique to these athletes.

In time, limitation of ankle dorsiflexion may force the foot and leg into a compensated position, creating biomechanical gait irregularities sufficient to effectively strain foot and knee structures. Arch pain, general metatarsalgia, heel pain, and other symptoms develop as the foot compensates into a flat-footed, pronated position. In the leg, the knee may compensate by bowing backward, or it may suffer from medial malalignment syndrome.

Few conservative measures are available, and most treatment is aimed only at temporary symptomatic relief. Rest, ice, compression, and elevation are typically recommended. Heel lifts may increase freedom in the ankle joint for improved ankle motion. Above all, athletes in the high-risk sports should carefully monitor this condition.

Professional treatment may include symptomatic treatment with anti-inflammatory medication, limited steroid injections, and physical therapy. Foot orthotic devices can help limit compensatory pronation and reduce strain in secondarily affected foot and leg structures. If symptoms continue, best long-term results are achieved by surgical excision of the bony growth.

Suggested Reading for "Anterior Ankle Impingement Syndrome"

Parkes et al. (1980)

See reading list at the end of the book for a complete source listing.

Ankle Sprains

Paul M. Taylor, D.P.M.

Ankle sprains are one of the most common acute athletic injuries. Unlike overuse injuries, which result from low-grade stresses applied repeatedly over long periods of time, acute injuries develop from sudden blows or twists.

Ankle sprains can affect either side of the ankle but most frequently damage the lateral (outside) ligaments. This occurs when the foot turns under the leg, stretching the ligaments to the point where they may tear or rupture (lateral ankle joint ligaments are shown in Figure 5.4).

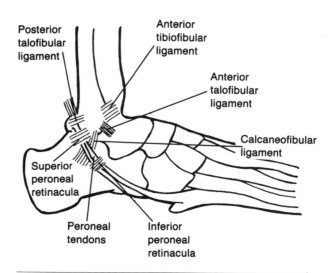

Figure 5.4 The lateral ankle ligaments are most frequently injured in ankle sprains.

Degree of Sprain

Sprains are graded as mild, moderate, or severe. A mild sprain usually affects only the anterior talofibular ligament, causing a partial rupture. A moderate sprain involves the anterior talofibular and calcaneofibular ligaments, resulting in increased damage to the structure of the ligaments. A severe sprain affects these two ligaments as well as the posterior talofibular ligament and may result in their complete rupture or, occasionally, a fracture of adjacent bones.

Treatment

The degree of sprain determines treatment necessary and how long it takes before resuming regular exercise. Although some mild sprains may allow a return to activity in 2 or 3 days, the seriousness of a moderate or severe ankle sprain should not be underestimated. Improper treatment may result in a chronically unstable ankle that is prone to repeated injury, forces limitation in sports activities, causes early arthritis in the ankle joint, and eventually results in the need for surgery. For the athlete to avoid these complications, each ankle injury should be evaluated and treated properly.

Mild Sprains

Mild ankle sprains cause some initial discomfort, mild swelling, and little or no bruising. Treatment should include immediate discontinuation of the physical activity, icing the ankle as soon as possible for 20 to 30 minutes, and applying an elastic wrap. The affected foot should be kept elevated as much as possible. If swelling persists, icing should be repeated several times a day. Make an ice "popsicle" by freezing water in plastic or paper cups and tearing away the sides to expose the ice. This initial treatment is referred to as RICE—rest, ice, compression, and elevation. With mild ankle sprains, RICE usually needs to be continued for only 2 or 3 days, followed by a gradual return to running.

Moderate Sprains

Moderate ankle sprains cause a greater amount of pain around the outside of the ankle than mild sprains as well as increased swelling and bruising within 12 to 24 hours. Initial treatment is the same as for mild sprains: using the RICE method. In addition, moderate sprains require increased protection, such as a soft cast, to allow proper healing of the ligaments. Anyone with a suspected moderate to severe sprain should seek professional help, because of possible ligament damage. X-rays should be taken to rule out any bony damage. Immobilization of the moderate ankle sprain may have to be continued for 2 or 3 weeks. After the ligaments have healed, exercise involving the ankle can gradually be resumed. (A rehabilitation program will be described later.)

Severe Sprains

A severe ankle sprain is a serious injury. A tearing or popping may be heard or felt. There is immediate pain, with swelling within 5 minutes of the injury. Although it may be possible to walk on the ankle immediately afterward, pain and swelling increase over the next 30 minutes, until it becomes difficult to walk. There may be extensive bruising over the outside of the ankle, foot, and leg. Walking or running right after a severe ankle injury worsens swelling and bruising, and more damage to the ligaments results.

Initial treatment, as with lesser ankle injuries, is RICE. Crutches may be necessary to help completely rest the injured ankle. A professional examination and x-rays should be obtained as quickly as possible. If there is a complete rupture of the ankle ligaments, surgical repair may be required. If all the ligaments have been damaged but the ankle is still stable (this can be determined by stressing the ankle while taking x-rays), a cast may be necessary for 4 to 6 weeks. After recovery from a severe ankle sprain, a period of rehabilitation is needed.

Ankle Rehabilitation

An ankle rehabilitation program should be started after the ankle ligaments have had adequate time to heal, a period determined by the severity of the ankle sprain. Following the program below, begin with the first exercise and do not proceed to the next until the first can be done without pain. If you have any doubt about whether you can perform these exercises, check with your doctor.

1. Range-of-motion exercises without resistance. While sitting, move your foot up and down at the ankle 30 to 40 times. Then, invert (turn the foot in) and evert (turn the foot out) 30 to 40 times. This should be repeated three or four times daily.

2. Inversion-eversion exercises while standing. While standing with your feet 12 to 18 inches apart, alternate raising the inside and outside of the feet with your knees slightly bent. Repeat 20 to 30 times, three to four times a day.

3. Peroneal muscle strengthening. Place a large rubber band, cut from an inner tube or thick elastic material, over your toes while sitting on the floor with your legs straight. With the rubber band providing resistance, evert your foot (see Figure 5.5). Ankles should be 4 to 6 inches apart. Slowly allow the foot to invert (see Figure 5.6). This should be repeated 20 to 30 times, three times a day. If there is pain along the outside of the ankle, the exercises should be reduced in number so they can be done without pain, and then increased gradually.

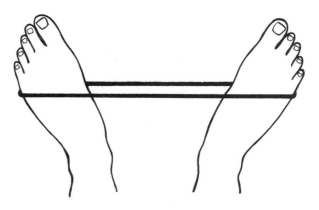

Figure 5.5 Use your feet and ankles to stretch the band out or evert your feet.

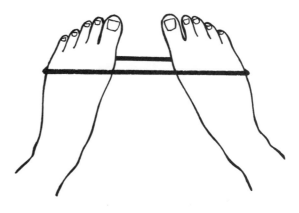

Figure 5.6 Use your feet and ankles to slowly release the band or invert your feet.

4. Toe walking, with shoes. Stand on your toes with your shoes on and walk around for as long as you can, or up to 5 minutes. Repeat two or three times a day.

5. Heel walking, with shoes. Walk on your heels with your shoes on for as long as you can, or up to 5 minutes. Repeat two or three times a day.

6. Gradual return to activity. As the exercises increase the strength in your ankles and the pain diminishes, you can gradually return to running and other normal fitness activities. When walking becomes comfortable, a slow jog can be started, including running large figure eights. Start with a large, slow figure eight, 20 to 30 yards in length, and gradually shorten the distance and tighten the turns. This helps to increase range of motion in the ankle and strengthen the surrounding stabilizing muscles.

As you increase your activity, some soreness may be noticed afterward. This can be reduced by applying heat for 5 minutes before exercising and ice afterward for 10 to 15 minutes.

Return to normal activity gradually. Exercises should be increased only if there is no pain. Returning too quickly may result in reinjury more serious than the original sprain, which will take even longer for recovery.

Prevention

A continued program for prevention of additional injuries should be carried out after your rehabilitation program. Tape or an elastic wrap should be used to support your ankle for 4 to 6 weeks after starting to exercise again. Strengthening exercises, particularly peroneal muscle strengthening, should be continued for 2 or 3 months. If you have had any history of repeated ankle sprains, exercises and the elastic ankle wrap should be continued indefinitely.

Ankle sprains are one of the most common injuries sustained by athletes. They should be taken seriously. Accurate diagnosis, a proper treatment program based on the severity of the injury, adequate rehabilitation, and preventive measures are all necessary for complete recovery from an ankle injury without later complications.

Suggested Reading for "Ankle Sprains"

Cetti (1982)

Crean (1981)

Hutson & Jackson (1982)

Kay (1985)

Laughlin et al. (1980)

Mack (1982)

Nemeth & Thrasher (1983)

Sando (1984)

Scheller et al. (1980)

Smith & Reischl (1986)

Stover (1980a, b)

Tropp et al. (1985)

Vesso & Harmon (1982)

Wilkerson (1985a, b)

See reading list at the end of the book for a complete source listing.

Subluxing Peroneal Tendon

Paul M. Taylor, D.P.M.

A subluxing peroneal tendon occurs when the tendon that passes behind the lateral malleolus (outside ankle bone) slips out of its groove and pops out on the side of the ankle. The peroneal muscles arise on the lateral (outer) side of the leg, and the peroneal tendon passes behind the lateral malleolus and attaches in the foot (Figure 5.7). There is a groove on the back of the lateral malleolus for the tendon to slide, and the tendon is held in place by fibrous tissue.

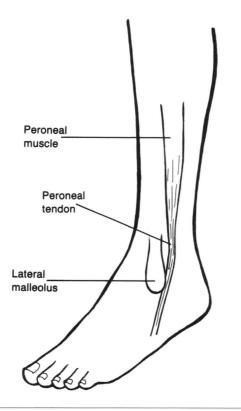

Figure 5.7 The peroneal tendon can sublux from its normal position behind the lateral malleolus.

The problem of the subluxing peroneal tendon may be acute, due to an ankle injury, or chronic, due to a congenital anomaly. The tendon can be displaced by an injury, such as an ankle sprain. In some cases, the subluxation is not noted immediately after an ankle sprain because of the pain and swelling of the ankle injury. When a chronic popping, swelling, or pain persists after an ankle sprain, it may be due to the subluxing peroneal tendon. Otherwise, there may be a congenital anomaly in which the groove is too shallow, allowing the tendon to easily slip out of place.

When repeated episodes of pain or popping occur on the outside of the ankle, a subluxing tendon should be suspected. You can diagnose this problem by attempting to evert or turn out the foot against resistance. When this is done, the tendon can be seen under the skin sliding over the lateral malleolus. If the peroneal tendon is allowed to continue slipping out of place, an inflammation with tendinitis and pain develops.

Initial treatment for this condition is to cut a felt "horseshoe" pad to fit around the lateral malleolus; hold this pad in place with an elastic wrap (Figure 5.8). This helps hold the tendon down in its normal position. If the area still

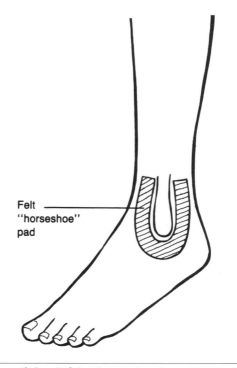

Figure 5.8 A felt "horseshoe" pad around the malleolus helps to stabilize the peroneal tendon.

becomes tender or swollen with activity, ice should be applied afterward. If the tendon continues to sublux and remains painful, surgical correction may be needed. This would require deepening the groove on the back of the malleolus or repairing the fibrous tissue that holds the tendon in place. There may be some residual swelling and tenderness persisting even after surgery, so this option should be considered carefully.

Prevention of the subluxing peroneal tendon involves carefully evaluating any ankle injury to be sure that the peroneal tendon has not been injured at the same time. The subluxing peroneal tendon is not a common injury and is therefore sometimes overlooked as a cause of lateral ankle pain.

Suggested Reading for "Subluxing Peroneal Tendon"

Arrowsmith et al. (1983)

Cohen et al. (1981)

Jackson & Gudas (1982)

_____

See reading list at the end of the book for a complete source listing.

CHAPTER 6

———

Leg Injuries

The leg, here defined as the portion of the lower extremity between the ankle and the knee, contains muscles that move the ankle and foot. These muscles get quite a workout during most fitness activities, both from putting out effort and from absorbing shock from the foot's impact with the activity surface. Sometimes the athlete relies upon the leg to handle too much of this stress, and injury can result. This chapter discusses several leg conditions that can interfere with the athlete's comfort or performance.

Shin Splints

David A. Bernstein, D.P.M.

Shin splints is a vague term used to describe pain in the lower leg that often results from participation in various athletic activities, including running. Two types of this condition exist, named for the location of the pain. Anterior shin splints occur in the front (anterior) portion of the shin bone (tibia). Pain from posterior shin splints is felt on the inside (medial) part of the leg, along the tibia (Figure 6.1).

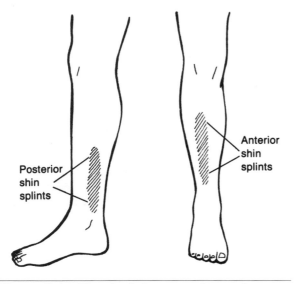

Figure 6.1   The shaded areas indicate the most common locations for shin splints.

Shin splints are caused by very small tears in the leg muscles at their points of attachment to the shin. The athlete may first notice a pulling or vague aching sensation after running. If ignored and allowed to continue, this aching may become more intense and could occur even during walking. Tender areas can usually be felt as one or more small bumps along either side of the shin bone.

Causes

Anterior shin splints are due to muscular imbalances, insufficient shock absorption, toe running, or excessive pronation of the foot. Posterior muscle groups located in the back of the lower leg are primarily responsible for propelling the body forward. Generally, they are much stronger than muscles in the front part of the lower leg, thus creating a muscle imbalance. In running, anterior leg muscles lift the foot upward toward the leg, allowing it to clear the ground and swing forward. These muscles also prepare the foot to strike the running surface. Any tightness in the opposing (posterior) leg muscles places unnecessary strain on the anterior muscles and may contribute to shin splints.

Insufficient shock absorption can cause anterior shin splints. Anterior leg muscles prepare the foot to strike the ground by helping reduce the amount of shock transferred through the foot to the rest of the body. Running or other athletic activity on hard surfaces such as concrete or asphalt roads increases this stress. Softer surfaces, such as grass, dirt trails, or cinder tracks, are capable of absorbing more shock and therefore transfer less to the shins. Old shoes may need to be replaced. All shoe cushioning materials tend to compress and lose resiliency after an extended period of wear. Shock-absorbing insoles, sold at running stores, and running or aerobic shoes specially made for landing on hard surfaces, also decrease shock to the legs.

Toe running occurs when the athlete lands only on the balls of the feet, without the normal heel contact. This inefficient method places the gastrocnemius and soleus muscles in continuous contractions.

Excessive pronation contributes to both anterior and posterior shin splints. Pronation is a complex motion of the foot, affecting the position and range of motion of almost every joint in the lower extremities. Understood simply as the flattening of the arch, pronation allows the foot to better absorb shock and adapt to uneven terrain. Though some pronation is necessary for normal joint function, too much produces an extremely unstable foot that may lead to an injury.

Instability occurring with excessive pronation results from misalignment of the joints of the foot. This causes the ankle, knee, and hip joints as well as joints of the lower back to undergo unnecessary, and often injurious, ranges of motion. As the muscles of the foot and leg overwork in an attempt to stabilize the foot, increased stress is transmitted to their attachments in the leg. Repeated stress may create very small tears at the points where leg muscles attach to the shin bone. Efforts to relieve this condition must be directed toward the excessive pronation.

Treatment

With a little basic medical knowledge and some common sense, many athletes can successfully treat themselves. Aspirin is a very effective anti-inflammatory medication and can be used in relieving pain from shin splints. If it can be taken without stomach irritation or other medical problems, two tablets with each meal (six per day) are recommended. Questions about aspirin safety can be answered by a family physician.

Ice massage also is helpful in treating shin splints. Immediately after running, firmly massage tender areas with ice for 10 to 15 minutes. Freeze a small styrofoam or paper cup filled with water, then peel away the top part of the cup. You should always do icing after running, never before.

A reduction in daily mileage and a change in running course may also be beneficial to the runner. By reducing mileage 50 percent for at least a week and avoiding hills and hard running surfaces, you may prevent further injury.

If you believe your feet are pronating too much, athletic shoes with a varus wedge may help. This wedge lifts up the inside part of the foot and reduces the amount of pronation. Custom-fitted orthotic devices may be necessary for more extreme cases.

Exercises

Most athletes with anterior shin splints improve with the use of weight-training programs to strengthen the muscles in the front of the lower leg. These exercises are also good prevention against shin splints. If weight equipment is not available, household items, such as a handbag filled with rocks or a few large books bound together with rope, can be used (see Strength Exercise 25 in chapter 12). Exercise with both legs, even if shin splints are present in only one leg.

It is also important to stretch the leg muscles in the back part of the leg and thigh gently as part of your recovery program (see calf stretching exercises in chapter 12). Strengthening and stretching exercises should be done only in the absence of pain.

Specialists

Persistent problems may necessitate a visit to a sportsmedicine specialist who deals with the foot and its function as it relates to the rest of the body. A biomechanical examination—including a study of your body structure, muscle strength, flexibility, and ranges of joint motion—as well as an evaluation of how you walk and run, may be performed. Strengthening and flexibility programs may be designed to correct muscular imbalance. Recommendations for shoes, training schedules, running surfaces, and courses often are provided. If you pronate excessively, orthotic devices may be suggested. Oral anti-inflammatory medications may be prescribed. Physical therapy such as ice massage, ultrasound, electro-stimuli, and heat are also commonly used to reduce inflammation and pain.

The Best Prevention

Maintaining good muscle strength and flexibility is the best way to prevent serious athletic injuries. Remember, small aches often grow into large pains. Running through an injury without proper medical advice and common sense can be a big mistake.

Suggested Reading for "Shin Splints"

Brody (1980)

Sloan (1980)

Viitasalo & Kvist (1983)

See reading list at the end of the book for a complete source listing.

Muscle Pulls and Muscle Tears

Paul M. Taylor, D.P.M.

A muscle pull is an overstretching of the fibers within the muscle. If there is an even greater force, the muscle fibers tear, and, in some cases, a complete rupture of the muscle can occur. The degree of pain and loss of mobility depend on the extent of the injury. A slight muscle pull causes local tenderness and discomfort during activity. A moderate tear brings sudden pain with loss of muscle strength and swelling; bruising develops later. A rupture of a muscle causes severe pain immediately with swelling, bruising, and loss of function of the muscle.

Pulls and tears occur usually when muscles are rapidly contracting against resistance. Any muscle can be involved; however, certain muscles are more prone to these injuries. A pulled calf muscle is frequently seen in sports that require jumping. Pulled hamstrings (muscles in the back of the thighs) occur frequently in sprinters. Sports requiring rapid changes in direction may cause groin muscle injuries. Swimmers develop muscle injuries of the shoulder. Whenever a muscle is forcibly contracted and there is resistance or pull in the opposite direction, a muscle pull or tear can develop.

There are certain conditions that may predispose a person to muscle injuries. These include a muscular imbalance secondary to overdeveloped muscle groups, inadequate warm-up, developing an exercise program too rapidly, accidents in which the foot slips and the muscle tries to pull back to keep the athlete from falling, and lack of flexibility.

The treatment for a muscle pull or tear depends on the degree of the injury. A mild muscle pull—which may develop gradually during exercise, without the athlete's recollection of a specific, acute injury—can be self-treated. Initially, the level of activity should be reduced, heat should be applied prior to activity, and ice and compression should be applied afterward. If continuing activity causes increased pain, the activity should be stopped. If relief is not obtained in 7 to 10 days, professional help should be obtained. Minor muscle pulls should not be ignored, because continued stress on these muscles may cause more serious injuries.

A moderate muscle tear requires immediate cessation of activity, applying ice, compression, and elevation. The ice should be continued for 15 to 20 minutes, three or four times a day for 2 or 3 days. The use of ice, compression, and elevation initially stops the internal bleeding in the muscle belly. Decreasing the amount of bleeding in the tissues allows for a quicker return to activity. After using the ice for the first 2 to 3 days, change to applications of heat for 20 to 30 minutes, 3 times a day. Follow each heat application with gentle range-of-motion exercises. This type of exercise consists of moving the injured part as far as possible. This should be done initially without weights; when there is no pain, gradually use increasingly heavy weights. As the muscle pain subsides, a gradual return to full activity can be started.

For a severe muscle pull or rupture, in which a defect may be palpated in the muscle, immediate medical help should be obtained. This type of injury is not very common. When it does occur, though, surgical repair of the muscle is usually required. Following this type of injury, an extensive rehabilitation program under the direction of a therapist is necessary.

The athlete who has sustained a muscle pull should determine if he or she has any of the predisposing factors listed above and should attempt to eliminate these prior to returning to full activity. This may require a stretching program to increase flexibility and a strengthening program to maintain better muscle balance (many sports emphasize using certain muscle groups, which begin to dominate opposing muscle groups, causing an imbalance). A reevaluation of training techniques, in order to avoid excessive stress on the muscle, and improved warm-up and cool-down periods may be needed. Once a muscle has been injured, it is tighter than before; a concentrated flexibility program is needed for that muscle.

Following the proper program for returning to exercise prevents potential complications from developing after muscle injuries. Loss of motion and strength, and development of scar formation or calcifications within the muscle can occur after this type of injury (see "Myositis Ossificans" section in chapter 15).

Muscle pulls or tears can range from minor nuisances causing a few days of tenderness to rather debilitating injuries. Through appropriate treatment of these injuries, the damage to the muscle can be minimized, and the return to injury-free activity can be assured.

[Note: This section deals with general aspects of muscle injuries. Some of the muscle pulls or tears that occur frequently are covered in more detail in the following articles: "Tennis Leg" (chapter 6), "Hamstring Injuries" (chapter 8), "Groin Pull" (chapter 8), and "Brachial Plexus Injury" (chapter 11).]

Suggested Reading for "Muscle Pulls and Muscle Tears"

Mazer (1983)

See reading list at the end of the book for a complete source listing.

Muscle Cramps

Paul M. Taylor, D.P.M.

Muscle cramps are a common athletic problem, involving sudden, involuntary contractions of muscle fibers. These may be minor cramps, involving only part of the fibers within a muscle, or severe cramps, affecting most of the fibers. When a cramp happens, it can temporarily incapacitate the athlete. A cramp can involve any muscle within the body; however, the muscles of the leg and foot are most frequently affected. The muscle cramp develops during or after activity, and occasionally occurs while the athlete is asleep.

The cause of muscle cramps is poorly understood. There are apparently several contributing factors. When the muscle begins to fatigue and is placed under a sudden stretch, the muscle can contract and cramp. There are both mechanical and chemical causes contributing to the muscle cramp. If the muscle is at a biomechanical disadvantage because of a malalignment of the lower extremity, or if the muscle is too tight, a cramp may result. Deficiencies of certain minerals within the body are also felt to contribute to muscle cramping. These include sodium, potassium, calcium, magnesium, and phosphorus. In some cases, there may also be a limitation of adequate blood supply to the muscle, which can result in the muscle cramping during exercise.

The immediate treatment for a muscle cramp is to gently stretch the muscle and to massage or simply grasp the muscle belly. When the cramp occurs in the calf, the athlete can pull back on the toes with one hand while massaging the muscle with the other hand. When the cramp occurs in the upper extremity or other parts of the body, it may be necessary to have a partner help work out the cramp. Such local treatment may be all that's necessary if the cramps occur only rarely.

If cramps occur frequently, an attempt should be made to identify and treat any of the contributing factors. These can include such biomechanical problems as a tight calf muscle, a leg length discrepancy, or excessive pronation or supination. Nutritional deficiencies should also be investigated; an increase of fruits and vegetables in the diet may help to restore any depletion of minerals. In the past, salt tablets were frequently recommended for helping to prevent muscle cramps during exercise in hot weather; however, recent studies have shown that salt tablets do not help and, in fact, may be detrimental.

Prevention of muscle cramps requires treating any biomechanical problems; maintaining a diet that includes fruits and vegetables, in order to maintain levels of minerals; and drinking fluids while participating in long events, especially in hot weather. If the athlete suffers from repeated muscle cramps, an evaluation by a physician is necessary to determine whether there is any undetected disease or illness that may be causing the cramps.

Almost every athlete sustains a muscle cramp at one time or another. A cramp is usually a normal physiological response by the body, but it may indicate that other, undesired mechanical or chemical changes are present in the body.

Suggested Reading for "Muscle Cramps"

Kotoske (1983)

Sheehan (1982, July)

Stamford (1986)

"The story of charley horse, . . ." (1982)

See reading list at the end of the book for a complete source listing.

Tennis Leg

Denis R. Harris, M.D.

During exercise, muscle fibers can be torn. If a major portion of the fibers becomes disrupted, severe pain may result. Tennis leg is just such a case—muscle fibers acutely rupture in the calf, with pain and swelling occurring immediately thereafter. The sensation is much like being kicked in the calf. Any muscle tear in the calf may be implicated; however, the plantaris muscle is thought of the most frequently. Quick exertion or stretching may cause the plantaris to tear. The plantaris is a muscle beginning just above the knee and extending to the heel, joining the Achilles tendon. The plantaris has no vital function, because two other muscles (the gastrocnemius and soleus) provide most of the strength in the Achilles tendon.

There is one other rupture that may mimic the plantaris—the Achilles tendon may tear and also cause calf pain. The main difference between the two is that the Achilles tear causes functional impairment to the limb. Without the strength of the calf muscles transmitted through the Achilles tendon, push-off from the foot is limited.

To differentiate between the two conditions, squeeze the calf muscles, watching to see whether the foot moves down toward the floor (first check your good calf to see whether you are doing the test correctly). The foot should move, with the toes pointing more toward the floor. If there is any doubt, medical evaluation is mandatory because, should the Achilles tendon be torn, immobilization or surgical intervention is necessary.

Once Achilles tear has been ruled out, immediate treatment for tennis leg is as follows:

1. Elevation
2. Rest
3. Compression

All of these reduce the immediate swelling. Remember that when a muscle is torn, it bleeds. The black-and-blue area seen after an injury is from this bleeding.

A heel lift also rests the muscles. Felt may be cut and tucked into the heel area of the shoe. Lastly, anti-inflammatory medication can reduce the body's response to trauma. Advil® and Nuprin® (consisting of ibuprofen) are among the nonprescription medications that can be helpful.

Once the acute inflammation has subsided, strengthening and stretching the calf muscles is necessary before the athlete returns to normal activities (see chapter 12, Stretch Exercises 2, 3, and 4; and Strength Exercise 24).

Leg Length Discrepancies

David L. Berman, D.P.M.

Leg length discrepancy, also known as short limb syndrome, is very common. For the athlete, this differential in leg length can cause any of a multitude of symptoms that, if not detected and treated, may result in injuries, leading to a cessation of activity at worst or, at best, to discomfort during activity.

With even a slight, ¼-inch limb length discrepancy, the athlete can develop extreme symptoms and disability from the body trying to compensate for the difference. This is a direct result of stress (three to four times the normal body weight is put upon the legs while running) and the difference in the running gait as opposed to the normal walking gait.

There are two types of limb length discrepancies. The first type is the structural or anatomical shortage, an actual shortening in the length of the femur (thigh bone) or the tibia (lower leg bone). The other type is a functional shortage, a positional change in the bones during running or walking. The athlete can have a combination of both deformities. They usually result in the same symptoms but are treated differently.

Causes

A structural or anatomical shortening can be the result of a fracture in the thigh or leg bone. In the child or adolescent, this usually results in a longer limb on the injured side, due to a stimulation in growth. Injuries to the epiphyseal plate (growth areas) of bones in children can result in leg length inequalities. Poliomyelitis, once the most common cause of leg length discrepancies, is rarely seen now but may be the cause in older patients. Most other structural inequalities are due to congenital abnormalities.

The functional leg discrepancy is usually the result of one foot being in a more pronated (flattened) position than the other foot. Pronation causes the arch to fall, leading the leg and thigh to rotate inward. As the foot, leg, and thigh turn, the pelvis drops downward on the same side, causing a functional shortage of this leg, compared to the opposite leg.

Most symptoms of a limb length discrepancy are caused by the body's attempt to compensate for the unequal leg length. This compensation leads to postural and structural changes in the spine, pelvis, hips, knees, and feet. An example of no structural or positional changes with a short right leg is shown in Figure 6.2.

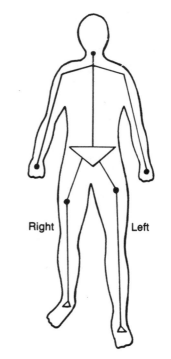

Right   Left

Figure 6.2   Short right leg without structural or positional changes.

Structural changes in the lower back are the most common. The pelvis rotates toward the long side and drops down or tilts to the short side. This results in a change in the spinal column. A scoliosis (curvature) develops in the spine, most often resulting in a convexity on the side of the short leg (Figure 6.3). This curvature allows the head to function in the erect

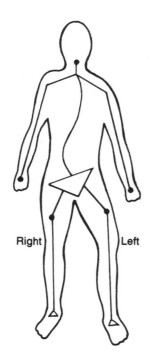

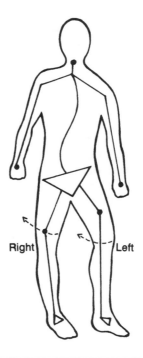

Figure 6.3 Short right leg with compensation including pelvic tilt to the short side, curvature in lower spine with convexity to the short side, and higher shoulder on short side.

Figure 6.4 The short leg, on the right, is externally rotated with the foot supinated. The long leg, on the left, is internally rotated, with the foot pronated.

position. The shoulder on the short side appears higher, and the arm on the longer side appears lower, when observed during walking or running. Due to the pelvic rotation, there is more contact and stress on the hip joint of the longer leg.

In the structural limb length discrepancy, the longer leg compensates through pronation, whereas the short limb supinates or turns outward (Figure 6.4). These changes in function can be seen in relationship to the gait. During pronation, the foot flattens in the arch, resulting in a relative internal (inward) rotation of the leg, knee, and thigh. This rotation lowers the pelvis of the long side. The short limb supinates, raising the arch of the foot. The leg, knee, and thigh externally (outwardly) rotate, raising the pelvis on this side. These mechanisms all result from the body's attempt to equalize the limb length differentiation.

Symptoms

Symptoms caused by a limb length discrepancy can occur anywhere, from the foot up to the lower back. The majority of symptoms are usually found on the side of the longer limb, because it is in contact with the ground longer and thus absorbs a greater amount of pressure and stress. When running, there is a longer stride time for the contact of the long limb. Electromyographic recordings (measuring muscle electricity) have shown muscle activity on the side of the longer leg to be greater than that of the shorter leg. The greatest differences were observed in the high and low spinal muscles, the tensor fasciae latae (areas on the outside of the thighs), and the hamstring muscles.

Hip pain accompanying a leg length discrepancy is associated with positional and muscular changes. The bones of the hip joint are not properly aligned, because of the altered functional position. Muscles around the hip joint are also under a greater amount of tension—especially the abductors (the muscles that rotate the hip outwardly).

Low back pain is usually associated in combinations with the other symptoms mentioned and often is located in the center of the lower back. Occasionally the symptoms may become more severe and result in sciatica, which causes the pain to radiate down the back or side of the thigh and possibly into the groin area. Sciatic pain also may radiate down the leg and into the foot.

The short limb also develops various symptoms. Shin splints usually are a result of the short leg overstriding while running. Most other short leg symptoms are due to the relatively supinated position of the foot resulting in a lack of shock absorption, with lateral (outside) foot, leg, knee, and hip pain developing.

Treatment

Treatment for the athlete with a structural or anatomical limb length discrepancy should be based on physical findings. Shoe lift therapy is instituted along with appropriate treatment for the corresponding symptoms. A gradual increase in the height of the lift should be made, usually starting with half of the leg length differential. This allows the patient to adapt to a gradual correction, necessary because of the structural and functional changes that have developed over the years.

For structural changes of ¼ inch or less, a lift under only the heel of the short side is appropriate. If the discrepancy is greater than that, the lift should be placed under the entire foot. In this latter instance, the lift should be of maximum height at the heel and be tapered toward the forefoot.

If a correction of over ½ inch is required, the lift is best placed on the outside of the shoe. Total amount of the lift can be distributed (e.g., half of the correction in the shoe and half on the outside of the shoe). Also, the height of the shoe on the longer side can be reduced, keeping the lift on the shorter side to a minimum— for example, removing ⅛ inch from the shoe of the long side and adding ⅜ inch to a shoe on the short side, thus equaling a lift of ½ inch.

If a limb length discrepancy is discovered at an early age, and the proper treatment is instituted, the compensatory curvature of the spine often disappears.

A functional discrepancy is treated with the use of orthotic devices. The orthotic device realigns the position and structure of the limb, resulting in an equal limb length and a leveling of the pelvis.

Functional and structural limb length discrepancies may exist in combination. In such instances, it usually is necessary to use orthotic devices to correct the positional changes on the long limb, and a lift for the correction of the short limb.

Immediate symptoms are treated with a combination of flexibility and strength exercises, ice massage, and anti-inflammatory medication. Increasing flexibility of your back muscles, strengthening abdominal muscles, and stretching the hamstrings are a must. Do isometric and isotonic exercises to help strengthen the knee joint musculature. (Isometric exercises are characterized by a contraction of the muscles, but without moving joints or the extremities, e.g., contracting and relaxing your biceps while you stand in front of a mirror, or pulling up on a chair in which you are sitting. Isotonic exercises, on the other hand, involve contraction of a muscle and movement of a joint, an extremity, or both in the process of contraction, e.g., weightlifting.)

Leg and foot symptoms are treated with strength and flexibility exercises, strapping, and ice. Orthotic devices may help prevent these symptoms from recurring.

Stretching and Strengthening Exercises

The following stretching and strengthening exercises, which are described in detail in chapter 12, should be done:

Increased Back Flexibility and Hamstring Stretching:
- Bent-Knee Toe-Touches (Stretch Exercise 12)
- Side Reaches (Stretch Exercise 21)
- Trunk Flex (Stretch Exercise 13)

Strengthening the Abdominals:
- Abdominal Curls (for upper abdominals) (Strength Exercise 14b)
- Leg lifts (Strength Exercise 14c)

Strengthening the Knee Muscles:
- Leg Extensions (Strength Exercise 18b or 18c)

Foot Strengthening, Flexibility:
- Toe Lifts (Strength Exercise 25)

Conclusion

Although limb length discrepancies are very common and occur in 75 to 80 percent of the population, they usually are not symptomatic in nonathletes. With the additional forces on the limbs and the need for symmetrical function in athletics, postural changes associated with differences in leg length can result in a great amount of stress for the athlete with such a discrepancy. Shortening of one limb creates compensatory changes on the other limb, along with changes in structure and function from the back of the body down to the feet. If these discrepancies are discovered early enough, a reversal in some structural changes is possible. With the proper use of lift and orthotic therapy, the athlete usually is able to function free of symptoms.

Suggested Reading for "Leg Length Discrepancies"

Sheehan (1984)

———————————

See reading list at the end of the book for a complete source listing.

Compartment Syndromes

Anthony H. Woodward, M.D.

Problems of the lower leg between the knee and ankle are common in athletes. Sometimes pain is due to a compartment syndrome.

Anatomy

Beneath the skin there is a layer of subcutaneous fat (sometimes more than we wish). Beneath this adipose blanket there is, as it were, a second skin made of fascia, which surrounds and supports the soft muscles. One can think of this fascia as a light stocking stretched from the ankle to the knee. Fascia is a strong, unyielding white sheet made up of the same connective tissue as tendons and ligaments. Further sheets of this fascia form vertical walls inside the tubular stocking, dividing the lower leg into compartments. Each compartment contains two or three muscles, blood vessels, and, very significantly, nerves. These compartments are surrounded by unyielding walls of fascia and bone.

Classically, four compartments are described in the lower leg (Figure 6.5). The anterior compartment is perhaps the best known. It contains the tibialis anterior muscle, which pulls the ankle up, and the extensor muscles, which do the same for the toes. Its nerve is the deep peroneal nerve, which is responsible for sensation in the skin between the first and second toes. This compartment is easily felt on the front of the leg just to the outside of the tibia (shin bone).

The lateral compartment, on the outer side of the leg, contains the peroneal muscles, which evert the foot, and the superficial peroneal nerve, which supplies sensation to the top of the foot.

The bulky muscles that form the calf are divided into two posterior compartments. The superficial posterior compartment holds the large gastrocnemius and soleus muscles, which you contract to raise yourself up on tiptoe. The deep posterior compartment is getting a lot of attention recently for its possible role in shin splints. This compartment contains the flexor muscles of the toes and the tibialis posterior muscles, which help to invert the foot. This last muscle is surrounded by fairly thick fascia of its own; sometimes considered to have its own compartment. The nerve of the deep posterior compartment, the tibial nerve, supplies sensation to the side of the foot.

Definition

A compartment syndrome occurs when the pressure within one or more of these anatomical spaces increases so much that the circulation and function of the muscles and nerves in the compartment are compromised.

Causes

As you can see from the definition, anything that causes a rise in pressure can precipitate a compartment syndrome. The most common cause is a broken tibia. For the athletes, though, that is not the usual problem. When

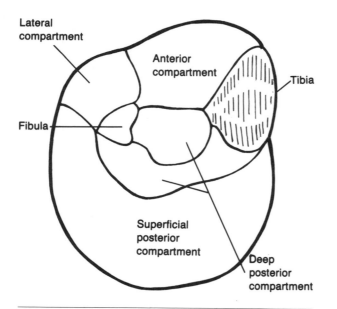

Figure 6.5   A compartment syndrome may involve any of the muscle groups of the leg.

they are exercised, muscles swell, increasing their volume by 20 percent. Within the fairly rigid compartment, this swelling increases the pressure and squeezes the tiny blood vessels that carry oxygen and nutrients to all the tissues in that compartment, most importantly the nerves and muscles. Normally, between muscle contractions the pressure falls and blood flow is restored. Occasionally, however, the pressure remains high, and circulation is impaired. The muscle responds by further swelling, and a vicious cycle is set up with progressively increasing intracompartmental pressure.

Although exertion is the usual cause in the athlete, rarely a blow or a tear of the muscle can cause a compartment syndrome. Such a tear occurring in tennis leg or after a severe ankle sprain can cause bleeding within the compartment, initiating a pressure rise.

Classification

Compartment syndromes are either acute or, more commonly in the athlete, chronic. They can also be classified on the basis of which compartment is involved, although one must remember that two or more compartments can be affected simultaneously.

Chronic Compartment Syndromes

The hallmark of a chronic compartment syndrome is pain occurring with exercise. The pain comes after a particular distance is run, forcing the sufferer to reduce the intensity of exercise or to rest completely. The pain is usually aching, or occasionally sharp or stabbing, in character. A sensation of tightness is common. There may be associated with the pain a feeling of weakness and disturbances of sensation, such as numbness or tingling in the legs. More than three fourths of patients have symptoms in both legs. The examination of a sufferer of chronic compartment syndrome is usually unrewarding. There may be a little tenderness over the involved muscle(s), but everything else usually checks out as normal. This explains why the average patient has seen several doctors and has tried (with little success, be it noted) a variety of remedies before the true problem is identified.

The diagnosis is best established by measurement of the pressure within the compartment. There are a number of ways to do this; usually a slit catheter or a wick catheter is inserted, under local anesthesia, into the muscle and connected to a device that can record the intercompartmental pressure. At rest the pressure in a normal compartment is about 4 millimeters (mm) of mercury (normal blood pressure is 120/80 mm of mercury). In the patient with chronic compartment syndrome, the pressure is high even at rest; with exercise it rises to far higher levels than normal and takes longer to fall after the exercise is stopped.

There are only two treatments for chronic compartment syndrome: the patient must reduce activity or have an operation. The operation is called a *fasciotomy*—dividing the constricting layer to allow the muscles to swell without increasing the compartment pressure. Fasciotomy is usually quite successful in relieving symptoms and allowing the athlete to enjoy his or her sport.

Acute Compartment Syndromes

Although chronic compartment syndromes are annoying and their surgical treatment entirely elective, acute compartment syndromes can be devastating and their treatment true surgical emergencies.

Fortunately the acute syndrome is much less common in the athlete. It occurs usually during or after exercise of unaccustomed severity, whereas the chronic syndromes are seen more often in the well-trained athlete. Acute pain starts during exercise, then gets worse and worse, despite stopping all activity. Weakness and numbness rapidly ensue. Examination reveals dramatic abnormalities. There is swelling, redness, and tenderness over the involved compartment. Even passive stretching of the injured muscles exacerbates the pain. Decreased sensation may be present, and weakness can be hard to determine because of the severity of the pain. Circulation in the foot is still good, even though the muscle in the leg is literally dying for lack of blood.

Measurement reveals the increased compartment pressure. In the acute case a pressure above 30 mm of mercury is considered dangerous and a pressure above 45 mm is an indication for immediate surgery. If the apparatus necessary for compartment pressure measurements is not readily available, surgery should be performed on clinical grounds. Again, the operation required is a fasciotomy. If this is performed within a few hours, full recovery can be expected. However, after several hours of intense compartment pressure, the muscle and nerve damage may be irreversible.

Medial Tibial Syndrome

A common site for chronic postexercise pain in the athlete is the inner side of the lower leg, a few inches above the ankle. This symptom has been attributed to a stress fracture or to perostitis—a stress reaction of bone, or strain of the tibialis posterior muscle-tendon unit. Other physicians feel that such pain is due to a chronic compartment syndrome affecting the deep posterior compartment, which, as you recall, does contain the tibialis posterior muscle. Some of these patients suffer from raised compartment pressures and get relief from fasciotomy.

Conclusions

Compartment syndromes are uncommon causes of lower leg pain in the athlete. The diagnosis can be suspected because of characteristic pain patterns and confirmed by measurement of the compartment pressures. They are among the very few disorders in the athlete that are best treated by surgery.

CHAPTER 7

Knee Injuries

The knee, a hinge joint, primarily allows the movements of flexion and extension in the sagittal plane. In many athletic activities, forces may push the knee into moving beyond its structural capabilities. Acute trauma—especially when force is applied perpendicular to the knee's natural plane of movement—and overuse can result in damage to many different knee tissues. This chapter examines several conditions that can afflict the athlete's vulnerable knee.

Patellar Tendinitis (Jumper's Knee)

Vincent G. Desiderio, Jr., M.D.

The patellar tendon connects the patella, or kneecap, to the lower leg, or tibia (Figure 7.1). It is a very strong and heavily stressed tendon, particularly in runners or jumpers, and is vital for good knee and leg function. Patellar tendinitis, sometimes called *jumper's knee*, is an overuse syndrome of that tendon. Typically, the athlete with patellar tendinitis complains of pain just below the kneecap after a vigorous workout. Often, participation in an activity such as volleyball or basketball, in which there is a great deal of up-and-down movement, causes the pain. The pain often is insidious in nature, and there is rarely an acute injury noted. A soccer player may notice trouble kicking the ball, for instance. Pain also may develop with other types of activity, such as

rock climbing, in which the knee is put under excessive bending stress. The area may become so sensitive that the sufferer is unable to kneel.

The athlete with patellar tendinitis frequently has point tenderness and some swelling just below the kneecap. At times a small defect can be noted in the tendon. There may be pain when the tendon is stressed. This can be reproduced by the physician bending the knee to approximately 90 degrees and asking the athlete to extend or straighten the leg.

Treatment is the same as for most overuse syndromes: rest, heat, and anti-inflammatory medication, such as aspirin. Often it is quite helpful to apply heat to the area just before exercising, and ice afterward. More specifically, a patellar tendon brace, an orthotic device that places pressure over that area, can be quite helpful. It is also important that the athlete refrains from vigorous athletic activity that puts stress on this area.

Unfortunately, the patellar tendon has a very poor blood supply, and a chronic condition can evolve, which may require surgery. Surgery in this instance involves removing the degenerated and inflamed portion of the tendon and, if necessary, reattaching the tendon to the kneecap. Results of surgery in this circumstance are reasonable. At times, cortisone shots are helpful; however, because the tendon may already be deteriorated and cortisone itself weakens tissue, it is possible to weaken the tendon significantly enough to rupture it. If a rupture does occur, surgery is mandatory if the athlete is to regain full function.

Obviously, prevention of tendinitis is important. If you notice pain in the patella tendon, it would be advantageous not to be so vigorous in the activities that cause pain—typically, jumping and kicking. Ice, heat, and anti-inflammatories, when used early, are often sufficient to cure the problem.

In summary, patellar tendinitis, or jumper's knee, is an overuse syndrome of the tendon

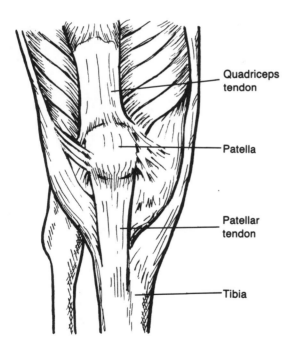

Figure 7.1 The patellar tendon extends from the kneecap (patella) to insert into the leg bone (tibia).

just below the kneecap. It is somewhat different than other overuse syndromes in that the problem does not always resolve with routine care. This has to do with the amount of stress placed on the area and the poor vascular supply to the tendon. The athlete, particularly one who participates in jumping activities, should be very cautious when experiencing pain in the knee and treat it with due respect.

Suggested Reading for "Patellar Tendinitis (Jumper's Knee)"

Ferretti et al. (1983, 1985)

Kelly et al. (1984)

Maddox & Garth (1986)

See reading list at the end of the book for a complete source listing.

Chondromalacia Patella

Lloyd Nesbitt, D.P.M.

Chondromalacia patella, commonly known as *runner's knee*, is an increasingly prevalent condition. This is a problem in which repeated stress on the knee causes inflammation and an eventual softening of the cartilage under the patella (kneecap). This adversely affects the normal, smooth gliding of the kneecap (patella) over the end of the femur (thigh bone); a roughness, pain, and swelling of the knee develops.

Many causes of this problem have been cited in the literature. One of the deformities most commonly associated with runner's knee is a pronated foot. This biomechanically unstable foot, which flattens out and rolls in with running, results in a lower leg that rotates inward; hence, the kneecap slides from side to side. The underside of the kneecap should be smooth like marble and ride inside the femoral groove (a groove on the thigh bone). However, when the kneecap is pulled sideways, it rubs against the chondyle of the femur, becoming rough, much like sandpaper, and symptoms result. It is often aggravated by prolonged sitting or flexion of the knee, because as the knee becomes flexed, the kneecap presses against the femur much more (sometimes called a "movie sign").

Another cause for runner's knee can be a weak thigh muscle (quadriceps), which normally aids in proper tracking of the kneecap. Muscle imbalance, direct or repeated trauma, a neglected ligament injury, and even nutritive changes can also be causative factors, although these are less common. Anatomical factors may play a role, because some people have kneecaps that are predisposed to more injury because of shape or position.

Incidence

This pain syndrome comprises up to 25 percent of overuse injuries seen in many sports clinics. It occurs most commonly in teenage girls; however, any active person from age 14 onward can be affected.

The pain in cases of chondromalacia patella can vary, and provoking factors are inconsistent. The patient may complain of sore or "trick" knees or arthritis. The condition usually starts with pain that builds gradually, often throughout a year or longer, and finally becomes severe enough that the athlete seeks medical attention.

Symptoms usually occur beneath or on both sides of the kneecap, but can sometimes be felt throughout the knee. Pain can be aggravated by a short run, squatting, jumping, or other activities. Sometimes stiffness occurs simply from prolonged sitting (e.g., watching too many movies, or the movie sign) or going down stairs.

Athletes who always run on the same side of the road may experience pain in one knee resulting from the tilt of the road and the consequent accentuation of the flattening or pronation of the foot.

Often, athletes suffering from runner's knee continue to participate in their normal activities—and suffer for it later. In most cases, proper diagnosis and physiotherapy—exercises combined with proper mechanical foot control—can alleviate the pain and allow resumption of the full athletic routine.

Treatment

A sportsmedicine specialist definitely should be consulted for this problem. It may well be worthwhile to see a podiatrist along with an orthopedic surgeon or a family doctor who is interested in sportsmedicine. Conservative management is recommended, and one of the most important factors is time! Young people often grow out of this, yet they immediately need to calm down symptoms and correct the causes. Pain should be your guide; if it is aggravated by activity, you must decrease your activity and consider swimming or cycling instead. Mild discomfort should not be too much of a cause for concern, but definite pain warrants proper examination.

Rest is important, especially when the knee is painful and swollen. Ice is helpful; you can apply an ice pack to the knee for 15 minutes two times a day and after any activity. This reduces pain and inflammation. Medications, such as coated aspirin, can be helpful, but check with your doctor first, because more sophisticated anti-inflammatory medications may be recommended.

Physiotherapy is the key to long-term success. Exercises can be done to strengthen the thigh muscles, such as straight leg raises, which also help with kneecap mechanics. Stretching exercises may be recommended as well (see chapter 12, Stretch Exercises 2, 3, 5, and 6 and Strength Exercises 18a and 18c). Cortisone injections are never recommended for this problem. Correction of abnormal foot mechanics is a must; a sports-minded podiatrist should do a complete gait evaluation and biomechanical analysis of your foot function. Orthotic devices may be helpful if pronated feet are a cause. Orthotic devices work very well when combined with physiotherapy and proper exercise techniques.

Chondromalacia patella should not keep the athlete from activity, as long as appropriate steps are taken to treat the causes of the problem.

Suggested Reading for "Chondromalacia Patella"

Allman (1983)

Block (1982)

Pretorius et al. (1986)

See reading list at the end of the book for a complete source listing.

Pes Anserinus Bursitis

Anthony H. Woodward, M.D.

A bursa is a fluid-filled sac positioned between two structures that move against each other. The fluid is a lubricant similar to joint fluid and normally is present in microscopic quantities only. Bursitis—inflammation of the bursa—can be caused by friction, by a direct blow, or by infection with bacteria.

There are dozens of bursae scattered about the body, including several—14, by one count—around the knee. The pes anserinus bursa, or anserine bursa, is situated near the front of the knee, just below the joint line itself, on the medial (inner) aspect of the tibia (shin bone). This bursa facilitates the movement of a triad of tendons over the tibial collateral ligament. These are the tendons of the sartorius, gracilis, and semitendinous thigh muscles. These tendons together are attached to the upper part of the tibia. They spread out on the surface of the tibia like the three webbed toes of a goose's foot, which in Latin is pes anserinus—hence the peculiar name of the related bursa.

Although anserine bursitis may be induced by a direct blow squashing the bursa against the hard bone, it is usually caused by friction. Like other overuse syndromes, in the athlete anserine bursitis is more likely to occur when mileage or speed is being increased. It can also be associated with osteoarthritis of the knee in older people.

Symptoms are pain and tenderness localized to the upper medial surface of the tibia. Pain is aggravated by movement of the knee.

Anserine bursitis often responds very nicely to an injection of a corticosteroid (with local anesthetic). Other treatments that have been reported to be helpful are immobilization, heat, nonsteroidal anti-inflammatory drugs, and ultrasound. If symptoms do not respond to these measures, a more serious condition—such as a torn medial meniscus or stress fracture of the tibia—should be suspected as the true cause of the pain.

Popliteal Cysts (Baker's Cysts)

Anthony H. Woodward, M.D.

The popliteal space is the soft area behind the knee that is bounded above by the hamstring tendons as they diverge to each side of the knee, and bounded below by the swelling belly of the gastrocnemius (calf) muscle. Lumps in the popliteal space can be as simple as overgrown pieces of fat or as dangerous as aneurysms or malignant tumors, but most often they are popliteal cysts.

Anatomy

Bursae are sacs, filled with the same type of fluid as joints, that separate two moving parts. There are many bursae throughout the body, but the one we are concerned with is found in the popliteal area, lying between the overlapping tendons of the semimembranosus (the largest of the hamstring muscles on the inner side of the knee) and gastrocnemius muscles. This semimembranosus bursa connects with another bursa, located between the gastrocnemius tendons and the back of the knee joint itself, to form the gastrocnemio-semimembranosus bursa. Anatomical dissections have shown that there is usually a hole in the knee joint capsule, allowing fluid to pass between the joint and this composite bursa.

Causes

At least some, and perhaps all, popliteal cysts are really distensions of this composite bursa. Some disorder within the knee joint inflames the synovium—the inner lining of the joint—to produce excess fluid. Movement of the knee raises the pressure within the joint quite markedly and forces the fluid through the capsule hole and into the bursa, blowing it up like a balloon. The overlapping muscle may act as a valve, preventing the fluid from returning, so that the bursa can never deflate. Another possible mechanism of cyst formation is that the high pressure in the knee joint forces the soft inner lining out through a weakness in the joint capsule to form a popliteal cyst in exactly the same way as an inner tube could bulge out through a tear in the outer tire.

Whatever the exact mechanism may be, it is important to realize that a popliteal cyst is usually a secondary problem: it is a consequence of something wrong in the knee joint itself. The knee diseases implicated vary with the age of the patient. In younger adults, the commonest problem is a torn meniscus (cartilage). One investigator found that the tear is most often of the posterior horn (the back end, as it were) of the medial meniscus. In older patients, arthritis is a more common cause.

Clinical Findings

A swelling in the popliteal space is the most common, and sometimes the only, complaint. Aching pain and a feeling of tightness may occur. Usually, of course, there are also the signs and symptoms of the underlying knee disorder. Often a popliteal cyst is found incidentally during investigation for another knee problem.

In the old days, the only test for a popliteal cyst was to turn the lights out and shine a flashlight against the lump to see the red glow around it, which proved that the lump was indeed a fluid-filled cyst. Today there are several ways to show up a popliteal cyst. Arthrography is an x-ray examination in which *dye*, a liquid opaque to x-rays, is injected into the front of the knee joint. If there is a popliteal cyst communicating with the joint, dye flows into the cyst and outlines it on the subsequent x-rays. A cyst can also be detected by ultrasound scanning. In this test, a picture of the structures of the back of the knee is produced in the same way that sonar is used to detect a submarine or school of fish. The sound waves will be reflected differently from different types of tissues. A receiver will detect these differences and project an image of the cyst on a screen. Popliteal cysts can also be detected by injecting radioactive compounds into the bloodstream.

Treatment

Once a popliteal cyst has been found, the first thing to do is to try to find the causative knee disorder and treat that. Usually, successful treatment of the underlying disease allows the popliteal cyst to disappear. If not, the cyst can be excised by a surgical operation, if it produces sufficiently bothersome symptoms (a few cysts recur even after surgical removal). Sometimes the popliteal cysts associated with arthritis of the knee can be relieved by corticosteroid injections.

Popliteal Cysts in Children

Popliteal cysts are not uncommon in children, particularly boys. Such swellings, though usually painless, worry parents. The situation in children seems to differ from that in adults. There is usually no problem within the knee joint; indeed, the cyst is less likely to communicate with the joint. However, the most important difference is that most children's cysts disappear without any treatment at all. If the child does have an operation, there is a 40 percent chance that the cyst will come back.

Conclusion

A lump at the back of the knee is most likely a popliteal cyst. In young adults, it is usually due to a torn meniscus and resolves with treatment of the causative knee problem. In children, a popliteal cyst is best managed by observation only.

Iliotibial Band Syndrome

Denis R. Harris, M.D.

Runner's knee has become a catchall term for afflictions ranging from arthritis to tendinitis and bursitis. Symptoms can be caused by anatomical abnormalities as well as poor training habits. A leading cause of lateral (outside) knee pain in runners is iliotibial band friction syndrome (ITBFS), the result of both anatomical abnormalities and poor training.

The iliotibial band is a superficial thickening of tissue on the outside of the thigh and leg (Figure 7.2). The band begins on the outside of the pelvis and runs over the outside of the hip and knee, inserting just below the knee.

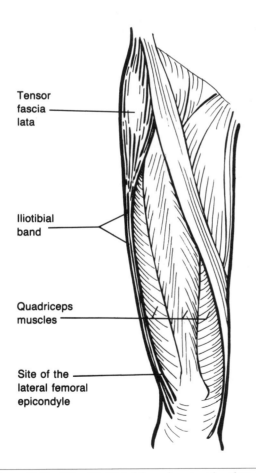

Tensor fascia lata

Iliotibial band

Quadriceps muscles

Site of the lateral femoral epicondyle

Figure 7.2 The iliotibial band extends along the outside of the thigh to just below the knee. It is at the outside of the knee that the iliotibial band syndrome occurs.

Causes of ITBFS

During running—particularly long-distance runs—your iliotibial band works very hard. It plays an important role in stabilizing the knee. Prior to, and during, foot strike, the band helps rotate the leg inward, stabilizing the leg during that phase of running. As the knee bends and the foot pushes off, the iliotibial band moves from behind a prominence of the femur (lateral femoral epicondyle) and to the front of it. It is this continual rubbing of the band over the bony prominence that can cause problems, especially if you have a tight iliotibial band. The repeated flexion and extension of the knee during running, combined with a rubbing of the iliotibial band over the femur, can cause the bursa at that site to become inflamed. Also, the iliotibial band itself may become irritated. The athlete with bowlegs or a tightness about the iliotibial band is predisposed to such problems.

Training errors can create the same problems. For example, when you run on a banked surface, such as an indoor track or the shoulder of a road, the downhill leg is bent slightly inward, causing an increased stretching of the iliotibial band against the femur. This friction can cause pain and tenderness. Improper warm-up and cool-down also may overwork and injure your iliotibial band.

Symptoms

Pain usually does not register immediately, but occurs as a stinging sensation later into your activity and may persist afterward. The pain most often is felt just above the knee joint, on the outer side of the knee, but it also may radiate all along the iliotibial band. Swelling may be present, and you may notice a thickening of the tissue at the spot where the band rubs over the femur. Pain worsens when your foot strikes the ground if you overstride or run downhill. It can be aggravated by running an excessive distance in a single workout or by increasing your weekly mileage too quickly.

If you stop running and walk slowly with your leg held straight, the pain usually subsides.

Treatment

To correct this painful rubbing of the iliotibial band over the lateral femoral epicondyle, you need to be concerned with both structural and functional abnormalities. If you have a natural tightness of the band, stretching it every day, especially before you work out, helps make the band more flexible and less prone to injury. Refer to chapter 12 for Stretch Exercises 9 and 10 for the iliotibial band.

Treating Functional Problems

In addition to stretching to help alleviate structural abnormalities, you can do several things to treat functional errors:

- Decrease your mileage. If the knee hurts, apply ice after you run. Take aspirin to help reduce or eliminate pain.
- If you run on a pitched surface (a track or shoulder of a road), frequently alternate the pitched surface upon which you run; for example, change your road route, and/or run clockwise as well as counter-clockwise on a circular track. This will keep you from putting too much stress on the iliotibial band of just one leg.
- Put a lateral sole wedge (bought over-the-counter or specially made by your sports physician) in your shoe. A lateral sole wedge is built up higher on the outer edge, which helps relieve undue pressure on the knee.

Last Resort

Not all tightness of the iliotibial band responds to conservative training measures, shoe inserts, or stretching. In such cases, additional examination by a sports-oriented orthopedist is in order. In rare instances, your last resort may be partial surgical release of the tight band.

Suggested Reading for "Iliotibial Band Syndrome"

McNichol et al. (1981)

Terry et al. (1986)

See reading list at the end of the book for a complete source listing.

Knee Sprain

Anthony H. Woodward, M.D.

A sprain is a ligament injury caused by tensile stress. (Ligaments are bands of connective tissue which connect bones together at joints.)

The knee is the largest joint in the body and has a very complex anatomy. At the knee, the two rounded, cam-shaped condyles at the end of the femur (thigh bone) rest on the almost dome-shaped upper surface of the tibia (shin bone). In contrast to a joint such as the hip joint in which the articulating bones form a ball and socket, the contour of the bones at the knee provide no stability. Instead, the stability of the knee joint depends entirely on soft tissues.

The menisci, or cartilages, are two crescent-like wedges at each side of the knee that slightly deepen the socket for the femoral condyles (see Figures 7.3 and 7.4 in next article titled "Meniscal Injuries"). The bones are connected by a sleeve of tissue called the *capsule*, which is attached to the femur, the tibia, and the menisci. The capsule is strengthened by thickening in places, particularly posteriorly and at the inner posterior corner.

The capsule is further helped in its function of stabilizing the joint by two ligaments, one at each side of the knee, which allow the knee to flex and extend, but prevent sideways motion. On the inner side of the knee is the medial (tibial) collateral ligament, attached above to a bony prominence of the femur, and attached below to a 2-inch long strip of tibia. On the outer side, the lateral (fibular) collateral ligament is a rounded cord stretching from the femur above to the head of the fibula below (the head of the fibula is the bony prominence easily felt on the outer side of the knee). There are two other vitally important ligaments holding the femur and tibia together; however, these—the anterior and posterior cruciate ligaments—are actually inside the center of the knee joint. The muscles of the thigh—the quadriceps and hamstrings—as well as the popliteal muscle provide dynamic stability to the knee, augmenting the stability supplied by the capsule and ligaments.

Thus the stability of the knee, essential for athletic activities, depends on the integrity and strength of the menisci, capsule, ligaments, muscles, and tendons. Yet the knee joint between the two longest bones of the body—femur and tibia—is at the center of two long lever arms; thus, it can be subjected to very large stresses. Sprains of the knee are common in contact sports and skiing but, fortunately, are rare in running. The running athlete may sustain a sprain by a misstep on an uneven surface or possibly by tripping and falling forward, forcing the knee into hyperextension.

Sprains come in three grades of severity. A first-degree, or mild, sprain is one in which only a few ligamentous fibers are damaged. There is pain, mild tenderness, minimal swelling and bleeding, and, above all, no abnormal laxity. The medial collateral ligament is the most commonly injured. A minor sprain can be treated by ice initially and by the sufferer using crutches if needed, with rapid advance to weight bearing, full range of motion, and return to athletics.

A second-degree, or moderate, sprain is due to a greater ligament disruption, but one that is not yet a complete rupture. Pain, tenderness, swelling, and bleeding are more evident, but the key feature is the presence of some instability of the joint. If the medial collateral ligament is injured, the knee can be forced open medially by pulling the lower leg laterally. The degree of laxity depends on the amount of ligament that has been torn. If there is just a slight opening, treatment is the same as for a first-degree injury. More marked laxity requires more aggressive treatment: cast immobilization for 4 to 5 weeks, followed by a formal rehabilitation program of quadriceps strengthening and range-of-motion exercises. A significant second-degree sprain keeps the athlete away from leg-intensive activity for 8 weeks or more.

A third-degree, or severe, sprain is due to a complete rupture of the ligament and is associated with marked disability. In the knee, a complete rupture of one ligament only too often means a tear in another ligament and a meniscal injury also. The rare isolated ligament rupture may be treated by cast immobilization. However, combined injuries, in the athlete at least, usually demand surgical repair.

Injuries to the anterior cruciate ligament are uncommon in the athlete unless he or she trips and falls. Posterior cruciate ligament ruptures are generally only seen in falls or automobile accidents. Due to the ligament being inside the knee, the injury becomes evident only if there has been enough damage to cause bleeding into the joint. A so-called isolated rupture of the anterior cruciate ligament may be treated by cast immobilization. When this rupture is combined with injuries to other knee structures, though, surgery is usually recommended for the athlete.

Suggested Reading for "Knee Sprain"

Hede et al. (1985)

Jensen et al. (1985)

Noyes et al. (1980)

See reading list at the end of the book for a complete source listing.

Meniscal Injuries

Vincent G. Desiderio, Jr., M.D.

The knee's cartilage, which is referred to at times as a *meniscus*, is often injured by athletes. This particular cartilage is different from the articular cartilage of the knee in both its function and its structure. The articular cartilage is the smooth glistening tissue in the knee that allows the joint to move freely. It has the appearance of white marble and the consistency of semirigid plastic. The meniscal cartilage, on the other hand, is designed as a cushion and is constructed in a C-shaped fashion to lie between the articular cartilage of the femur (thigh bone) and the tibia (lower leg bone) in the knee. There are two meniscal cartilages in each knee, which form a shallow cup arrangement serving as a stabilizer as well as a cushion (Figures 7.3 and 7.4).

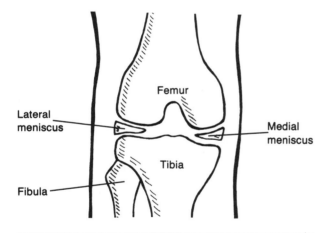

Figure 7.3   The menisci act as cushions between the tibia and femur in the knee joint.

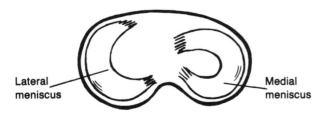

Figure 7.4   A top view of the knee joint shows the shape of the two menisci.

The usual mode of injury to a cartilage is a sudden twisting and compression injury to the knee. It commonly happens to a football or soccer player who has his foot planted in one direction and suddenly suffers an exaggerated twisting stress to his knee, such as inflicted by a collision with another player or even by a simple, sharp change of direction of running. Often there is a pop heard or felt by the athlete, whose leg experiences pain, either in the front or side. If there is even further stress to the knee, the ligaments of the knee can be torn as well.

The most common sports in which a meniscal injury occurs are basketball, soccer, football, and lacrosse. All of these sports involve sudden cutting and twisting of the knee while the athlete is running at high speeds. Runners, as well, may have meniscal injuries; however, this is unusual and occurs mainly when there is a misstep, such as from an unexpected dip in the road.

Many meniscal injuries are small, and the athlete does not seek medical attention. A common complaint in this circumstance is that the leg swells after exercise, with pain on either the inside or outside of the knee joint. There may be a phenomenon of locking: The knee does not come out straight, but after it is jiggled, eventually extends fully. Finally, a common symptom is the knee giving way: The athlete feels his knee give out underneath him while he is doing a relatively simple maneuver; this is sometimes called a *trick knee*.

Treatment for a torn meniscus is varied. Many times, resting the knee with a splint for a few days relieves the symptoms and there can be a return to routine activities in a few weeks, with no further problems. Other times, the symptoms are not relieved, and further treatment is necessary. To understand the rationale behind the treatment of a torn meniscus, one must understand some of its anatomy. In order for a structure to heal, it must have a blood supply. Only the outer peripheral rim of the meniscus has blood supply. Therefore, if the athlete has a torn cartilage around the rim of the meniscus, where there are blood vessels, the chances for healing that tear are good. If, on the other hand, the tear is in the area of the meniscus that does not have the blood supply, that area will never heal; consequently, if it is giving the athlete trouble, it must be removed to alleviate his symptoms.

A physician treating the athlete with a torn meniscus usually obtains an arthrogram to determine whether the meniscus is torn. If it is, and the patient is having significant symptoms, the doctor would recommend excision. An arthrogram is still a valuable diagnostic test, but the arthroscope has changed things dramatically. The arthroscope is an instrument that allows the physician to look inside the knee to examine the cartilage for tears via a small incision. If it is the doctor's opinion that the tear in the meniscus is such that it cannot heal, he can remove it by the use of arthroscopic instruments. (These very small instruments are inserted in the knee; their movements are observed with the arthroscope.) On the other hand, if the physician sees a tear in the portion of the meniscus that has a good blood supply, the periphery, an attempted repair of that meniscus may be pos-sible. At times, both procedures require a larger incision in the knee; however, the new techniques using an arthroscope are proving valuable.

In summary, the meniscus is a structure vital to the knee. It provides a cushioning effect as well as stabilization for the knee function. It is torn usually by a rotatory type of injury to the knee, such as can occur in a clip in football. Treatment of a small tear centers around resting the knee to allow it to heal. If symptoms persist, arthroscopic intervention may be needed. The arthroscope is first used to define the tear. Then it is used either to remove the portion of the cartilage that cannot heal or to attempt to repair a tear that has a good blood supply.

Suggested Reading for "Meniscal Injuries"

Baker et al. (1985)

Jensen et al. (1985)

Puddu et al. (1984)

See reading list at the end of the book for a complete source listing.

Popliteal Tendinitis

Anthony H. Woodward, M.D.

Popliteal tendinitis is a cause of lateral knee pain in runners and other athletes. Many athletes seem to know about chondromalacia ("runner's knee") and other problems of the kneecap, but not all cases of runner's knee are due to disorders of the patella. Pain on the lateral, or outer, side of the knee in particular may come from different conditions, including popliteal tendinitis.

The popliteus is a relatively small muscle at the back of the tibia, the larger bone of the lower leg. Its tendon winds gradually upward around the lateral side of the knee to attach itself to the femur (thigh bone) just above the outside of the knee (lateral epicondyle). The popliteus tendon comes into immediate contact with a number of important structures of the knee. It adheres to the capsule, the sleeve of tissue that connects the two bones—the femur and tibia—that form the knee joint. The tendon passes through a deep indentation in the lateral meniscus—the cartilage on the outer side of the knee—then runs underneath

the lateral ligament of the joint before it reaches the femur, where it lies in a groove in the bone (see Figure 7.5).

With each movement of the knee, the popliteus tendon has to glide around all these other knee parts, which may irritate it. Chronic irritation leads to inflammation of the tendon and the surrounding structures, with the gradual development of popliteal tendinitis.

Popliteal tendinitis causes pain in the outer side of the knee, usually most noticeably when the athlete is running downhill. The pain seems located deep in the knee. When the knee is examined, tenderness is found in the area below the lateral epicondyle and above the line of the knee joint. The painful symptoms can be reproduced by the sufferer standing on the affected leg and bending the knee about 20 degrees. Another test is performed while you are lying on your back. Bend the knee to a right angle and rest the ankle of the affected leg on the opposite shin. If the popliteus tendon is inflamed, this maneuver is painful.

The athlete afflicted with popliteal tendinitis should reduce both the time spent in working out and the stress put on the body. If these simple measures are unsucessful, total abstinence from exercise may be necessary for 10 to 14 days. The local use of heat, applied for 20 to 30 minutes, 2 to 3 times a day, may be helpful.

If local treatment and rest do not resolve the tendinitis, professional help may be necessary. The use of nonsteroidal anti-inflammatory agents can be tried initially. For persistent cases, cautious injections of corticosteroids may be helpful. X-ray evaluation helps to confirm the diagnosis and rule out any other problems.

Popliteal tendinitis is an infrequent cause of knee pain in the athlete but needs to be recognized in order to be successfully treated.

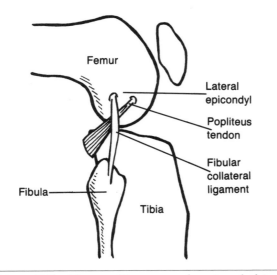

Figure 7.5 The popliteus muscle arises behind the knee, then the related tendon passes under the ligament on the outside (lateral) of the knee.

Biceps Femoris Tendinitis

Paul M. Taylor, D.P.M.

Biceps femoris tendinitis is an inflammation of the tendon of the biceps femoris muscle. This muscle, along with the semitendinous and semimembranous, make up the group of muscles commonly referred to as the *hamstrings*. These muscles are used primarily to flex, or bend, the knee, but they also assist in extending the hip. The biceps femoris muscle arises from two muscle bellies that attach to the pelvis and the femur. They combine to form a single tendon, which attaches to the fibula just behind, and on the outside of, the knee. This tendon can be seen bowing under the skin on the outer, back portion of the knee during a partial deep knee bend. It may occasionally cause lateral knee pain in the athlete. If there is pain on squeezing the tendon, this is most likely a biceps femoris tendinitis.

Initial treatment of a biceps femoris tendinitis includes reduction of the level of activity and applying ice after activity for 10 to 15 minutes. Also, oral anti-inflammatories, such as aspirin or ibuprofen, taken for 7 to 10 days, may be needed. If this does not resolve the pain, complete rest, and application of moist heat for 15 to 20 minutes, 2 or 3 times a day, may be necessary.

Prevention of this tendinitis includes stretching the hamstrings (see chapter 12, Stretch Exercises 5 and 6) and avoiding speed work and hill training. If it is necessary to incorporate these techniques in a training program, they should be incorporated gradually.

If pain on the outside of the knee persists, professional help should be obtained, because there are a number of other causes for pain in this area.

Biceps femoris tendinitis is not a common injury in the athlete. The related muscle is more frequently involved in hamstring pulls. When pain occurs on this tendon, though, this tendinitis should be suspected.

Plica Syndrome of the Knee

Vincent G. Desiderio, Jr., M.D.

The plica syndrome is caused by a thickened lining of the knee joint, usually localized just inside the upper border of the patella, or kneecap. The lining of all joints is composed of tissue called *synovium*. The synovium produces a lubricating liquid called *synovial fluid*. If there is a thickening in this lining, it can then rub across certain areas of the knee, particularly the inner portion of the femoral condyle (the lower end of the thigh bone), and cause pain and irritation.

The typical person with plica syndrome is the runner who feels pain on the inside of the knee. Some individuals will feel pain sooner than others. There is more pain when running up hills, because the knee may be more flexed, or bent, in that circumstance. Many of the symptoms are the same as those of chondromalacia patella, or runner's knee.

In the athlete with plica syndrome, there is tenderness, and possibly some thickening, just inside and above the kneecap. At times there is a feeling of snapping or grinding as the knee is bent either during a physical exam or running. Diagnosing this problem can be somewhat difficult at times, because the plicas may be symptomatic only during activity. Therefore, a diagnostic problem often is seen with the athlete with plica syndrome.

Rest, anti-inflammatory drugs, and possibly a steroid injection cure the problem some- times. Often, an arthroscopic evaluation of the knee (looking inside the knee through a periscopelike device) can identify and treat the problem quite readily. It must be remembered that not all plicas are symptomatic; also, not all of them are localized to the upper inner side of the knee, although this is the most frequent place. Furthermore, of the many patients who have patella pain, only a very small percentage are afflicted by a synovial plica.

In summary, the plica syndrome is a relatively rare condition. The lining of the knee joint becomes thickened; this thickening generally rubs and irritates the inner upper portion of the lower femur. Treatment is usually surgical through the arthroscope, by which the plica can be cut and the area smoothed. The major problem with the plica syndrome is diagnostic; at times it can be perplexing to both the athlete and the professional treating it.

Suggested Reading for "Plica Syndrome of the Knee"

Rovere & Adalh (1985)

See reading list at the end of the book for a complete source listing.

Dislocating Patella

Vincent G. Desiderio, Jr., M.D.

The patella, or kneecap, acts as a fulcrum by which the quadriceps, or thigh muscles, gain mechanical advantage to provide power to straighten out the leg (the quadriceps is a major muscle group that stabilizes the leg). Clearly, the kneecap is necessary for high-level athletic activities that put demands on the lower extremities. The patella is a disk-shaped bone that sits at the end of the femur, or thigh bone. The femur has a groove at its end, in which the patella rides when the knee is bent (Figure 7.6). If the patella comes out of this groove and shifts to one side or the other, it has become dislocated. A variant of dislocation is subluxation, in which the kneecap does not come all the way out but slides slightly to one side, producing pain and apprehension that the patella may dislocate.

Typically, the athlete who dislocates the kneecap is performing some twisting activity, such as side-stepping or swinging a baseball bat. In these circumstances, the rear leg rotates inward, and the kneecap shifts to the outside (the vast majority of patella dislocations occur with the kneecap shifting to the outside). The athlete has severe pain in the knee and is unable to straighten it. When examined, the kneecap is still dislocated on the outside of the knee.

A dislocated patella should be treated by a professional. An x-ray is necessary because of the potential for bone fragmentation. Generally, the patella can be correctly relocated with some gentle sedation—possibly a local anesthetic. This relocation consists of a maneuver in which the knee is extended (straight) and the kneecap is pushed back in place. Thereafter, the athlete should have the knee immobilized for several weeks, followed by rehabilitation exercises. Some professionals feel that operative intervention is indicated in acute circumstances, because the inside ligaments of the knee have been severely stretched and torn.

A subluxing patella may result from an acute dislocation or in the athlete whose patella alignment is such that the patella has a tendency to slide to the outside. This person notes pain when climbing stairs or when doing activity in which the knees twist regularly. There is a feeling of instability in the kneecap and difficulty in doing daily activities such as walking.

Upon physical examination, there is tenderness under the kneecap and a positive apprehension sign. When the kneecap is pushed to the outside by an examiner, pain is not necessarily experienced, but the athlete feels very anxious that the kneecap may shift out of place.

Treatment first includes thigh-strengthening exercises that do not stress the kneecap. These are generally done with the knee in extension or in only slight flexion (bent): See Strength Exercises 18a and 18c in chapter 12. A patellar stabilizing brace, holding the kneecap in the groove, is often valuable. If persistent symptoms occur despite an adequate trial

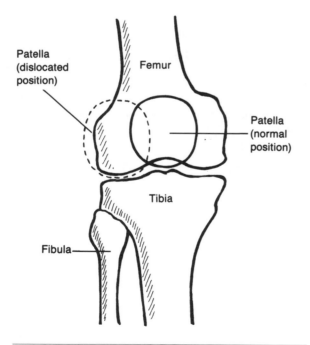

Figure 7.6 The solid line shows the normal position of the patella. The dotted line indicates the direction of the dislocating patella.

of exercises, brace, and so forth, operative intervention to realign the kneecap is indicated. There are various surgical procedures that are designed for such realignment.

In summary, a dislocated patella is an acute injury in which the kneecap is shifted to the outside. It is necessary to have professional care in relocating the kneecap, because fractures can occur both during the dislocation and in the relocating process. Treatment afterward should at least include immobilization for several weeks, and possibly surgery in an acute phase. At times, acute injury may lead to a subluxing patella, or a subluxing patella may result even without an acute episode. In such a case, quadriceps-strengthening exer-

cises with the leg in extension, a patellar brace, and, possibly, athletic modifications (e.g., a reduction in activity, and a change to less strenuous sports) can solve the problem. If symptoms persist, operative intervention to realign the kneecap so that it stays in its groove may be indicated.

Suggested Reading for "Dislocating Patella"

Jensen et al. (1985)

See reading list at the end of the book for a complete source listing.

Extensor Mechanism Malalignment (Malicious Malalignment Syndrome)

Paul M. Taylor, D.P.M.

Malicious malalignment syndrome is a combination of biomechanical imbalances within the lower extremity that predisposes a person to injury. This condition has been referred to by various authors as *malicious malalignment syndrome, miserable malalignment syndrome,* or *extensor mechanism malalignment.* This syndrome consists of an internal rotation of the hip, inward-directed kneecaps (squinting patellae), knock-knees, and sometimes a bowing of the lower leg (tibia) and flatfeet (excessive pronation).

This particular combination of anatomical variations is of concern to the athlete because it places excessive stress on the lower extremity, especially the knee. This condition is most commonly diagnosed in young females; they usually complain of knee pain developing with increased activity. This syndrome can also cause pain in the lower back, hips, legs, ankles, or feet.

The knee is susceptible to injury because the positional changes of the lower extremity force the kneecap to be pulled laterally off its normal track. The amount of deviation can be determined by measuring the "Q" angle (Figure 7.7). This angle is measured by drawing one line from the center of the kneecap to the anterior-superior spine of the pelvis, and another line bisecting the patella tendon. The angle formed by these two lines is the "Q" angle. It is considered excessive if it exceeds 20 degrees.

This is a hereditary condition and it usually cannot be avoided. However, there are various treatments that can help reduce the stress on the lower extremity resulting from the malalignment syndrome. Strengthening exercises should be done for the quadriceps muscles, with special attention to developing the vastus medialis muscle (this muscle, which is part of the quadriceps, helps to stabilize the kneecap) (see chapter 12, Strength Exercise 18). Stretching exercises for the hamstring muscles should be done, also (see chapter 12,

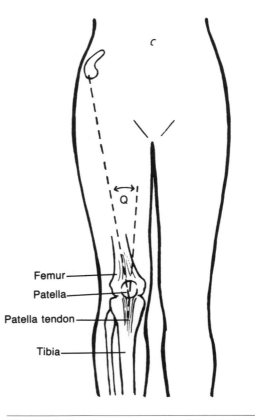

Figure 7.7   Measurements of the "Q" angle determine a person's potential for developing an extensor malalignment problem. The higher the "Q" angle, the greater the potential for injury.

Stretch Exercises 5, 6, 7, 12, 13, and 15). If the knee is painful, activity should be reduced or temporarily stopped. If exercise is continued, ice should be applied to the tender area for 5 to 10 minutes afterward. Aspirin or other anti-inflammatories can be used to reduce the inflammation. Shoes that provide good pronation control should be worn. Additional shoe inserts to reduce pronation can be tried, also.

If such self-treatment does not provide relief, professional help may be needed.

Professional measures could expand on the self-treatment and provide additional help.

Physical therapy can be utilized to more accurately determine any muscle weakness and set up a more specific exercise program. Muscle stimulation could be utilized to aid development of particular muscle groups, such as the vastus medialis. Orthotic devices may be prescribed to control the excessive pronation and relieve some of the stress from the knee. Stronger anti-inflammatories may be prescribed; cortisone injections may be considered. It is also important to thoroughly evaluate the lower extremity to rule out any other causes for the pain. In addition to aggravating the knee, this syndrome may also cause other problems to flare up. A neoprene knee brace, which helps to stabilize the kneecap, may also be recommended. This may help by holding the kneecap in its normal groove so that it glides more smoothly without excessive pressure on its undersurface.

Since this syndrome involves multiple structures, successful treatment requires addressing all of the components; any one treatment by itself will not work. In order to obtain relief, it is necessary to use a combination therapy utilizing a strengthening and stretching program, physical therapy modalities, anti-inflammatories, orthotic devices, and modification of the exercise program. In the rare cases in which this approach does not succeed, it may be necessary to consider surgical correction. This may involve various procedures to stabilize the kneecap or improve its alignment with the leg. Unfortunately, this only helps one element of a complex align-ment problem. However, in most cases, relief can be obtained through conservative measures.

Because the malalignment syndrome is actually an anatomical variation, it is never completely corrected; treatment merely provides relief of symptoms. Therefore, preventing the symptoms from recurring requires continuing with the treatments. This especially refers to the stretching and strengthening exercises, and the orthotic devices. The anti-inflammatory medication should be used for the acute stage only and should not be continued on a permanent basis.

The malicious malalignment syndrome is a compound anatomical variation that places an inordinate amount of stress on the lower extremity, especially the knee. However, with proper, continuing treatment, this problem can be overcome and the athlete can continue in his or her sports activities.

Suggested Reading for "Extensor Mechanism Malalignment (Malicious Malalignment Syndrome)"

Brody (1980)
James et al. (1978)
Roy & Irvin (1983)

See reading list at the end of the book for a complete source listing.

Anterior Cruciate Ligament Injury

Wayne B. Leadbetter, M.D.

The anterior cruciate ligament is found within the knee and is critically valuable in performance of sports requiring sudden changes in direction and velocity. Football, skiing, and court sports, such as tennis and basketball, especially require this movement. Ligaments hold bones together. The anterior cruciate ligament is a tough band of tissue approximately the diameter of the ring finger. It cannot be felt or seen, but lies deep inside the knee and joins the femur and the tibia. By definition, it is the front crossed internal ligament of the knee. (There is also a posterior cruciate ligament, which functions to balance the anterior cruciate ligament, and is also important [Figure 7.8]). No other anatomical structure has been more glamorized than the anterior cruciate ligament, because of the prevalence of injury to it in professional football.

The loss of the anterior cruciate ligament results in a serious disability to the knee in the vast majority of affected athletes. Injury to the anterior cruciate ligament is caused either by sudden dynamic overload on the fibers by a torque (twist) or extension of the knee, or by a direct blow. For example, hooking the edge of a ski without proper binding release or changing direction suddenly while running can result in the twist. In football, being hit (clipped) on the outside and rear of the knee can result in this injury.

The athlete may feel a sudden tearing sensation or hear an audible pop, which is statistically highly correlated with injury to the anterior cruciate ligament. Rapid swelling, which invariably means bleeding internally in the knee from torn blood vessels, is accompanied by an inability to continue play. A prominent limp and inability to move the knee without pain are the cardinal signs of serious internal knee injury, to the anterior cruciate ligament in particular. The anterior cruciate ligament is often injured in coincidence with other structures, such as a cartilage or another ligament, making the trauma to the knee even more serious.

Although the athlete usually notices when this injury occurs, in a few cases the injury causes very little swelling; the swelling that does arise may resolve quickly, deceiving the athlete into continuing activity until a second injury happens. Any injury to the knee that results in dramatic swelling, limp, or inability to continue play should be evaluated by a physician with x-rays and physical examination to determine the extent of the damage.

An injury causing loss of a ligament is significant because such a loss results either in excess, abnormal motion or in laxity between the two bones that should be held—in this case, the femur and tibia. Rotatory instability occurs when the anterior cruciate ligament is lost, making it difficult for the athlete to recover the ability to change direction without having the knee give way, buckle, swell, or cause pain. The athlete often reports the feeling that the knee is shifting. This shifting sensation may occur simply by turning around on a stairway, or it may occur only during the

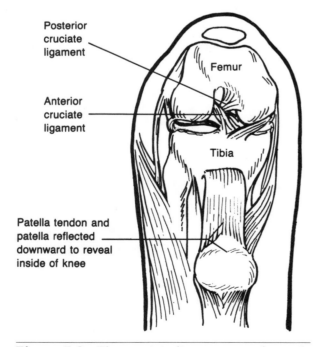

Figure 7.8   The cruciate ligaments are located deep inside the knee.

most active phases of the sport. The athlete is at most risk during changes of direction, cutting, jumping (because of the hazard in landing), or high-velocity sports, such as downhill skiing or waterskiing.

Once the diagnosis of an anterior cruciate ligament injury has been established, the potential for further sports or fitness activity depends on several variables. Athletes who are willing to give up substantial ranges of activity will be okay, but athletes who continue high-level activity with anterior cruciate ligament injury or deficiency of the knee invariably develop disabling symptoms. Studies have revealed that over 50 percent of these latter athletes suffer pain, swelling, and giving way during strenuous sports. Also, more than half have the probability of developing over several years additional injuries to the knee, because of repetitive trauma that leads to damage of the joint surfaces or to arthritis. Clearly, the anterior cruciate ligament injury is a significant dilemma and requires early diagnosis, protection, and, in many cases, surgical repair in order that the athlete avoid long-term disability or changes in lifestyle.

There are a few encouraging options for the injured athlete. He can pursue such activities as jogging that do not impose twisting stress on the knee. Also, activities that do not require repetitive loading of the knee, such as swimming or bicycling, are aerobic and fitness alternatives that do not run as great a risk of reinjuring the knee.

For the athlete unwilling to make such compromises, evaluation requires arthroscopic diagnosis of the knee by the orthopedic surgeon, followed by attempts at surgical measures to correct the instability. It should be emphasized that the goal of the athlete with anterior cruciate ligament deficient knee is to avoid reinjury either by protected activity (with external brace support), or by having ligament function resupplied by surgical treatment.

Any participation in sports that continues to aggravate or reinjure the knee leads to the knee's destruction and to long-term pain and disability even in daily activity. In this regard, at no time is recurrent swelling or pain in the knee acceptable as a side effect of an exercise—it implies ongoing damage.

Suggested Reading for "Anterior Cruciate Ligament Injury"

Gray et al. (1985)

Halperin et al. (1983)

Hede et al. (1985)

Jensen et al. (1985)

Lipscomb & Anderson (1982)

Odensten et al. (1985)

Puddu et al. (1984)

See reading list at the end of the book for a complete source listing.

CHAPTER 8

Thigh and Hip Injuries

The thigh is the portion of the lower extremity between the knee and the hip. The hip connects the lower extremity to the torso. Because the hip joint is a ball-and-socket joint, movements of the thigh and hip, as well as the spine, are interrelated. The thigh and hip each consist of many structures that work very hard in movement and stabilization during the athlete's participation in fitness activities. This chapter looks at several overuse and acute conditions that can befall the athlete's thigh and hip.

Hip Pointer

Wayne B. Leadbetter, M.D.

A hip pointer is a painful bruise resulting from a blow along the outer margin of the pelvis, typically at the belt line, where pelvic bony structures are most prominent. Because a bruise represents bleeding underneath the skin, this injury is painful and interferes with running and walking. It is an injury sustained primarily in contact field athletics, such as football and soccer.

Occasionally, the injury involves a blow to the outer aspect of the hip itself, known as the greater trochanter (see Figure 8.1 in "Hip Bursitis"). Muscle strains or tears may accompany these blows and compound the disability. The circumstances of the injury, accompanied by signs of bruising on the skin, warmth, swelling, and direct tenderness, confirm the diagnosis.

Treatment is similar to any other soft tissue injury and initially consists of RICE (*rest, ice, compression,* and *elevation*), followed by protective padding for return to sports. This is generally not a serious injury unless it is accompanied by injury to the underlying bone structures, but it can represent a formidable interference with competitive goals and pursuit of activity. As such, it should be respected and treated early to reduce discomfort.

Hip Bursitis (Hip Tendinitis)

Vincent G. Desiderio, Jr., M.D.

Hip pain commonly results from trochanteric, or hip bursitis. Early recognition and appropriate treatment of the problem can reduce suffering and time lost from athletic participation.

A bursa is a fluid-filled sac that allows the smooth, friction-free gliding of one body part over another (e.g., tendon over bone). Looking like a small, partly deflated balloon, a bursa is made of special cells that produce clear, protein-rich synovial fluid to lubricate joints and tendons.

When inflamed or irritated, the bursa produces additional synovial fluid and expands, resulting in increasing, self-perpetuating pressure on the sac. The more fluid, the more pressure, and the joint area swells and develops a very painful condition known as *bursitis.*

There are many bursa in the body, including the greater trochanteric or hip bursa, located between the iliotibial band muscle on the outside of the thigh (running from hip to knee) and the most prominent outer knob (greater trochanter) of the thigh bone (femur). You can locate your greater trochanteric joint and bursa by placing your hand at the most prominent part of the pelvis, at the top of the hip. Reach down about 4 inches to the most prominent knob of the femur; that's the trochanter (Figure 8.1).

The greater trochanteric region gets quite a workout during running and is susceptible to irritation when overexerted.

Muscles called the gluteus medius and gluteus minimus (see chapter 9, "Low Back Pain," Figure 9.3) attach to the greater trochanter and lift the femur away from the torso. In addition to this, the glutei muscles stabilize the pelvis, keeping it level when you run. Overall, then, the hip sustains a wide range of motion and pressure, with the iliotibial band shifting over the greater trochanter. Overexertion and undue or unbalanced pressure can irritate the related bursa.

Unequal leg lengths and other structural variations (one foot flatter than the other, creating a situation like a leg-length discrepancy) can make the athlete susceptible to hip bursitis. Running on banked surfaces produces an uneven pelvic level and may irritate the bursa. A tight iliotibial band or tendinitis of other hip muscles, such as the gluteus medius or piriformis (see chapter 8, "Piriformis Syndrome"), can cause or aggravate the problem. Frequently, a careful physical exam is required to differentiate between bursitis or tendinitis of one of the hip muscles.

Symptoms of trochanteric bursitis include pain over the outer edge of the hip, exacerbated by getting out of a chair or running on a banked surface. The pain may radiate down the outer leg to the knee, but does not reach beyond the knee. The athlete, particularly if suffering from chronic hip bursitis, may feel a snapping in the hip and an uneasy suspicion that it is out of joint.

To diagnose hip bursitis, the physician manipulates the leg and places pressure on the bursa. If it is inflamed, pain occurs. The doctor examines the hip to rule out a problem in the joint itself. In trochanteric bursitis, the hip joint moves smoothly and fully.

The best preventive medicine is to avoid overextension that can lead to hip bursitis. Don't push yourself severely. Never increase mileage and pace simultaneously.

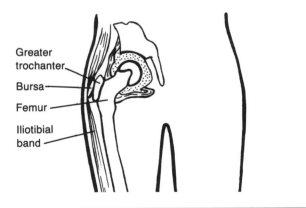

Greater trochanter

Bursa

Femur

Iliotibial band

Figure 8.1 Hip bursitis develops from inflammation of the bursa between the iliotibial band and the greater trochanter of the femur.

Doing appropriate stretching and strengthening exercises can be preventive as well as therapeutic. Do stretching exercises to loosen the iliotibial band and relieve stress placed on a bursitis-prone hip. Stretching and strengthening exercises for the lower back and buttock muscles help keep the hips and pelvis level, relieving unnecessary stressful motion in the hip joints as you walk or run.

The following exercises (described in chapter 12) loosen, stretch, or strengthen muscles in the hip area and may prevent and treat bursitis:

1. For the iliotibial band, follow Stretch Exercises 9 and 10.
2. For hip extension follow Strength Exercise 17.

Piriformis Syndrome

Denis R. Harris, M.D.

The piriformis syndrome is a cause of pain felt in the thigh and buttock from irritation to the sciatic nerve. Usually, the sciatic nerve is irritated as it exits the back, but it also may become compressed as it enters the thigh from the pelvis. As it travels this route, it passes around one of the hip muscles—the piriformis. If the piriformis becomes inflamed and swollen, the sciatic nerve, too, may become inflamed.

The piriformis syndrome is associated with pain felt in the buttock and thigh. Tenderness may be felt in the sciatic notch—the soft area in the posterior gluteal area (see chapter 2, "Injury Identification by Anatomic Location," Figure 2.14). Because piriformis rotates the hip, rotation of the hip may increase the discomfort. Symptoms rarely radiate to below the knee. Pain occurs after activities and is not associated with back pain.

Anti-inflammatory medicine (especially ibuprofen) can be beneficial. Local heat before exercise, and ice afterward, should be used. Stretch the hamstring muscles and rotators. Once the initial pain has subsided, work on strengthening the hip rotators and extensors (see chapter 12, Stretch Exercises 12, 13, and 15, and Strength Exercises 17, 19, and 20). As with all rehabilitation, begin the exercise program slowly, to ensure that the pain and inflammation do not return.

Hamstring Injuries

Vincent G. Desiderio, Jr., M.D.

The hamstring muscles are a frequently injured structure in the athlete—in particular, the runner. The hamstrings comprise a group of three muscles that have their attachment at the base of the buttock, in the bone on which we sit, called the *ischium*. These muscles travel down the back of the leg and attach to the upper portion of the lower leg bones, the tibia and fibula (Figure 8.2).

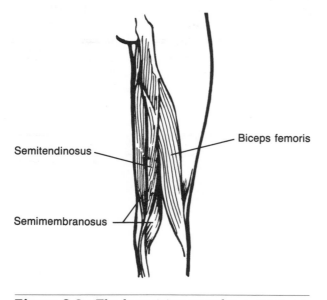

Semitendinosus

Biceps femoris

Semimembranosus

Figure 8.2   The hamstring muscles comprise a group of three muscles.

Because the hamstrings cross two joints—the knee and hip—their function is varied. When the hamstrings contract, the hip extends—that is, the thigh goes from a position of being bent in front of the body to one of being in line with the torso. Thus, the hamstrings are used very commonly in everyday activity, such as in getting out of a chair or climbing stairs, both of which extend the hip. During normal walking, the hamstrings also bend the knee. In athletic activities, the hamstrings are particularly important when the athlete goes from a crouched position to an erect position—such as with a sprinter, whose front leg in the starting position takes the brunt of the start.

The muscles opposed to the hamstrings are the quadriceps. These are in front of the thigh and extend the knee (bring it out straight from a bent position). The quads tend to be the most powerful muscles in the body. In many athletes, they are much stronger than the hamstrings.

Hamstring injuries are fairly common. One can cause a nagging problem for the athlete. Most injuries to hamstring muscles are classified as strains. The word *strain* is sometimes confusing; when used to describe a hamstring injury (commonly called a pulled hamstring), it refers to a partial tear of the hamstring muscles.

Strains frequently afflict athletes whose legs undergo sudden, explosive motions, such as sprinters. One may also befall the athlete who has frequent contractions of the hamstrings, such as a long-distance runner. In the acutely injured sprinter, the hamstrings contract against the very strong pull of the quadriceps, producing sudden hamstring stress, thus tearing their fibers. You often see a sprinter grab the back of his thigh about 3 to 4 seconds after the start of a race. In the long-distance runner pain occurs in the same area, but develops gradually.

Hamstring injuries may be very minor, with only a small tear of the muscle, or can be substantial, wherein an entire muscle is ruptured and separated in its midportion. Occasionally, the muscles can completely pull off of the bone, particularly in adolescents. This usually occurs at the attachment of the muscle to the ischium.

At times, treatment for hamstring injuries can be very frustrating. The best treatment for such problems is prevention. The hamstrings are probably the muscles in the body whose stretching prior to physical activity is the most important. The reason that this muscle group is so susceptible to injury is because it is shortened and tightened during most daily activities. Most recreational athletes spend most of the day sitting, either at a desk or some other site. In sitting, the hamstrings are in a contracted state and often tighten up and shorten. The body may compensate by increasing the tilt of the pelvis, thus arching the back. The most commonly prescribed stretching exercise for the hamstrings is the hurdler's stretch (see chapter 12, Stretch Exercises 5 and 6). To establish whether your hamstrings are at the appropriate length, you should be able to lie flat on your back with the hip flexed to 90 degrees and the knee fully extended comfortably.

For the athlete who has the misfortune of sustaining injury to the hamstrings, treatment consists primarily of rest, followed by rehabilitation. In the case of severely injured hamstrings, it is imperative that the extremity be rested extensively. Depending on the extent of the injury, ice is often initially helpful. Some form of wrapping device helps support the muscle as it heals; often this is composed of ace bandages and tape. If the injury is severe enough, crutches may be warranted. Most of the time, anti-inflammatory drugs help limit inflammation and swelling from injury; aspirin tends to be very effective for this purpose.

In the case of chronic tendinitis, as often occurs in the long-distance runner, the treatment involves a few days of rest, followed by a good stretching program. On resumption of running, distance and speed should be reduced, so as not to have the injury recur. At times, it is required that the long-distance runner refrain from stressing the muscles for several weeks prior to resuming activity.

Once the acute phase of the hamstring injury has subsided, gentle stretching exercises should be undertaken along with a mild strengthening program. The stretching is often facilitated by the use of heat prior to the exercise, followed by ice to the affected area after stretching.

When the athlete has regained the full length of the muscles and has minimal pain, more vigorous strengthening exercises can be undertaken (see chapter 12, Strength Exercise 22). A good way to strengthen the hamstring muscles is through bicycling. The exception to the rule that athletes have much stronger quads than hamstrings is the competitive cyclist.

It is often reasonable to use a support for the thigh, such as the wrap mentioned previously or a commercially available thigh sleeve, on resuming activity. Again, gradual increase in activity is usually recommended. It is imperative that the athlete faithfully stretch the hamstrings prior to the resumption of vigorous activity. Other modes of treatment include various physical therapy modalities, such as ultrasound. Occasionally, a steroid injection can be of benefit, although it is not nearly as effective in hamstrings as it is in other parts of the body. The unfortunate aspect of a hamstring injury is that it can be a nagging problem, significantly limiting the ability of the athlete to perform. Also, at times it is unresponsive to treatment.

In summary, hamstring injuries are a frequent, and often nagging, problem to both the amateur and professional athlete. The best treatment tends to be prevention with stretching exercises, which should be done faithfully, to maintain the appropriate length of the muscles.

Groin Pull

Wayne B. Leadbetter, M.D.

Groin pull injuries involve acute tears of muscles fibers located on the inner aspect of the thigh. As such, the athlete does not injure the groin, which is an anatomic area, but rather the specific groin muscles located on the inner aspect of the thigh—notably, the adductors of the leg. A *pull* is a lay term for a tearing of a muscle and is technically known as a *strain*. Strains vary in severity from grades 1 and 2, representing small fiber disruption, to grade 3, a complete and severe injury.

Muscle pulls are characterized by sudden pain in the area, usually during a moment of dynamic stress, as when the athlete suddenly sprints or spreads the legs to reach for a ball. The athlete is usually stopped from continuing play, and within 24 to 48 hours notices warmth, swelling, and often, bruising—which show up in the inside of the thigh along the margin of the pelvis and crotch. This bruising often gravitates down the inner thigh toward the knee, creating concern to the athlete because it seems the injury is spreading. This concern is unfounded; in reality, the bruise's apparent spreading is due only to gravity pulling on the bleeding site of the trauma.

The treatment for pulls is the same as for any other muscle injury: RICE (*rest, ice, compression, and elevation*). The decrease of pain and swelling may be followed by return to activity. The waiting period in a grade 1 strain can be as short as a week. However, a grade 3 strain may require 6 weeks or longer before a return to stressful sports activity.

Most important in the recovery of strains or pulls of muscles is the rehabilitation and further protection during return to activity. Runners and field athletes who suffer groin injuries need to wrap the thigh carefully with elastic wraps, in combination with commercially available Neoprene® thigh sleeves, to counteract the distracting pull of the muscles during activity and to give dynamic support. Locally applied pads are helpful. Icing after activity may be required for several months. Heat is generally not used during the acute phase when swelling and tenderness are apparent; however, as swelling disappears, and the early stages of inflammation are no longer present, using a moist heat pad in the evening may be a practical measure to relieve aching and discomfort.

Muscle injuries invariably imply a preexisting vulnerability or improper conditioning. The adductor muscles are responsible in running activity for assisting in the change of direction from side to side, as well as in straight-ahead running. This stress must be prepared for by proper strengthening exercises, involving lifting weights in a cross-legged fashion (see chapter 12, Strength Exercise 20a) or involving resistance machines now currently available in many health clubs, in order to strengthen the inner aspect of the thigh. A simple measure is to squeeze a small ball between the knees (see chapter 12, Strength Exercise 20b).

Flexibility is also critical in avoiding further injury. Because injured muscles especially tend to shorten during the healing process, they must be stretched gradually to proper resting length to avoid reinjury and cramping (see chapter 12, Stretch Exercises 7 and 8).

Returning to activity requires a cautious program of increasing exposure to the stresses of the chosen sport, usually over a period of several weeks. Small amounts of discomfort during a return to activity are to be expected.

Stress Fracture

Wayne B. Leadbetter, M.D.

Any bone exposed to repeated overloading may develop a stress fracture. Although a *fracture* technically is any discontinuity or coming apart of a bone, that is, a break, most stress fractures in recreational athletes do not progress to that point before they are diagnosed. Stress fractures can occur in both the upper and lower extremities; statistically, they are most common in the foot, due to the magnification of force produced by jumping or running. As such, these weaknesses in bone structure have been described in ski jumpers, joggers, all types of running athletes, and hikers; in military recruits, they are termed *march fractures.*

Stress fractures are overuse injuries, produced by the repetitive cyclic loading of the bone structures. The classic example of a failure of a material due to recurrent load is the bending of a paper clip. Bone, though, has the advantage of being a living structure, with cells that can respond to the exposure of excessive activity by attempting to rebuild the bone. The bone is made even stronger, thereby increasing the athlete's endurance in the stressful activity.

Unfortunately, pain is not always present as an early warning, or it is ignored by the athlete, and the bone cells cannot rebuild as fast as the loading damages them. The result is deterioration at the site of weakness, thereby creating a true microfracture in the involved bone. Rarely is there an underlying disease creating weakness in bone structure, although women can suffer from osteoporosis. Most stress fractures occur in normal bone that is exposed to excessively intense training. This fact is underscored by their occurring in only three competitive animals: race dogs, racehorses, and humans.

The diagnosis is confirmed by complaints of pain, accompanied by direct bone tenderness at the site, often producing a limp or an inability to participate in physical activity. When this condition is found in the shin area, it is often confused with shin splints, which is another overuse injury. Eventually, disability leads to a medical evaluation, which should include an x-ray. This may not reveal the microfracture in its early stages, but rules out other concerns—such as possible malignancy and infection—which mimic the signs of a stress fracture. A bone scan is a sophisticated isotope test in which a low-dose radioactive substance is injected into the patient. The material circulates in the bloodstream for a short period of time and becomes more concentrated where tissue is inflamed at the site of the injury, where it can be recorded by a Geiger counter and camera (the radioactive substance is totally excreted in a matter of hours). This test is highly accurate in identifying the microfractures before they can show up on x-rays.

Treatment begins with rest but does not necessarily require total abstinence from sports. Evaluation must include a search for underlying structural causes that load individual bones excessively during activity; examples are one leg being longer than another, an excessively high arch, and flatfoot. Dynamic factors include asymmetric stride length and obvious training mistakes.

Especially when occurring around the hips and pelvis, stress fractures presenting with pain can be indistinguishable from a variety of more serious causes and should be followed with a physician's help until recovery is clearly occurring.

Returning to activity in the face of a healing stress fracture is a highly individual matter, dependent on the skill of the participant and the exact sport that is being performed. A substitute sport, such as bicycling or swimming, may be required to maintain cardiovascular fitness during this healing phase. Full recovery is usually achieved, but this may require several months in the case of larger bones. Ultimately, the involved repaired bone is stronger than it originally was, representing, in most cases, an adaptation of the body to increased physical demand.

When stress fractures are ignored, serious complications can result. These include complete breaks of the bone, especially in the hip area, resulting in surgical treatment and prolonged disability.

Suggested Reading for "Stress Fracture"

Abel (1985)

Shangold (1983)

Sullivan et al. (1984)

See reading list at the end of the book for a complete source listing.

Jock Itch

Paul M. Taylor, D.P.M.

Jock itch is a frequent complaint among athletes. It commonly refers to a redness and itching of the skin in the groin area. Jock itch may be due to irritation, contact dermatitis, or a fungus or Candida infection.

The chafing that occurs from moisture and rubbing between the thighs, or against seams in shorts or a "jock strap" (athletic supporter), is the most common form of jock itch. This can be treated by wearing clothing that fits better and does not have seams that can irritate the area. Drying the area well after bathing or showering and applying powder help to resolve the redness.

Other than simple irritation, there are more serious causes of redness and itching in the groin area. Fungus or monilial (Candida) infections can occur in this area. The fungus causes redness, itching, small blisters, and drainage, with crusting on the skin. Candida infections cause shiny, red areas that are well demarcated; itching, which may be severe, and, sometimes, drainage with scaly areas. There are over-the-counter medications for treating jock itch caused by a fungus. However, if the condition does not improve in 7 to 10 days, or gets worse during use of the medication, professional help should be obtained.

Another cause of jock itch is contact dermatitis. The physical changes are the same as with other types of jock itch. However, this type is caused by an allergy to clothing, detergent used in washing clothes, or medication used to self-treat the jock itch. Again, professional help may be needed to identify the allergen and to establish a proper treatment plan.

Jock itch, when caused by a simple irritation, can usually be adequately self-treated. However, when the problem persists, professional help should be obtained, because there are other, more serious causes of this common malady of the athlete.

Suggested Reading for "Jock Itch"

Andrews & Domonkos (1964)

See reading list at the end of the book for a complete source listing.

CHAPTER 9

Low Back Injuries

The lower back (the lumbar region) provides strength to the torso as well as to the hips and thighs. Also, the crucially important nerves of the spinal cord travel through the backbone, exiting along its length, each to serve its own area of responsibility. Bending, twisting, shock absorption—overuse of the lower back by the athlete can not only make back muscles sore, but it can also impinge on the freedom of some of these nerves to perform without pain. This chapter examines some of the causes and treatments of low back pain. Many of the principles in this chapter apply to the upper back and neck (thoracic and cervical portions, respectively, of the spinal column) as well, though overuse pain in these regions is much rarer.

Low Back Pain

Wayne B. Leadbetter, M.D.

Low back pain affects many people. In sports the problem is seen most frequently in activities such as gymnastics, ballet, or basketball, in which there is great stress on the back. Surveys of running-related injuries reveal that low back pain is not one of the most common injuries among runners. To prevent or cope with this kind of avoidable pain, many athletes need help in establishing an accurate diagnosis and redirection of conditioning programs.

What Is the Back?

Knowledge of the anatomy of the back is essential to understanding low back pain and its treatment. To most people, the back is a mysterious blend of bones, muscles, ligaments, and nerves, to which are added curious structures called *disks*. In one sense, the back conjures an image of strength—Atlas holding up the earth with his back. On the other hand, the back is seen as a vulnerable and capricious structure, notorious for causing disability in sedentary societies.

The basic functional unit of the back consists of two adjacent structures, the vertebrae, separated by a disk (Figure 9.1). This unit bears the brunt of the impact during running. The disk is a shock absorber shaped like a water-filled balloon that has been compressed. It is filled with a gelatinous substance called *matrix* (nucleus pulposus). Matrix is 80 percent water at birth but, with aging, gradually changes in chemical character, becoming more brittle—and more likely to rupture or fragment.

The "slipped" disk is a frequently cited back ailment, in which pain is caused by pressure on nerve roots. However, disks do not literally slip as often as they bulge or protrude into the foramen, openings in each vertebra through which nerve roots pass from the spinal cord (Figure 9.1). Although much attention is paid to the possibility of a slipped or ruptured disk—one of the most serious and persistent types of pain in the low back—this is not

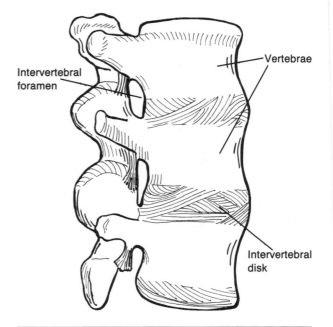

Figure 9.1   The spinal column is composed of bones called *vertebrae* that are separated by the disks. Nerve roots exit from the vertebrae through openings called *foramen*.

statistically the runner's most common cause of back pain and soreness.

The guiding portion of the vertebrae-disk unit consists of facet joints that guide the motion of the lower (lumbar) spine during running. Facets fit together in a way that prevents pronounced rotation of the spine but allows bending and extension (Figure 9.2). These small joints can become arthritic—just like other joints (such as the knee) can become inflamed—and are not an uncommon source of inflammation and soreness.

The site where the vertebral column meets the pelvis is called the lumbosacral junction. The rhythm established between bending motions of the spine and motions of the pelvis and lower legs constitutes one of the major influences on the lower back and plays an important role in determining undesired symptoms that may develop.

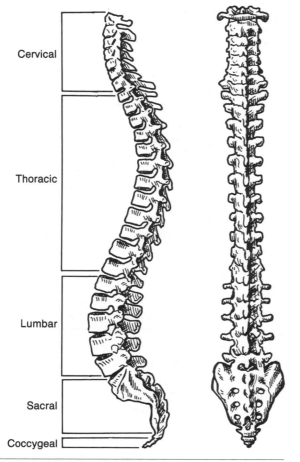

Figure 9.2 The multiple vertebrae that compose the backbone allow for support, strength, and flexibility.

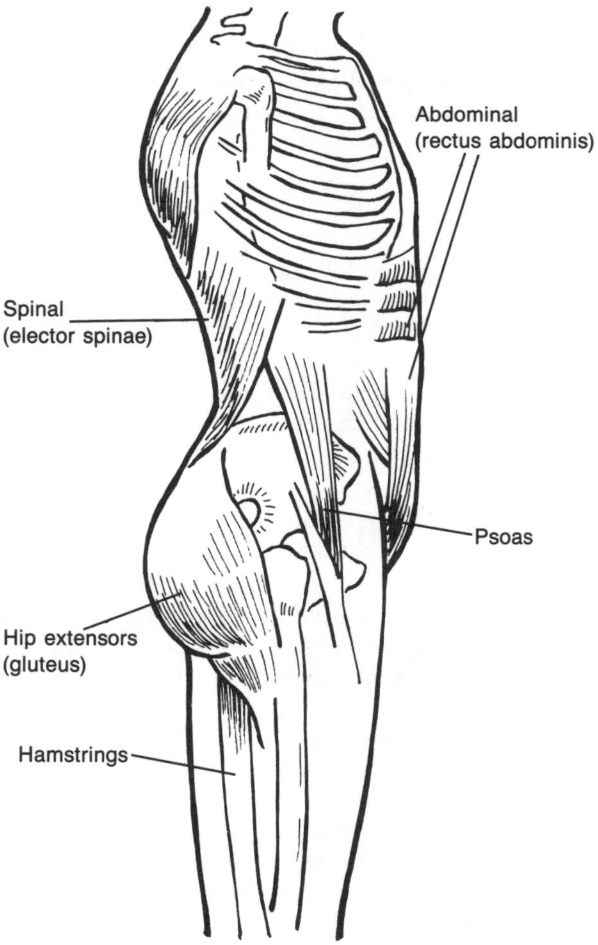

Figure 9.3 The muscle groups of the back and abdomen support the back and maintain the posture.

Muscles

Muscles, more than any other part of the back, are most responsive to the effects of conditioning programs and physical exercise. In the lumbosacral region, five muscle groups are important: abdominal (rectus abdominis), psoas (iliopsoas), spinal (erector spinas), hamstring, and hip extensor (gluteus) (Figure 9.3). The balancing and pulling of these muscle groups against each other is needed to maintain an upright posture, one of the requirements for an efficient gait. The abdominal muscle group is balanced by the erector, or supporting, spinal muscle system behind it.

The psoas muscle—often mentioned, but commonly misunderstood as to its origin and function in running—begins in the lower spine and passes through the pelvic area to attach to the femur, the thigh bone, which extends from the pelvis to the knee. The psoas muscle has the most influence in bending the hip. A contraction of this muscle produces an increased curvature of the lower back (a condition called *lordosis*), places increased stress on the vertebral column, and decreases the space in the foramen, through which the nerve roots pass. It also makes other supporting muscles work harder to maintain an upright posture, producing a greater tendency toward fatigue.

Tight hamstring muscles, a common result of distance running, place undue stress on the lower vertebrae and contribute to low back problems by flexing the knee—preventing forward rotation of the pelvis—during bending and stretching. Tight hamstrings also create problems during the swing phase of running, in which the leg reaches forward before the heelstrike and transmits excessive stress to both the lower back muscles and hamstrings, resulting in a possible muscle tear (see "Hamstring Injuries" in chapter 8).

Nerves

Nerves are the pathway for pain, and in the back there are a variety of nerves that can send this warning. Two types of pain can be identified. One is not localized or sensitive in any particular area. Dull aching, the general back pain known as *lumbago*, falls into this category and is caused by small nerve endings stimulating the facet joints or the muscles.

The second type of pain is specific and probably the most feared—sciatica. In this case, pain radiates downward through the lower leg from the sciatic nerve, the main nerve consisting of nerve roots from the lower vertebral levels of the spinal cord.

Role of Posture

From a purely biomechanical point of view, the goal of running is to move the athlete's center of gravity—in front of the second sacral vertebra—from point A to point B in as straight a line as possible. The perfect role model is a wheel, which has a center of gravity at its hub and does not shift sideways or up and down as the wheel moves from point to point.

The athlete's case is different. The athlete's center of gravity, moving from point to point, forms an undulating up-and-down curve when followed from the side. The best the human body can do is try to limit side-to-side and up-and-down deviations as much as possible. There are three factors that determine the path of the athlete's center of gravity by affecting the movement of the pelvis and lower spine: The tilting, forward-and-back rotation, and side-to-side shifting of the pelvis—even by a few degrees or centimeters—provide a dampening effect on what would otherwise be a rigid, robotlike gait.

The running athlete does not swing the leg forward from the hip joint like a hinge during the swing phase. Instead, there is a complex forward swinging motion that combines forward rotation of the pelvis as well. The net effect is to create a bending back-and-forth and sideways at the lumbosacral junction, a mo-

tion not unlike the repeated bending of a paper clip.

The key for tolerating repetitive bending stresses, reducing energy consumption and resulting fatigue, and improving performance, is to maintain good posture. With the spine, pelvis, and leg aligned, the effort required to stand and to support the frame of the body is minimized. Excessive swayback—often due to wearing high-heeled shoes or to the pot-bellied, weak abdominal posture of a non-exerciser—results in a forward shifting of the center of gravity, an imbalance in skeletal alignment, and an increase in the amount of work necessary to walk or run. Additional stress on the other supporting back muscles occurs and can cause backache.

A knock-kneed stance can lead to forward tilt of the pelvis. Runners with such a characteristic appear to be running in a crouch and are identifiable not only by an outside whipping motion of the lower leg but also by a forward lean to the trunk of the body. This is tiring and produces a complex of symptoms related to the lower back as well as to the lower leg. Elevation of the arch of the foot by inserting an arch support or orthotic device in the shoe can, in some cases, have the effect of straightening the knee and correcting the forward tilt of the pelvis.

Effects of Exercise

The basic argument for participating in an athletic activity is that your body benefits from physiological changes it undergoes. Stress is the body's response to exercise. Most responses to exercise are beneficial: improved cardiovascular function, lower blood pressure, more efficient use of oxygen, increased calorie burning, and greater physical stamina.

It is foolish, however, to think that the stress response to exercise is without problems. Muscle imbalance due to excessive shortening of one muscle group is the underlying reason for many overuse injuries. In running, the psoas muscle is shortened from repeated and pronounced activity. This can lead to a loss of balance or improper posture. Such a muscle imbalance is aggravated by occupations characterized by sitting, which allow the psoas to shorten and contract further.

This is not said to discourage running, but rather to emphasize that running alone does not correct postural imbalance, but actually aggravates it. It is conditioning—the preparation for running—that is the most beneficial. For example, because the abdominal muscles are not strengthened much by running, in comparison to the psoas muscle, conditioning through exercise is needed to strengthen the muscle and maintain spinal balance.

Stress From Impact

The other obvious effect on the spinal column from exercise is impact caused by repetitive heelstrikes. Disk pressures rise precipitously because of the increased downward force that occurs when the foot strikes the ground—three times the body's weight. Hundreds of pounds of force, therefore, can be imparted to the vertebral column. The greatest amount of stress is centered at the lumbosacral junction. It is not a coincidence, then, that this is where most disk protrusions occur.

Any measure that decreases the stress of impact—improving heel and sole cushioning, decreasing body weight, avoiding excessive bouncing while running—often prevent the onset of low back pain.

Recognition of the Problem

Most backaches and soreness associated with exercise respond to rest and improved conditioning. Ironically, because many low back problems originate from work-related emotional tensions, exercise is often a good prescription for alleviation of backaches.

One of the low back ailments athletes suffer from is sciatica, in which pain radiates downward from the sciatic nerve; related numbness can occur in the back of the thigh, calf, or toes. This usually is caused by a ruptured disk; the suffering athlete should see a physician.

Dull, aching pain in the low back is the most common kind of back problem among athletes. However, not all backaches originate in the back, and pains transmitted from pelvic organs such as the ovary, uterus, colon, and prostate, or from major blood vessels, are conditions to be wary of, especially in older persons. Rarely, interosseus tumors can masquerade as backache.

Also, the hip can be a listening post for lumbar disk disease or other problems. Hip pain can be transmitted from other parts of the body through nerve roots.

Vulnerable Athletes

Although serious back complaints may not be common in the general population, certain groups of athletes are particularly susceptible to low back pain. Obviously, any history of injury or degenerative disease increases vulnerability. Athletes with x-ray evidence of advanced arthritis, vertebral misalignment with nerve root encroachment, or previous trauma with fractures may not be able to tolerate the effects of exercise.

The overweight person risks developing a protruding disk. This person may have to engage in an aggressive walking program and other activities, such as swimming, before attempting more strenuous, high-impact activities.

Any prior imbalance of the spinal alignment, such as adolescent spinal curvature (scoliosis), places facet joints in an incongruous alignment and may cause pain. However, many childhood spinal curvatures are not painful. Exercise has not been shown to be harmful to the athlete who wishes to exercise with a curvature condition.

The competitive runner who is in transition in a training program often experiences backache due to muscle imbalance from overuse. Common occurrences after a marathon, a variety of severe low back and psoas muscle spasms usually are temporary and respond to rest and alterations in training patterns. The child runner, especially, should be cautious since it has been recognized that the vertical growth of children produces an imbalance of the lumbar fascia and muscle system, creating tightness of the spinal muscles, accentuating swayback of the spine, and producing backache (see chapter 16).

Treatment and Prevention

At the onset of low back discomfort, the athlete should assess posture. Errors in training are responsible for approximately 60 percent of all running injuries, the most common mistake being excessive mileage. Most spinal curvatures and leg length differences greater than ¼ inch can be dealt with by altering shoes.

Table 9.1   Pain Classification and Prevention

Category and symptoms	Treatment
Treat yourself	
First degree	
No limitation of motion.	No great change in routine, other than a more thorough warm-up.
Low-grade pain at start, decreasing as run progresses.	Work past the pain before undertaking heavy exertion.
Pain reappears after running.	
Second degree	
Little effect on running form.	Eliminate activity that causes pain to increase, such as races, hard speedwork, and very long training runs.
Pain constant or increasing as run goes on.	
Consult a sports orthopedist	
Third degree	
Mild pain on easy runs.	Start slowly and cautiously.
Severe pain on hard runs with disturbance of running form.	When pain builds to form-disturbing level, slow to a walk or do stretching exercises.
	Run, walk, run, walk, etc.
Fourth degree	
Impossible to run without great pain and a pronounced limp.	Substitute an activity that causes no pain, such as walking or swimming. According to Dr. Kenneth Cooper, 2½ miles of walking or ¼ mile of swimming produce the aerobic benefits of 1 mile of running.

Posture problems are best controlled through exercise programs (see Table 9.1).

As with all muscle imbalance caused by overuse, a strengthening and stretching program often is supplemented by other forms of treatment, such as ice massage after exercise, moist heat during sleep, massage, heat liniments, sauna, whirlpool, and others. All relieve muscle pain.

As a rule, more serious pain does not respond to these measures and is a warning signal to consult an orthopedist. Symptoms persisting for longer than a week to 10 days should be evaluated carefully. An x-ray is warranted in such cases and may reveal an underlying skeletal cause for the discomfort, such as degenerative arthritis, a stress fracture with spondylolisthesis (forward slipping of a vertebral body) or other congenital abnormalities.

In the case of a protruded disk that produces unmanageable pain or worsening neurological problems, surgery may lead to a successful return to activity, although this depends on the individual and is somewhat unpredictable. If the earlier recommendations are followed, however, surgery rarely is required for the athlete with low back pain.

As Ronald Lawrence, M.D., notes, "Good posture should not be taken for granted by runners. . . . Good posture is good physical balance and is the key to effective movement. No one has perfect posture, and running only amplifies minor postural imperfections. You may get away with these imperfections if you pursue only the daily activities of walking, standing, and sitting, but the flaws must be corrected if you run daily."

Exercises

There are five basic exercises for maintaining good posture. The following exercises should be performed to prevent back problems. Refer to chapter 12 for specific methods.

1. Bent knee sit-ups for abdominals (Strength Exercise 14b)
2. Low back extension (Stretch Exercise 14)
3. Lower back and hamstring stretch (Stretch Exercises 13 and 15)
4. Starting line stretch (Stretch Exercise 16)
5. Back flattener (Strength Exercise 14a)

Suggested Reading for "Low Back Pain"

Blake & Fettig (1983)

Keene (1983)

Mozee & Prokop (1984)

Spencer & Jackson (1983)

———————

See reading list at the end of the book for a complete source listing.

CHAPTER 10

Chest and Abdomen Injuries

The abdomen and chest, besides carrying important muscles, contain and protect most of the body's vital organs. Some of these muscles and organs are directly and adversely affected by athletic overuse. On the other hand, special congenital and acquired conditions of some of these organs can limit the athlete's participation in physical activities. This chapter discusses some aspects of abdominal and chest structures that are of interest to the athlete.

Side Stitches

Paul M. Taylor, D.P.M.

Side stitches or pain, usually occurring in the upper right quadrant of the abdomen during exercise, is common in athletes. Although most athletes have experienced this, medically the condition is poorly understood. Generally, it is not serious, but it can be annoying, especially if it occurs during competition.

Various explanations have been offered as to the cause of side stitches, including air or gas trapped in the intestines, constipation, and exercising after eating. A commonly accepted theory relates to intestinal ischemia. The *ischemia* refers to inadequate blood supply to the abdominal muscles, the diaphragm, or the muscles between the ribs. During exercise, the body redirects blood from the organs in the abdomen to the large skeletal muscle groups. If this occurs too quickly, there may be inadequate blood to the above muscles, which are needed for respiration. This ischemic condition then results in pain from cramping of these muscles.

Because the mechanism of the side stitch is poorly understood, there is no standard treatment. If the athlete is prone to side stitches, he or she may be able to reduce them by improved breathing techniques. Belly breathing should be practiced, in which the stomach should expand with the inspiration, or breathing in. This allows a deeper breath and takes pressure off the diaphragm. Rapid shallow breaths should be avoided. If the stitch continues, the intensity of running or other exercise has to be reduced. In some cases, the exercise has to be discontinued.

Because the cause and extent of the stitch varies considerably between individuals, it may be necessary to experiment to find the best way to relieve the stitch. It may be necessary to avoid eating before exercising or at least to avoid certain foods that produce more gas or are more constipating. Try different breathing techniques. Start slower and gradually build up the level of exercise. When the stitch occurs, it sometimes helps to bend over and apply pressure over the area with the hands or to place the arm of the affected side over your head.

Side stitches are not usually a serious problem. However, if they occur frequently and do not appear to be lessening as the level of training increases, a medical evaluation should be done to be certain that there is no other underlying problem.

Suggested Reading for "Side Stitches"

Stamford (1985)

See reading list at the end of the book for a complete source listing.

Palpitations (Premature Beats; Premature Ventricular Contractions, or PVCs)

James R. Snyder, M.D.

Palpitations, premature beats, and premature ventricular contractions (PVCs) are all events that sometimes occur in normal people with otherwise regular heart rhythms. Medical terms are often clumsy and difficult to remember, but words such as *premature, rhythm, rate*, and *regularity* are in common usage. These terms all refer to normal heart functions. With some understanding of basic facts about the heart, it becomes easier to understand the deviations. The most important thing for the athlete is to understand his or her own heart functions and not to be afraid of them.

The average resting heart beats about 70 times per minute. This measurement—beats per minute—is termed the *heart rate*. The heart rate and the pulse rate are essentially the same. The heart rate requires an electrocardiograph, but the pulse rate can be felt by the fingertips on any large artery, such as the radial artery in the wrist and the femoral artery in the groin. The carotid arteries in the neck are large and easily felt, but nerve reflexes may be caused by fingertip pressure, making the carotids poor for giving an accurate pulse rate.

Information from the arterial pulse consists of pulse rate (beats per minute) and the rhythm and regularity of the beats. The pulse rate requires a full minute of counting, not only 10 seconds of beats multiplied by 6. Feeling the pulse for an additional minute detects any irregularities in the rhythm of the pulse.

The pulse rate changes with breathing, eating, excitement, exercise, medicine, alcohol, smoking, and everything else. However, the rhythm can be observed at fast or slow rates. People should know what their pulse rates are at rest, walking, during exercise and recovery, and after eating.

Palpitations is an ambiguous term that refers to a sensation of heavy throbbing, beating, or pounding in the chest. Measurement of the pulse rate and rhythm is especially impor-

tant to the diagnosis when palpitations are the complaint. It is not uncommon for people to not want to record their pulse; they would rather not know. However, this reduces their chances of understanding the heart rhythm and thereby being reassured through information.

Pulse irregularities, such as occur with premature beats or PVCs, are superimposed upon a regular rhythm; an electrocardiogram can show the sequence of regular beats and the occurrence of early, or premature, beats. On the electrocardiogram, the premature beat has a distinctive form that makes it readily distinguishable from the normal beat.

When premature beats or PVCs occur, the person may feel a palpitation within the chest. When the pulse is being taken, the premature beat is not felt by the fingertips. The premature heartbeat does not create a pulse wave; therefore, a skip in the pulse is the diagnostic feature. However, the premature beat is seen on the electrocardiogram as multiple heart contractions. This may be difficult to understand, but remember that taking the pulse is feeling the blood flow; when multiple beats occur, the heart does not have time to be refilled by blood, so a strong, new pulse wave is not generated. Because the electrocardiogram measures electrical changes and not pulse waves, it records the premature beat. Still, the pulse is valuable in providing information relating to heart rate and premature beats.

The skip in the pulse and the sensation of a palpitation in the chest usually happens when the person is at rest, such as lying down to sleep. The heart rate is at its slowest at this time, and the chances for a PVC are the greatest. Getting a drink of water increases the heart rate, making the premature beats cease.

Rhythm changes can occur in normal, healthy people. Patients with heart disease may have more complicated heart rhythm disorders for which treatment is required. People who ask about rhythm changes such as palpitations are usually really asking whether they have heart disease.

Learning how to take a pulse accurately is important in defining any form of heart irregularity, for first aid care, and as a help in fitness work. Measuring the pulse, temperature, body weight, and blood pressure—the body's vital signs—is simple to learn.

Mitral Valve Prolapse

James R. Snyder, M.D.

Mitral valve prolapse (MVP) has become a common medical diagnosis over the past 10 years, with young adults who exercise regularly as prime candidates for MVP syndrome. In order to understand this problem, some knowledge of the anatomy of the heart is helpful. The heart has four valves and four chambers. All the pumping and movement of blood is accomplished by the two lower chambers, the right and left ventricles. Each ventricle has an inflow and an outflow valve. The mitral valve is the inflow valve of the left ventricle.

The right and left ventricular outflow valves are identical. Each consists of three components neatly attached to a cartilage skeleton on two sides, analogous to a sail's attachment to the mast and boom. The side that is free can collapse or fill depending on the direction of the pressure.

The right and left inflow valves are larger, with less precise form. The right inflow valve consists of three components, whereas the left, or mitral, valve has two parts. A partial analogy for the mitral valve would be a parachute, whose outer edge is held in position by many small cords; the mitral valve is anchored to the inside muscular tissue of the left ventricle. The outer edge of the mitral's two components is attached to the heart tissue making up the inflow tract of the left ventricle. When the ventricle pumps, a pressure wave fills the mitral valve's two parachutelike components; they come together, closing the inflow area while the ventricle empties through the now-collapsed outflow valve. Though there is always a certain amount of prolapse, or billowing, of the mitral valve when its parachutelike components close, excessive prolapse is part of the diagnosis for MVP. Other aspects for diagnosis are whether the tissue and timing of the mitral valve closure are normal.

MVP is not a disease or sickness. It is a syndrome that occurs in people between 20 and 40, more often in women than men, and rarely will it develop in people over 60. People with MVP tend to be thin, with normal circulation, and with small to normal heart size. The MVP patient comes to the cardiologist complaining of chest pain, anxiety, and shortness of breath. The cardiologist listens to the heart with a stethoscope and runs a variety of tests to rule out coronary artery disease, rheumatic heart disease, and valve infections. People with MVP have normal electrocardiograms and stress tests. However, through the stethoscope the doctor can hear clicking sounds over the mitral valve.

There is no record of deaths caused by MVP; thus, pathologists have been unable to study the tissue of people with MVP. In the future, as people with diagnosed MVP die from other causes, researchers will be able to study the condition to a greater extent.

Treatment

Treatment for the MVP syndrome is directed toward control of the several different, related symptoms. Because the problem is not serious, treatment should be simple and safe. Most people who develop MVP are stressed, Type A achievers; it is important that this problem not cause them to worry, which would induce even more anxiety. The assurance received by the patient from seeing a normal heart on an x-ray, a normal ECG, and a normal stress test is usually helpful. Exercise is recommended because it not only strengthens the heart and lungs but also helps relieve stress. Although MVP is not a cardiac risk factor, it still is imperative for MVP patients to maintain a healthy weight, not smoke, reduce salt and alcohol consumption, and eat a low-fat diet. Also, medicine to reduce anxiety and tension in the upper gastro-intestinal tract is prescribed for some MVP patients.

Though MVP is not serious, the patient should visit the doctor at 6-month intervals to make sure the mitral valve continues to show no evidence of disease, inadequate valve closure, or leakage. Because many symptoms of MVP are similar to coronary artery disease, updates with the cardiologist can rule out disease as the cause of the symptoms.

Effects of Endurance Training on the Heart

Richard L. Jones, M.D.
Karen Lenz Jones, B.A.

One of the most strongly held beliefs of this athletic era is that regular exercise—especially regular aerobic exercise—produces cumulative and beneficial effects in cardiac function. Because of superficial similarities between the athletically trained heart and the diseased heart, however, doctors often mistake the healthy athlete for a person with a chronic heart ailment.

Cardiac Questions

Surprised? Ask yourself these questions:

1. Is your resting heart rate less than 60 beats a minute?
2. Can you feel or see your chest wall throb as your heart beats?
3. Has your doctor said you have a heart murmur or that your heart appears to be enlarged?
4. Do you experience brief lightheadedness when you move quickly from a sitting to a standing position?
5. Do you occasionally perceive an extra or skipped heartbeat?

If you can answer yes to one or more of these questions, you may have the athletic heart syndrome.

Basic Physiology

Understanding how and why the athlete's heart at rest appears so similar to the heart with chronic heart disease requires a basic knowledge of how the heart adapts to physical stress.

The heart is not one, but two, pumps, anatomically attached to one another but working in series, each with a chamber that receives blood (atrium) and a chamber that pumps blood (ventricle). The right side of the heart receives blood from the body and distributes it to the lungs. The left side receives blood from the lungs and pumps it to the different organs of the body.

The heart is only a servant in the circulatory system. It responds to signals from elsewhere that regulate its actions. Pressure receptors in arteries of the neck, blood-borne hormones, and nerve-induced changes in blood vessels of the various organs are only a few sources of the heart's instructions. The heart responds by changing its rate and strength of contraction.

The amount of blood pumped by each ventricle during each beat, termed the *stroke volume*, is about 80 cubic centimeters (nearly 3 fluid ounces) in the average resting male. Cardiac output (stroke volume) times heart rate results in about 5.5 liters (5.8 quarts) per minute in the average resting male. During strenuous exercise, the heart can increase its cardiac output up to 700 percent of normal, or 35 to 40 liters of blood each minute.

Stress Adaptation

Healthy hearts adapt to repeated physical stress by increasing the amount of blood pumped with each beat. This increase in stroke volume results in more blood pumped with each heartbeat; in turn, fewer strokes are required to deliver the necessary volume of blood to the body. The result is that the trained athlete has a lower resting heart rate than the untrained person, indicating a more efficient pump. Generally speaking, early morning resting heart rates of 40 to 60 beats a minute confirm an athletically trained heart, if no underlying heart disease exists.

Dizziness and Extra Beats

This lower heart rate, at any level of physical work, explains why dizziness may occur in athletes upon a change in position. A temporary drop in blood pressure, the cause of this lightheadedness, is much more likely with lower heart rates (see chapter 10, "Orthostatic Hypotension").

Extra beats, or unusual heart rhythms, may also be caused by a low resting heart rate. These extra beats and irregular rhythm patterns can be disconcerting to both the athlete and the physician because these types of alterations seen on electrocardiograms (ECGs) are similar to, or the same as, those seen with diseased hearts. The key difference, however, is that with an increase in heart rate during exercise, the athlete's ECG abnormalities disappear, whereas those of the diseased heart may worsen.

Enlarged Heart Muscle

To achieve an increased stroke volume, the heart must increase in weight and mass in a manner not unlike muscle buildup seen in weight lifters. This increase in size is restricted to the left ventricle only. Upon physical examination, ECG, and chest x-ray, the athlete's heart appears enlarged, with a prominent chest wall impulse, ECG readings that confirm increased left ventricular wall thickness, and a large heart shadow on the chest x-ray. These findings are similar to those of people with long-standing hypertension as well as other forms of chronic heart disease. The major difference upon examination, however, is that the athlete has normal or lower blood pressure.

Heart murmurs, often reported in the athlete, are the result of an increased volume of blood ejected from the left ventricle. The larger volume of blood pumped with each beat is thought to increase turbulence, which often is presumed to produce murmurs.

Physicians Take Note

Physicians may find, then, that the endurance-trained athlete and the patient with chronic heart disease look distressingly similar in the resting state. Both may have evidence of an enlarged, possibly failing heart, extra heart sounds and murmurs, and ECG rhythm abnormalities. Physicians must note, however, that the athlete also has a slower heart rate, normal blood pressure, healthy appearance, and no other signs of heart disease, such as recurring chest pain, shortness of breath, or skin blueness.

Important Difference

The endurance-trained athlete may appear, upon initial examination, to be a person with a dying heart, in need of medical attention—but there is one distinct and very important difference: The athlete has developed the athletic heart syndrome, a physiological condition developed through regular conditioning of the heart muscle, resulting in increased cardiac reserve; the patient with progressive heart disease has used up the cardiac reserve and possesses a dilated, enlarged, and failing heart.

Suggested Reading for "Effects of Endurance Training on the Heart"

Burton (1980)

Hauser et al. (1985)

See reading list at the end of the book for a complete source listing.

Coronary Heart Disease and Exercise

James R. Snyder, M.D.

Coronary heart disease (CHD) is also known as *arteriosclerotic heart disease* and *ischemic heart disease*. Along with angina pectoris, myocardial infarction, and sudden death, CHD is a disease of our century; it was uncommon prior to 1900. Mortality due to CHD rose steadily, reaching a peak in the late fifties and beginning to decline in the sixties. The decrease in mortality during the past 2 decades has been an astounding 36 percent. This look at the incidence of deaths from such a widespread disease, demonstrating large changes over only a few decades, is even more striking because no specific cause has been found, and no specific treatment has been introduced.

Two questions logically follow this information. First, why has such an epidemic fallen upon us? Second, why is it getting better? The cause of the epidemic has never been easy to understand. It appears to be related to a number of factors that are associated with a type of blockage of the coronary, or heart, arteries. Major factors are hypertension, cigarette smoking, and high serum cholesterol. Lack of exercise and body weight are less important factors.

Many people die with their first heart attack, which may also be the first sign of their coronary heart disease. Angina pectoris, or chest pain, can be a more stable and treatable symptom; patients may survive for decades with recurrent chest pain.

Because exercise is thought to play a minor role in the development of CHD, its benefit in prevention remains questionable. Exercise is not known to be helpful in reducing the mortality and morbidity of patients with known CHD.

The mortality from CHD has been dropping steadily for 2 decades. What role has exercise played? The general changes in lifestyle Americans have recently experienced are considered to be important parts of this improvement. Exercise reinforces these changes, which include a reduction in cigarette smoking, more attention to blood pressure, reduced serum cholesterol, and a lower body weight. Exercise also improves stamina and enhances a feeling of accomplishment and well-being.

Although lack of exercise may not be an important risk factor for CHD when cited as a single variable, it is important as part of a healthy lifestyle. The influence of exercise on diet, alcohol intake, cigarette smoking, and body weight makes it a significant part of good health.

Orthostatic Hypotension

Gabe Mirkin, M.D.

In the 1960s Frank Pflagging was one of the best distance runners in the country; now he is one of the best runners over 50 years of age. Whenever he raised himself rapidly from lying or sitting, he would feel dizzy. There is an interesting explanation for this. His training had given him a very strong heart that could pump a large amount of blood with each beat; when he was not exercising, his heart needed to beat only 30 times a minute. Thus, when he would raise himself up rapidly, gravity would pull the blood down from his brain before his next heartbeat arrived to pump the blood back up, and he would feel dizzy.

Such a condition is called *orthostatic hypotension* and is usually harmless. However, if you feel dizzy when you change position, you should check with your doctor. Dizziness can also be caused by an irregular heartbeat, and this can harm you. If your heart is susceptible to certain types of irregular heartbeats, it could stop pumping blood through your body, and you could die. If you have an irregular heartbeat that makes you dizzy, you may need to take medication to make your heart beat more regularly.

Fortunately, most cases of dizziness in the athlete changing position are due to orthostatic hypotension and are harmless.

Upper Respiratory Infections

Gabe Mirkin, M.D.

It's all right to exercise when you have a cold, provided that your muscles do not hurt and you do not have a fever. Certain viruses and bacteria that cause colds can affect your muscles, as well as your nose and throat. Muscles use carbohydrates and fat for energy. There are specific chemicals called *enzymes* in muscles to help the muscles convert fuel to energy. Some infectious agents that cause colds interfere with these enzymes so that the muscles cannot contract effectively and are more likely to tear. Fortunately, your muscles usually tell you when they are not functioning properly: They hurt.

It can be dangerous to exercise when you have a fever. Some germs that cause colds also cause a swelling in the heart muscle. This can interfere with the natural rhythm of the heart and cause it to beat irregularly.

Your heart also has to work much harder during exercise when you have a fever. Exercising muscles generate a tremendous amount of heat. To keep your body from overheating, your heart pumps large amounts of blood from the exercising muscles to the skin, where the heat can be dissipated. When you have a fever, your temperature is already high and your heart has to work much harder just to keep your body from overheating.

As a general rule, you do not have to check with your doctor every time you have a cold. However, you *should* check with your doctor when you have yellow or green mucus, your throat is sore, or the infection lingers more than a couple of weeks. Discolored mucus often indicates that you have a bacterial infection that can be treated with an appropriate antibiotic. Lingering infections can be the result of a breakdown of your immunity, or they can be caused simply by bacteria that require specific treatment.

Allergies and Asthma

Richard L. Jones, M.D.

Runners, cyclists, and other outdoor enthusiasts cherish the spring and fall months as times of climatic moderation between the cold darkness of winter and the long, hot days of summer. Yet for many of the 35 million Americans with allergic diseases, spring and fall are harbingers of something else—allergic rhinitis (inflammation of the mucous membrane of the nose) and asthma, with the associated symptoms of sneezing, itching, nasal stuffiness, postnasal drip, sinus headaches, chronic tearing, cough, wheezing, irritability, fatigue, depression, and even anorexia.

Seventeen percent of all Americans have at least one allergic disease. Four percent have asthma, 7 percent have allergic rhinitis, and 6 percent have other allergic disorders. Many suffer from a combination of allergic problems.

Allergens Everywhere

Respiratory allergens—substances you're especially sensitive to—are the most frequent cause of allergic rhinitis and extrinsic asthma (asthma of external origin). These allergens (also called *antigens*) directly affect the mucosal cells lining the respiratory tract and are small (1/1,000 of a millimeter in diameter), water-soluble protein derivatives of such natural organic materials as pollens, mold spores, house dust, insect excrements, animal danders, and airborne pollutants.

Inhaled allergens may be seasonal or perennial, depending on whether they produce symptoms only during certain parts of the year or year-round. Tree and grass pollen wreak their havoc in the spring and early summer, whereas weed pollens, such as of ragweed, predominate in the late summer and fall. Contrary to popular folklore, flower pollens rarely cause allergic symptoms. Perennial (year-round, nonseasonal) allergens include house dust, animal danders, molds, foods, and some plant products.

House dust is a mixture of lint, particulate matter, fibers, danders, insect parts—and mites, which present evidence strongly suggests may be the principal allergen in dust.

The next time you vacuum or sweep the floor, take a look at the kinds of things we live around and inhale. It's almost enough to make you decide to wear a filtering mask.

Fungi (also called *molds*) are ubiquitous in the environment. *Alternaria* and others predominate outdoors, while our good friends *Penicillium, Aspergillus*, and others are found mainly indoors. High spore counts are found in clouds and mist, often leading to increased allergic symptoms in mold-sensitive persons during periods of high humidity. Usually it's the dry windy days that lead to dissemination of pollens and, thus, symptoms. Mother Nature gets us regardless of the weather conditions!

Respiratory allergens produce their impact with each breath you take in and expel. It is thought that these water-soluble antigens diffuse into the cells lining the respiratory tract and, under appropriate circumstances (in the genetically susceptible host), lead to the production of a certain type of antibody (these antibodies are termed IgE; antibodies serve as one of the body's major defenses against compounds perceived as foreign). They, in turn, sensitize the respiratory mucosal cells to respond to respiratory antigens (allergens) by releasing compounds that produce your allergic symptoms. Once symptoms have started, various trigger factors can lead to chronic symptoms. Nonspecific irritants, such as strong odors, air pollution, or climatic changes, also may trigger symptoms.

As mentioned above, dry windy days favor pollen dispersion. Likewise, episodes of symptoms in the early morning may be followed by improvement the rest of the day (with decreased exposure). Because the respiratory mucosa can be sensitized to produce the same symptoms in response to a variety of allergens, recognition of the seasonal influences of particular allergens may be difficult.

Self-Treatment

Solving the riddle of which allergen(s) cause the unwanted symptoms may not require a medical assessment if symptoms can be eliminated or minimized either by avoidance of the offending allergens or by use of over-the-counter (OTC) antihistamine-decongestant medications.

For the runner and other outdoor sports persons, avoidance of airborne allergens can be enhanced by carefully choosing when and where to exercise. An early morning or late afternoon workout, avoiding dry and windy weather (by working out indoors or cross-training with another sport), and minimizing of closeness to allergic sources (e.g., dusty roads or trails lined with trees and grasses) may decrease symptoms before and after exercising and minimize a reduction in performance.

Decreasing daily exposure to known offending allergens is important in lessening sensitization. Hence, removal of offending foods, drugs, and animals as well as an aggressive dust (i.e., mite) control program can lower exposure and, thus, sensitization. In practice, a few measures can improve allergic symptoms greatly. The use of car and home air conditioners and electrostatic air filters can lower your daily allergen dosage. If your livelihood permits, liberal scheduling of vacation time— or if your training schedule does not permit a large interruption, temporarily leaving the area during the peak of the allergy season— may be feasible.

Use of oral and nasal medications to decrease symptoms has to be balanced with the understanding that side effects may occur, for example, excessive drying and sedation; occasionally, if excessive amounts are used, personality changes such as disorientation and hallucinations result. A variety of nose drops and nasal sprays that contain drying agents are useful for short-term, intermittent control of nasal congestion and runny nose (e.g., rhinitis). Either a short-acting agent (phenylephrine hydrochloride) or two long-acting agents (oxymetazoline or xylometazoline, both as hydrochlorides) are available in a variety of OTC medications. Their long-term regular use (more than 3 or 4 consecutive days) is risky, because more severe nasal obstruction can result from rebound nasal recongestion. In addition, some users can become psychologically dependent on the stimulant side effects of the drugs.

Oral medications for allergic rhinitis usually contain a drying agent, either pseudoephedrine or phenylpropanolamine, in combination with one of a variety of antihistamines (it is histamine that is one of the compounds released in the body to produce allergic symptoms).

In choosing an OTC medication, several things should be remembered. They all produce sedation as a side effect (although the drying agent may counteract it to some degree), and they may lose their effectiveness after a period of time. In addition, they must be taken regularly to *prevent* symptoms, rather than taken to *relieve* ongoing symptoms. The rule of thumb should be as follows: Use the medication regularly for at least 7 to 10 days at the maximum recommended dosages before deciding that it doesn't work for you. If after several months of use your symptoms seem to recur despite regular use, try another agent. Balance symptom relief with reducing the side effects of drowsiness and excessive nasal drying. Try several nasal or oral preparations before resorting to a visit to your physician.

Professional Medical Treatment

When you consult a physician regarding suspected allergic problems, the type of physician you decide to see can be important. Seeing an allergist first—rather than an internist, family practitioner, or pediatrician—isn't necessary, because the allergist does little extra unless allergy testing is required.

When making an appointment, ask whether the physician handles suspected allergy problems. At the time of the visit, describe in detail what measures you have taken to avoid and ameliorate your allergic symptoms. If the physician's response is merely to hand you a prescription after a 5-minute physical, say, Thanks, but no thanks, and look elsewhere.

The possibility of coexisting infection (of the sinuses or elsewhere) as well as other associated problems should be investigated. On the other hand, if evaluation and treatment (with antihistamines *not* obtainable over-the-counter and other medications) have proved unsuccessful, allergy testing and subsequent immunotherapy (allergy shots) probably are necessary. Be prepared for a series of visits during the evaluation phase. Once allergy shots have begun, recognize that relief of symptoms occurs only gradually as desensitization builds.

Because the field of knowledge about allergies is rapidly expanding, unsubstantiated or quasi-scientific ideas may occasionally be passed on as fact. It is important that you, as a patient, understand what is being done and what the physician's conclusions are. Ask questions and make sure they are answered to your satisfaction.

Asthma and Allergies

Asthma in its various forms can seriously affect athletic performance. The word *asthma* has been used since ancient times and is derived from the Greek word for panting or breathlessness. Asthma is a disease that involves both large and small airways and is characterized by wheezing, breathlessness, and, sometimes, cough and mucus production. The basic defect in all asthmatics is partial obstruction to airflow in the airways, which can be reversed by medications.

Asthma is typically intermittent and is due to spasm of the smooth muscles that line the respiratory airways. The most recent term used for this condition is *reversible obstructive airway disease*. It is only with long-standing, recurrent episodes that produce chronic changes in the airways that asthma becomes partially irreversible.

Major types of asthma are listed in Table 10.1. It is IgE-mediated (intrinsic) asthma that results from allergic stimulation, although, as in allergic rhinitis, sensitization can lead to airway smooth-muscle spasm (bronchospasm) in response to nonspecific stimuli (see Table 10.2). Asthma can be a combination of intrinsic and extrinsic conditions, usually seen in the adult with a history of childhood allergies.

Exercise-induced asthma (EIA) is a recently recognized condition in at least ⅔ of asthmatics. Typically, it is seen in runners (but not swimmers or in participants in sports associated with brief periods of exercise), beginning 3 to 10 minutes after exercise and characterized by increased wheezing and breathlessness. It is presently believed that oral inhalation of cold air initiates bronchospasms. Fortunately for runners, there are several medications now available that can prevent

Table 10.1 Major Types of Asthma

Factor	IgE-mediated asthma (extrinsic asthma)	Non-IgE-mediated asthma (intrinsic asthma)
Age at onset	Usually childhood	Usually after age 25
Symptoms	Variable with environment, season	Unpredictable fluctuations, chronic
Associated conditions	Allergic rhinitis, atopic dermatitis	Bronchitis, sinusitis, nasal polyps
Family history of atopic disease	Strong	Asthma only (?)
Skin tests (wheal erythema)	Several positive, related to history	Usually negative
Total IgE	Often high	Normal
Eosinophilla in blood	High during allergen exposure	High
in secretions	High, often with bacteria	Variable, increased over neutrophils
Prognosis	Good, especially with allergen avoidance	Fair, remissions uncommon

Table 10.2　Agents Causing Asthma

Category	Active substance
Metal salts	Salts of platinum, nickel, chrome
Wood dusts	Oak, western red cedar (plicatic acid), redwood
Vegetable dusts	Grain (mite, weevil), flour, castor bean, green coffee, gums, cottonseed, cotton dust
Industrial chemicals, plastics	Toluene diisocyanate, polyvinyl chloride, phthalic and trimelletic anhydrides, ethylenediamine
Pharmaceutical agents	Penicillins, phenylglycine acid chloride, spiramycin
Biologic enzymes	*Bacillus subtilis*, pancreatic enzymes
Animal, insect materials	Animal dander, rat urine protein

EIA, such as cromolyn sodium (Intal®) and the so-called B-adrenergic drugs like albuterol (Proventil® and Ventolin®). All are available by prescription and are effective.

The possibility that asthma may exist in a person with intermittent wheezing or a chronic cough (in the nonsmoker) is increased if the person's history includes any of the following: (a) family history of asthma, allergic rhinitis, allergies of other types, or eczema; or (b) personal history of rhinitis, allergies, or eczema.

Evaluation by a physician is in order if asthma is suspected, because the symptoms of wheezing, breathlessness, and chronic cough can actually be due to other diseases. A family practitioner, internist, or pediatrician can adequately evaluate and treat the usual case of asthma. However, beware of advice that exercise must be terminated. Get a second opinion, preferably from a sportsmedicine physician.

The good news regarding allergies and asthma is that with appropriate evaluation (much of which can be done by you), the cause(s) of your itchy nose or wheezing can be identified and eliminated or treated with appropriate medications. Take it from one who has both rhinitis and asthma: Extensive exercise is still possible!

Bloody Urine, or Exercise-Induced Hematuria

Richard L. Jones, M.D.

Hematuria is defined by physicians as the presence in the urine of one to two red blood cells per high-power-microscope field in males and three to four red blood cells per high-power field in females. The higher count for females results from the close proximity of the vagina to the site of urination and the possible contamination of urine with menstrual blood. Catheterized urine samples, because they take urine directly from the bladder, should show no red blood cells in normal urine.

In most cases, blood in the urine indicates a serious urinary tract condition; with the athlete, however, other factors must be considered. Of chief concern is the blood's origin. Any athlete—male or female, young or old—can, as a result of extreme dehydration and physical activity, create a bodily environment ripe for development of hematuria.

Anatomy

The upper urinary tract consists of two kidneys, one on each side of the body, with a ureter coming from each. The lower urinary tract is made up of the bladder and urethra.

The kidneys are located in the rear of the abdominal cavity, just above the hip bones, situated in an area called the *retro peritoneal space*. They filter by-products of metabolism from the blood, including lactic acid, organic acids, and other waste products.

Each kidney consists of millions of microscopic filters (glomeruli) that normally keep formed elements of the blood—such as red blood cells, white blood cells, and proteins—from leaving the bloodstream. During normal function, the kidneys produce a sterile, ultra-filtrate of blood, which we know as urine. In times of disease or injury, however, any or all these blood elements may pass directly into the urine.

Urine pools at the base of kidneys, exits through two ureters, and travels to the bladder. The ureters are rarely the source of red blood cells, unless they have been damaged by disease or injury.

Source of Blood

Red blood cells found in exercise-induced hematuria victims have been shown to come from the bladder—the small, expandable, balloonlike organ located directly behind the pubic bone. Urine is continuously produced by the kidneys and passed to the bladder at a rate of 2 to 3 milliliters per minute (4 to 6 ounces per hour). Because the bladder can expand, urination usually is necessary only once every few hours. The quantity of urine excreted depends on fluid intake, the amount of fluid already in the body, and fluid loss due to sweating.

Hematuria results from an empty bladder combined with inadequate urine production and heavy exercise. Under these conditions, empty bladder walls rub together and chafe and, if rubbed together for a long enough period, begin to bleed. This blood mixes with urine, turning it red. The process is not unlike the chafing runners experience between their thighs or under their armpits during a long run.

Superficial abrasions of the bladder wall have been shown to be the major cause of exercise-induced hematuria through a technique called *cystoscopy*, in which a fiber-optic viewing device is passed through the urethra and into the bladder. This technique has also shown that the urethra is not the origin of blood in exercise-induced hematuria.

Self-Diagnosis

How can the athlete determine whether blood in urine is the result of dehydration, an empty bladder, and heavy exercise—or due to a more serious condition, such as infection, serious injury, or tumor? Physicians can answer this readily through various medical procedures, but there are a few guidelines the athlete can follow to determine whether his or her condition is serious.

If you experience blood in the urine after activity, recount the events prior to it. Did you urinate immediately before the activity? Did you take inadequate fluids en route? Did you not urinate for several hours after the event? If you answered "yes" to all of the above questions, bloody urine that clears in 2 or 3 days is probably due to exercise-induced hematuria.

On the other hand, a history of urinary tract disease or a recent back or lower abdomen injury may indicate some other condition, and a trip to your doctor is advised. If urinalysis reveals only red blood cells that decrease to zero during the next week, shown through repeat urinalyses, exercise-induced hematuria is probably the correct diagnosis. The presence of other blood elements, such as white blood cells or protein, may indicate a more serious problem. Also, if the condition lasts for more than a week, and if it occurs more than once, a urinary tract evaluation is recommended.

Prevention

Exercise-induced hematuria can be avoided. The most important precaution is to drink plenty of fluids, especially during hot weather. This maintains fluid in the bladder and reduces the risk of irritation to bladder walls.

Minimum suggested fluid intake on a normal day is 8 ounces every 25 to 30 minutes. On extremely hot days, take fluids whenever they are available. Drink 8 ounces of water within the hour before you exercise and as much as you want afterward. It is almost impossible to overhydrate. These rules apply to training as well as competition; the body does not discriminate between the two.

Irregular Periods

Gabe Mirkin, M.D.

Twenty to 60 percent of women who engage in strenuous athletics develop irregular periods. All women who have irregular periods for more than 6 months need to check with their doctors, and almost all probably need to take hormones.

Most women menstruate every 28 days. Those who menstruate more often than every 25 days or less often than every 35 days have irregular periods. Some athletes stop having periods completely during strenuous training. This is called *athletic amenorrhea*, and its cause is not well understood.

Under normal conditions, a woman produces two primary hormones—estrogen and progesterone. Estrogen stimulates the inner lining of the uterus to grow, and progesterone stops the stimulation. Women who do not menstruate lack either progesterone or both estrogen and progesterone. If a woman lacks progesterone, her breasts and uterus are stimulated all the time; there is no progesterone to stop the stimulation from the estrogen. The continued stimulation can lead to uncontrolled growth, which is cancer. Women who lack estrogen are more likely to develop weak bones (osteoporosis) and vaginal dryness. It is estrogen that helps to keep the bones strong and the vagina thick and moist.

Women who lack either or both hormones need to be treated to prevent cancer and osteoporosis. There are some women who won't take hormones because they feel that doing so would not be natural. They should compare their condition to that of a diabetic: It is natural for a person to have insulin; when a person's body does not make insulin that person has diabetes and needs insulin to be healthy. Similar reasoning applies to women who are not normal because they lack estrogen or progesterone: Replacing the missing hormones makes them normal.

Suggested Reading for "Irregular Periods"

Dale & Goldberg (1982)

Gass et al. (1983)

Green et al. (1986)

Marcus et al. (1985)

Reynolds (1987)

See reading list at the end of the book for a complete source listing.

CHAPTER 11

———

Upper Extremity Injuries

The upper extremity is that part of the body including all the structures from the shoulder, and its attachment to the spine, to the tips of the fingers. The multiple bones, joints, muscles, ligaments, nerves, and blood vessels form a complex system that allows a person to lift heavy weights or work with delicate movements.

In athletics, these structures are subjected to a wide variety of potentially harmful forces. Injury can occur from direct trauma, such as falling on the shoulder, or from the repeated microtrauma of overuse injuries. This chapter looks at the most common problems that the athlete may face with the upper extremity.

Bowler's Thumb

Paul M. Taylor, D.P.M.

Bowler's thumb is a condition in which the digital nerve to the thumb becomes chronically irritated by repeated friction against the edge of the thumbhole in a bowling ball. If the irritation on the nerve continues long enough, a permanent fibrosis (thickened, fibrous tissue) of the nerve may result.

Initial treatment consists of simply enlarging the thumbhole or applying protective padding to the thumb. If the symptoms become severe enough, though, surgical freeing of the nerve may be necessary.

Suggested Reading for "Bowler's Thumb"

Dobyns et al. (1972)

Howell & Leach (1970)

See reading list at the end of the book for a complete source listing.

Gamekeeper's Thumb

Denis R. Harris, M.D.

Not all serious injuries around the thumb are fractures; one such injury is gamekeeper's thumb. Here, one of the major stabilizing ligaments of the thumb is ruptured. Understanding the thumb's anatomy is essential to understand the gamekeeper's injury (Figure 11.1).

Consider the drastic limitations of a hand without a thumb: you cannot pinch or easily hold onto anything without the thumb acting as a pillar on which to stabilize. At the MCP (metacarpal-phalangeal) joint (see Figure 11.1), the joint should only flex and extend because of these ligaments; the most important of these ligaments is the ulnar collateral, which stabilizes the joint in pinching.

In times of old, the gamekeeper commonly ruptured this ligament in his duties. Today, the skier frequently does it through catching his or her thumb in the ski pole's harness. In a fall, the thumb can be pulled against the ligament, causing it to rupture. X-rays can be normal if the bone is not injured. Pain is felt on the inside of the thumb at the MCP joint, and the pain is increased with attempts to pinch.

This injury should be treated by an orthopedic surgeon. Casting or surgical repair of the ligament may be necessary; delay in the diagnosis only makes the treatment more difficult.

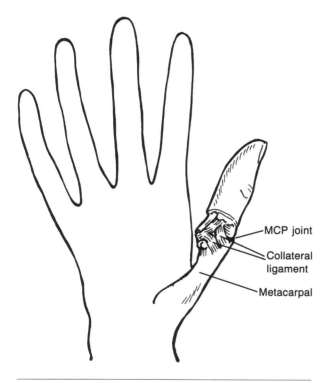

Figure 11.1 Gamekeeper's thumb results from a force that causes a rupture of the collateral ligament.

Handlebar Palsy

Paul M. Taylor, D.P.M.

Handlebar palsy is a symptom that develops in the bicyclist from pressure on a nerve in the hand resting against the handlebar. This can result in some numbness to part of the hand or, in some cases, to muscle weakness of the hand, also.

Treatment requires additional padding to the handlebars, gloves with more padding, and changing the position of the hands during riding.

Suggested Reading for "Handlebar Palsy"

Burke (1981)

Small (1975)

See reading list at the end of the book for a complete source listing.

Carpal Tunnel Syndrome

Vincent G. Desiderio, Jr., M.D.

Carpal tunnel syndrome results from compression of the median nerve, one of the major nerves to the hand, at the wrist. The carpal tunnel is composed of the bones of the wrist and lower arm, along with a very thick, strong ligament called the *transverse carpal ligament*. The tendons that control the fingers, as well as the median nerve, run through the tunnel (Figure 11.2). The median nerve provides sensation to the thumb and index, middle, and, partly, ring fingers. It also supplies most of the nerve supply to the muscles of the thumb.

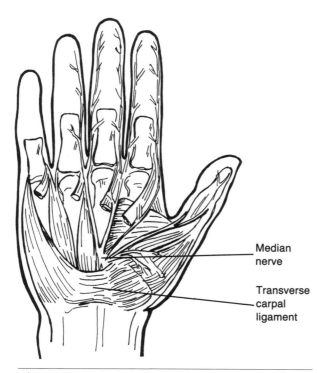

Median nerve

Transverse carpal ligament

Figure 11.2 Carpal tunnel syndrome occurs when the median nerve is irritated as it passes under the transverse carpal ligament.

Typically, the athlete with carpal tunnel syndrome experiences numbness and some loss of sensation to the thumb, middle, and index fingers and possibly some loss of pinch-

ing strength. Many times, symptoms do not occur during activity, but afterward; also, the hand may be painful or numb when the athlete wakes up. These symptoms are often relieved by shaking out the hand. The athletic events that typically produce such a problem include cycling, rowing, and other sports that produce swelling of the hands and wrist. This swelling applies pressure to the nerve, thus causing the symptoms of nerve compression.

On examination, the athlete has altered sensation in the fingers noted above. There may be weakness in pinching. A positive Tinel's sign—produced by tapping the median nerve on the lower surface of the wrist causing tingling and altered sensation going to the involved fingers—may be elicited. There also may be duplication of symptoms by holding the wrist in forced flexion (as far down as it can go) for approximately 30 seconds; this is called *Phalen's sign*.

The electromyogram (EMG) is a diagnostic aid in carpal tunnel syndrome. This is used in nerve conduction studies, in which the electrical impulses of the nerves and muscles can be measured. If the nerve is compromised, it is evident in these studies.

Treatment for this problem is to abstain from the activity that seems to cause it. (There are causes of carpal tunnel syndrome other than that seen in the athlete. One must be certain that a process unrelated to athletic activities is not causing the symptoms.) Many times, wearing a splint at night while sleeping holds the wrist back, alleviating most of the symptoms. Anti-inflammatory drugs, such as aspirin or ibuprofen, can also be helpful.

If the problem persists, professional evaluation should be sought. At times, cortisone injection into the carpal tunnel can relieve the problem. However, if the condition persists, unrelieved by usual measures, surgical intervention may be helpful. Surgery consists of cutting the transverse carpal ligament to relieve the pressure on the median nerve.

In summary, the carpal tunnel syndrome is a compression at the wrist of the median nerve, which provides innervation and sensation to the muscles of much of the hand. It is characterized by numbness and tingling in the thumb and index and middle fingers, and possibly by weakness in the hand. It usually responds to treatment of rest, a splint, and, occasionally, medication. If the problem persists for an extended period of time and is disabling, especially with daily activity, surgical intervention may be helpful.

Little League Elbow

Vincent G. Desiderio, Jr., M.D.

Little league elbow is an overuse syndrome in the young athlete's elbow, primarily seen in baseball pitchers. Because the anatomy of the growing child's bones is complex, this problem cannot be treated lightly. The bones grow at their ends and until growth has stopped, these growing areas (epiphyses) can be damaged either by an acute injury, such as a fracture, or from a chronic injury, such as little league elbow syndrome. The problem of an overuse syndrome in a child is significantly unlike an overuse syndrome in an adult because damage in the growth area may cause the child's bone to form in an abnormal fashion; this may result in the child having permanent impairment of that particular bone or joint.

In the throwing motion of both the mature and immature athlete, the elbow is put under tremendous stress. The force of nearly the entire body is transmitted through the elbow; there are compressive forces generated on the outside of the elbow and a stretching force to the inside of the elbow. Consequently, the growth area on the outside of the elbow (lateral epicondyle) can be injured, producing growth problems, while the inside of the elbow tends to develop severe tendinitis. This problem can be such that the outside aspect of the elbow may fragment with loose portions of bone and cartilage going into the joint. Also, the lower portion of the arm bone (humerus) in that area may undergo what is termed *avascular necrosis*. This means that the protuberant tip of the humerus—the capitellum—actually dies, and significant fragmenting and distortion occur. Again, this may also result in growth deficiency, in which the bone does not grow properly.

Typically, the adolescent with little league elbow is a pitcher who gradually develops pain on both the inside and outside of the elbow. He may have some mild swelling; if the problem persists for an extended period of time, he can develop severe pain.

On physical examination he may have tenderness in both the inside and the outside of the elbow. He usually lacks full motion at the elbow, particularly extension—that is, he can't put his arm out straight.

Initial treatment is rest. Many times, a splint may help settle the problem down, as does ice. Because these injuries are usually seen in very young patients, the rehabilitative time is relatively short because the stiffness, if caught early, does not become a serious problem.

The athlete with this condition should be evaluated by a professional, then should return to his athletic activity very gradually so as not to reproduce the problem. If the capitellum has fragmented, and loose bodies are seen on an x-ray, surgery may be indicated to remove these loose fragments.

Obviously, an ounce of prevention is worth a pound of cure with little league elbow. It is important that the amateur athlete is taught appropriate methods of warming up and conditioning and is coached in the proper body mechanics of throwing. Many youth sport officials emphasize that the pitcher who is from 9 to 14 years old should not pitch more than 6 innings per week and should be prohibited from throwing curve balls or other breaking pitches. Also, at the first sign of elbow pain and stiffness, the athlete should be rested until the symptoms subside. Obviously, the above rule should be modified somewhat if the pitcher throws a great many pitches in a particular game; possibly a more reasonable solution would be limiting the total number of pitches per week. Finally, often the star pitcher of a Little League team is also an excellent hitter and is played at other positions during the week. It is recommended that if this is done, he not be placed behind the plate, because catchers are also forced to throw vigorously.

In summary, little league elbow is an overuse syndrome seen in adolescents and in still-growing baseball players. This problem can range from mild tendinitis to severe destruction of the joint, leading to contractures, abnormal growth of the bone, and deformity. The treatment is initially rest, stretching exercises, and rehabilitation, with alteration of throwing mechanics, if needed. Surgical intervention may be necessary to remove loose fragments that may be present in the joint. Finally, since this is an overuse syndrome, strict guidelines for the pitcher in this category should be followed so as not to allow him to do severe—even permanent—damage to his arm.

Suggested Reading for "Little League Elbow"

Loomer (1982)

_____

See reading list at the end of the book for a complete source listing.

Tennis Elbow

Denis R. Harris, M.D.

Tennis elbow is part of a generalized problem found in many areas of the body. Basically, through overuse or degeneration, the origin of a muscle may tear. Because the muscle continues to be used, the tear propagates, and symptoms worsen.

The muscles that turn up (supinate) the palm and those that extend the fingers and wrist take their origin from the outside (lateral) aspect of the elbow. If these tear, any attempt to extend the wrist or fingers may be painful.

A typical history of tennis elbow may start from a backhand swing with a tennis racket. Normally, the forearm should provide the force needed to hit the ball. However, if the wrist slaps at the ball (such as in table tennis), the player may tear the wrist extensors from the origin at the elbow or tear the fibers nearby. Each succeeding swing only causes the symptoms to worsen and to delay healing.

Treatment consists of resting the area, reducing the inflammation, and, once the injury heals, strengthening the area so that future damage will not occur. Resting the area may simply mean stopping the offending actions. However, if the pain is considerable, splinting of the wrist may be necessary. This stops the wrist from moving and allows the wrist muscles to rest completely. Anti-inflammatory medication, such as ibuprofen, may help the process.

After the acute inflammation improves, the extensors and supinators of the forearm need to be strengthened. Start with a 2- to 4-pound weight in the hand; grasp the weight with the fist clenched, then flex and extend the wrist (see Strength Exercise 8, chapter 12). Do not overdo the exercises at first—start slowly, because it may take 4 to 6 weeks to regain a substantial amount of muscle mass. If improving, consider using a tennis elbow brace—basically a circumferential band around the forearm. The band reduces the forces on the muscle's origin.

Suggested Reading for "Tennis Elbow"

Block (1982)

Carroll (1981)

Gerberich & Priest (1985)

Kohn (1985)

Loomer (1982)

Nirschl (1981)

See reading list at the end of the book for a complete source listing.

Shoulder Bursitis and Supraspinatus Tendinitis

Denis R. Harris, M.D.

Shoulder bursitis is a common cause of shoulder pain. The pain is usually felt 2 to 4 inches down from the top of the shoulder. To understand its cause and treatment, an understanding of anatomy is useful.

The shoulder is a ball-and-socket joint: The arm bone (humerus) ends with a rounded surface that fits into the wingbone (scapula); the socket is very shallow. A group of muscles that cover the top of the shoulder and help to stabilize it are called the *rotator cuff*. In close proximity to the muscles is a lubricating sac of fluid—the bursa (Figure 11.3). For additional anatomy of the shoulder, see Figures 11.4 and 11.5.

When the arm is brought out to the side, the rotator cuff is needed to keep the ball in the socket. However, with this motion (abduction), the muscles and bursa of the rotator cuff are compressed between the humeral head and the acromion of the scapula. The bursa is the first structure to inflame (bursitis), followed by the muscles (tendinitis); finally, the rotator cuff may tear.

Following basic orthopedic advice, first rest the shoulder. Avoid abduction exercises. Use anti-inflammatory medicine to reduce inflammation. When the acute pain lessens, stretch the shoulder capsule and begin exercises as shown in chapter 12, Stretch Exercises 20, 21, and 22, and Strength Exercises 3, 4, 11, and 12.

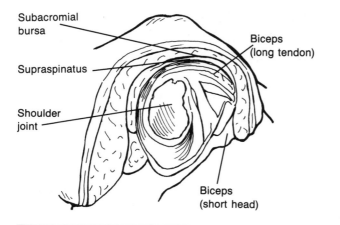

Figure 11.3 A side view of the shoulder, with the head to the top of the illustration, revealing the multiple structures involved in shoulder bursitis and supraspinatus tendinitis.

Rotator Cuff and Biceps Tendinitis

Vincent G. Desiderio, Jr., M.D.

Although injuries in athletes occur more frequently in the lower extremities, the upper extremities can also be involved in both chronic and acute conditions. Clearly the most frequently injured joint in the upper extremity is the shoulder, which is typically involved in throwing motions, such as in baseball, football, and the racquet sports.

The shoulder is a very complex joint. It is composed of a ball, known as the *humeral head*, and a very shallow socket, known as the *glenoid*. The ball is located at the upper end of the arm bone (humerus) and is generally slightly smaller than a tennis ball. The socket is saucer-shaped and measures approximately 1½ inches in diameter. The other joint of the shoulder is the acromioclavicular joint; this is made up of the outer end of the clavicle (collar bone) and the acromion, which is the most upper outer portion of the scapula (wing bone) (Figure 11.4). Because the shoulder moves through such large and varied ranges of motion—that is, it can move forward, backward, up, and around in various combinations—it is typically a very unstable joint. However, it has such versatility and wide range of motion that we may perform such activities as swimming and baseball.

Holding the joint together are various ligaments and the capsule. On top of these ligaments runs a group of muscles called the *rotator cuff*. They begin on the scapula and attach to the humeral head just outside the joint (Figure 11.5). These muscles control the

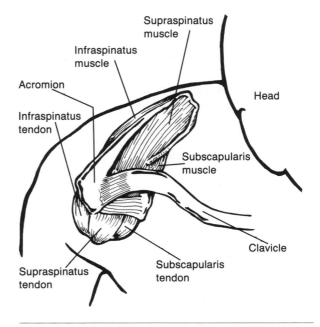

Figure 11.5 The rotator cuff muscles as they pass under the acromion, as seen by looking down on the shoulder.

rotation of the shoulder; they also hold the shoulder in place, by providing an adequate positioning of the humeral head in the glenoid, which allows the other muscles around the shoulder to function with better mechanical advantage. Another structure often involved with injuries in the shoulder is the bursa that lies between the acromion and the rotator cuff. Also sometimes affected is the biceps tendon, which is an extension of the biceps muscle on the upper arm that attaches inside the shoulder joint itself. There it becomes intimately involved with the rotator cuff and susceptible to shoulder injury.

Part of the shoulder's motion also takes place where the scapula attaches to the chest.

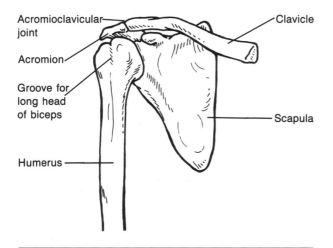

Figure 11.4 The shoulder joint is a ball-and-socket joint, which allows for its mobility. It is composed of three bones—the humerus, clavicle, and scapula.

As the arm is raised, the scapula rotates up and forward; this action allows the arm an extreme range of motion. The muscles that perform this particular motion are very strong and provide raw power to the shoulder, as opposed to the fine tuning that is more the function of the rotator cuff. The power muscles of the shoulders include the pectoralis, latissimus dorsi, and teres major, to name a few.

The rotator cuff muscles have a very difficult job. Not only must they rotate the humerus under various circumstances, but they also act as stabilizers and must work in a static, as well as dynamic, way. Not only are these muscles used rather vigorously during athletic activities, but also extensively in carrying out routine jobs of the arm and shoulder. Because of the location of these muscles underneath the acromion, they often become irritated by that bone; there often is attritional (frictional) fraying of the related tendons. In addition, the blood supply to these tendons is somewhat tenuous; therefore, the healing process is many times delayed.

The biceps tendon, because of its intimate involvement with the rotator cuff muscles, can also be irritated and, at times, can rupture after prolonged attrition and inflammation. The subacromial bursa, which lies between the rotator cuff and the acromion, often becomes inflamed when the rotator cuff tendons are involved; it can, in and of itself, lead to problems as well.

Tennis players often develop rotator cuff tendinitis from their frequent overhand serving motion, during which the humeral head places the rotator cuff in a position where it receives attritional wear from the acromion. This chronic wear and tear frays the tendon somewhat, weakening it. When the athlete uses the arm vigorously again, the tendon may tear very slightly. This subsequently produces an inflammatory response; the bursa may then become involved. The athlete then has pain with virtually any activity; this pain may persist for a long time.

If this sequence of movement (irritation, fraying, and inflammation) is repeated often enough, the rotator cuff tendons are at risk and may in fact rupture with a relatively minor stressful event. It is not uncommon for the doctor to speak to a patient who says that he or she has had intermittent shoulder pain for the last 2 years that usually resolved with some rest, heat, and aspirin. Then the athlete fell on the outstretched hand, and now complains of severe pain in the shoulder and is unable to raise the arm. More than likely, there is now a torn rotator cuff.

Thus, the common symptoms of rotator cuff tendinitis typically occur with overhead motions of the shoulder. They usually produce pain localized on the outside of the shoulder and sometimes go down the arm, but not past the elbow. Typically, the pain is worse at night while trying to sleep and certainly is exacerbated when the arm is raised above eye level. Some of the physical signs seen are tenderness with minimal swelling in the front of the shoulder and pain when the arm is put through its range of motion, particularly when it is moved from chest level to just above the head. If the problem has persisted for a while, there may be some subsequent stiffness of the shoulder, with limitation of motion. This itself can be quite disabling.

Treatment for such problems generally first involves resting the shoulder for a few days to allow the acute inflammation to settle down. This is followed by a course of physical therapy in which the shoulder is moved gently through various ranges of motion to prevent stiffness, but not moved so much as to aggravate the inflamed and slightly torn tendons. Once the pain and inflammation have settled down, then rehabilitative exercises to strengthen these tendons and muscles is generally indicated (see chapter 12, Strength Exercises 3, 6b, and 11). In addition to this, anti-inflammatory drugs, such as aspirin, ibuprofen, or more potent prescription agents, are prescribed. In certain circumstances, this regimen is not successful and steroid injections can be recommended. Steroid injections must be given with some caution, because they can wear away the rotator cuff and actually weaken the tendons in the area of poor vascularity. Finally, if all these measures have not been successful, and if a clear-cut diagnosis can be made, surgical intervention may be of value.

Obviously, prevention is the most effective measure to be taken by patients who may be at risk for developing rotator cuff problems. Good stretching exercises for the upper extremities and shoulders prior to participating in athletics are recommended. The athlete should be certain that throwing or racquet motion is physiologically sound, in order not to overstress these tendons. Finally, with the onset of significant shoulder pain, the athlete must refrain from that particular causative activity at least for a few days and try to do only stretching and strengthening exercises.

Unfortunately, the rotator cuff tendons can completely rupture, with even daily activities becoming significantly compromised. The treatment of this problem often is surgical and involves quite a prolonged rehabilitative effort, which is not always successful. Thus, it is important that the athlete pay careful attention to shoulder pain that suggests a rotator cuff involvement, and that he or she certainly see a doctor if the pain does not resolve readily with the above-mentioned measures.

The acromioclavicular joint also can contribute to irritation of the rotator cuff. This is the joint that is involved with the separated shoulder. Often people do not have a severely separated shoulder, but only a small sprain. This is incurred typically when a football player is tackled and falls on the shoulder directly. Often these sprains heal within a week and don't give any problems for many years. However, the healing process is such that the joint becomes somewhat irregular and may even give some significant arthritis eventually. Be-

cause of these secondary changes from the injury, the rotator cuff can become irritated. Lastly, the athlete must also consider neck injuries as a source of shoulder pain, because these occasionally cause referred pain to the shoulder.

In summary, the rotator cuff and biceps tendon are placed at risk with overhead motions of the arm and shoulder and can produce problems usually through attritional wear and tear. The treatment for these problems is initially conservative. However, if the problem becomes more pronounced, surgical intervention can be of help. The best course of treatment is prevention through stretching and strengthening. All athletes should pay careful attention to shoulder pain because it can lead to disabling problems.

Suggested Reading for "Rotator Cuff and Biceps Tendinitis"

McMaster (1986)

Nightingale (1982, May 3 & 1982, May 17)

See reading list at the end of the book for a complete source listing.

Brachial Plexus Injury

Denis R. Harris, M.D.

A common nerve injury is one that involves the brachial plexus, a collection of nerves that may be thought of as a switching area for information. For the innervation of the upper extremities, the nerves exit the spinal cord in the neck. They travel to the shoulder and axilla (armpit) where they interchange information with nerves from many different levels of the spinal cord; this interchange occurs in the nerve network called the *brachial plexus*. The nerves then exit the plexus and enter the upper extremities.

If the brachial plexus were to be stretched, the nerves that exit would not function properly. This stretching of the plexus happens frequently in athletics. For instance, in football, a player is brought down by his arm being grabbed; when the arm is pulled so, the brachial plexus is also pulled. The nerves in the brachial plexus may be stretched or torn.

Either way, the functions of the nerves are affected, and the arm may feel numb or weak. Nerves carry impulses that control the sensory and motor supply in the extremities. When nerves are not working properly, the functions they supply in turn do not work properly. If the nerve is just confused, function gradually returns. However, if the nerve has been severed, function may never return.

The immediate treatment is to rest the nerve by using a sling. To make sure the shoulder is not dislocated, it should be taken through a full range of motion; the shoulder should not look abnormal. Ice helps to reduce swelling. Once the immediate pain lessens, joint motion should be preserved by passive exercises. If symptoms do not improve quickly, x-rays and tests of the nerve function may be ordered. Rarely is surgical intervention warranted, except in case of severe symptoms.

Swimmer's Ear

Gabe Mirkin, M.D.

Pain, swelling, redness, and scaling in the outer ear canal is called *swimmer's ear*. There are many different treatments for this condition because there are many different causes. Most of the time, your doctor won't even find the precise one. The most common known cause is a bacterial infection due to pseudomonas, which can be cured with the appropriate antibiotic (geocillin). Swimmer's ear can also be due to chemicals in the water, skin diseases such as psoriasis and eczema, a maceration of the skin due to wetness, and, on the rarest of occasions, a fungus.

Pseudomonas cannot live in an acid media. Thus, people who are prone to develop swimmer's ear can often benefit by buying a squeeze bottle of acetic acid at the drugstore and squeezing a few drops into the ear canal immediately after swimming. Most of the common skin diseases that cause an irritation of the ear canal can be treated effectively with cortisone-type creams. As a general rule, plastic ear plugs are not effective in treating or preventing swimmer's ear—they all leak. You can, however, buy a special putty that can be put in the ear canal; this helps keep the canal dry.

Suggested Reading for "Swimmer's Ear"

Calderon & Mood (1982)

See reading list at the end of the book for a complete source listing.

CHAPTER 12

Exercises for Treating and Preventing Injuries

As the athlete continues to participate in sports, greater demands are placed on certain muscle groups than on others. The body responds to these demands by making these harder working muscle groups more powerful. This is a very positive adaptive change, because it allows for increased performance through training. However, there is a negative side to this. Because most sports emphasize certain muscle groups, this leads to an overdevelopment of these muscle groups and a relative weakness of opposing muscle groups.

A muscle group usually is a member of a pair. For example, the biceps muscle in the arm flexes the elbow, whereas the triceps extends the elbow. Such muscles, acting in opposite directions, are called *antagonistic muscles*. There are many such pairs of muscles in the body. A certain balance must be maintained between the muscles in order for the units to function efficiently. When an exercise program greatly overemphasizes one of the muscles in the pair, an injury usually develops. This injury can occur not only because one muscle becomes stronger but also because it becomes tighter.

However, an injury can develop in either the stronger or the weaker muscle. In the runner, the calf muscle generally becomes very strong, whereas the anterior tibial group of muscles in the front of the leg do not become as proportionately strong. With this imbalance, there is a potential for several injuries. As the calf muscle becomes stronger and tighter, it can contribute to a number of injuries, including Achilles tendinitis, muscle pulls, heel spurs, and calcaneal bursitis. The anterior tibial group of muscles may develop shin splints, myositis, or tendinitis.

Prevention of these injuries requires a stretching program for the muscles that become tight and a strengthening program for the muscle groups that do not receive adequate stimulation from the exercise program. In the example of the lower leg, the muscles in the calf need to be stretched, and the muscles in the front of the leg need to be strengthened.

Some people have claimed that stretching is not helpful and may lead to injury. However, the majority of experts still favor a stretching program. When injuries have resulted from stretching, they were probably due to stretching too aggressively or improperly. The first two articles in this chapter go into detail about stretching and strengthening. The exercises are designed for specific muscle groups.

One complaint frequently heard from the casual athlete is that he or she doesn't have time to develop a stretching and strengthening program. Some articles on this subject have been very inclusive, setting up programs that require 30 to 40 minutes a day. This may be necessary for the serious or professional athlete, but the athlete who runs 15 to 20 miles per week or the tennis player who plays only 6 or 7 hours a week does not need to use such an extensive program. Our article titled "Sport-Specific Exercises" gives tables of recommended stretching and strengthening exercises for various individual sports. Doing these recommended exercise routines daily helps prevent injuries that are common to these sports.

Suggested Reading for "Exercises for Treating and Preventing Injuries"

Anderson (1975)

Hatfield (1982)

Howard (1982)

Wallin (1979, 1985)

See reading list at the end of the book for a complete source listing.

Stretching Exercises

Paul M. Taylor, D.P.M.
Katherine A. Braun, R.P.T., A.T.C.

The regular use of stretching exercises has been proven effective in reducing injuries. Continuous exercise of a muscle tightens and shortens it, which can result in an injury to that muscle or its tendon when it is forced to stretch rapidly, as during exercise. A tight muscle also limits the range of motion of the joint it controls. Therefore, a tight muscle can also lead to increased joint injuries. A stretching program helps prevent tightness of muscle groups and maintain flexibility of the joints and aids in a warm-up program before strenuous exercise.

There are three basic types of stretching techniques: static stretching, ballistic stretching and proprioceptive neuromuscular facilitation (PNF). Static stretching is the technique most commonly used and generally recommended throughout this text. In static stretching, the muscle is gently stretched to the point of resistance or slight discomfort and held in this position for a period of time. The stretching exercise is then repeated several times for each muscle group.

Ballistic stretching is a more forceful stretch that utilizes repeated bouncing movements. Because the ballistic technique has an increased potential for muscle or tendon injury, it is usually *not* recommended for general use.

Proprioceptive neuromuscular facilitation is a technique used by physiatrists and physical therapists that takes into consideration the physiological responses of the nervous system, muscles, joints, and tendons. It is perhaps the most effective stretching technique. However, it has not gained much popular acceptance, because it is more difficult to understand and requires that the athlete have a partner. The general technique of PNF includes an initial stretch of the muscle, followed by an isometric muscle contraction (with resistance given by the partner), relaxation for a few seconds, and then a final passive stretch for several seconds. The passive stretch is done by the partner applying the pressure on the muscle.

There have been modifications of PNF methods, resulting in exercises that can be done without a partner. However, the athlete should not attempt these methods unless having first received instructions from qualified personnel. Therefore, with the above considerations, it is generally best for the athlete to continue to use the *static stretching techniques*. For more information on proprioceptive neuromuscular facilitation, refer to other sources listed in the beginning of this chapter.

In developing a stretching program, a standard routine should be followed. This would include a gradual warm-up, followed by the stretching exercises, a gradual increase in the activity, full activity, and then a gradual cooldown. This is the ideal situation; although it may not always be possible to follow this routine, it should be incorporated into the exercise program as much as possible.

The following pages describe specific stretching exercises for each muscle group, using the static stretching technique. Any stretching exercise recommended in the chapters on specific injuries can be found on the following pages. At the end of this chapter, there are tables of stretching and strengthening exercises that are the most beneficial for injury prevention for selected sports.

Descriptions and demonstrations of the stretches are general examples only; it may not be possible for an individual to do a stretch as demonstrated. These exercises should be done gently and without pain. Initially, do the stretching within your own limitations. As your program progresses, the stretching routine gradually improves. Everyone is different in natural flexibility: Some people can maintain their flexibility very easily, whereas others find it very difficult. Do not force the stretching exercises; work slowly and gently toward improving flexibility.

The times given for holding a stretch and the number of repetitions are guidelines only. The amount of stretching that is necessary is determined by each individual's body type. Also, if you have been plagued with a particularly tight muscle group, it requires more stretching—possibly two to three times per day. At times, it is necessary to emphasize such problem muscle groups in a stretching program.

Use the following guidelines when beginning a stretching program:

1. *Stretch slowly and gently.* Start slowly, and gently increase the stretch as the muscle relaxes.
2. *Do not bounce.* Bouncing initiates the reflex mechanism that tightens the muscle. This is counterproductive to effective stretching.
3. *Stretch regularly.* Stretching should be done daily, even if you are not participating in a sport.
4. *Breathe normally.* Do not hold your breath while stretching.
5. *Relax and enjoy.* Stretching is not only effective in reducing muscle tightness but also helps reduce emotional stress and contributes to an overall feeling of better health.

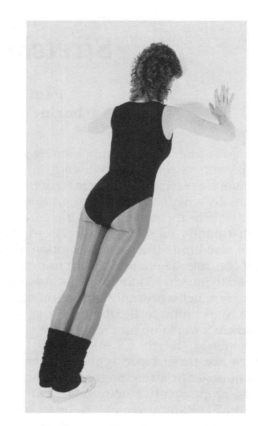

Stretch Exercise 2: Calf (gastrocnemius)

Wall push-up: Stand an arm's length away, facing a wall (or tree). With your hands on the wall, lean in, keeping your body straight and your heels flat on the floor. Hold the stretch for 15 to 20 seconds. Repeat 10 times.

(*Note.* There are two major muscles in the calf—the gastrocnemius and the soleus. Stretch 2 works primarily on the gastrocnemius, which inserts above the knee; Stretch 3 works primarily on the soleus, which inserts below the knee. Although both muscles arise at different locations, they combine at the lower portion of the leg to form the Achilles tendon, which inserts into the heel.)

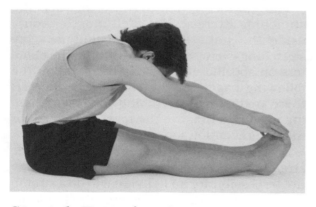

Stretch Exercise 1: Plantar Fascia

Sit on the floor with your legs outstretched. Grab hold of your toes and gently dorsiflex them toward you. If you cannot reach your toes in this position, then bend your knees until you can. Hold the stretch for 10 to 15 seconds, then relax. Repeat 10 times.

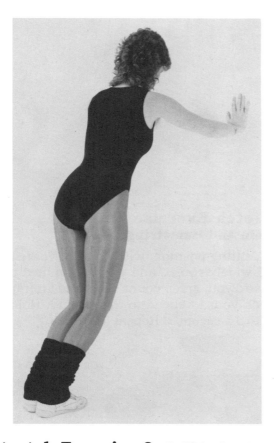

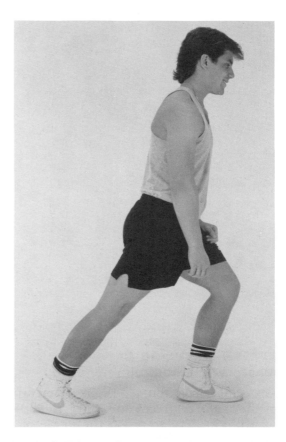

Stretch Exercise 3: Calf (soleus)

Assume the same initial position as in Exercise 2. While leaning into the wall, slightly bend your knees. Hold for 15 to 20 seconds. Repeat 10 times.

Stretch Exercise 4: Calf (modification of Exercise 2 and 3, for when no convenient wall or tree is available)

Stand with one foot 12 to 18 inches behind the other. Lean forward, keeping your heels on the ground. Stretch for 15 to 20 seconds. Switch the positions of your feet and repeat the stretch. Repeat this sequence 10 times.

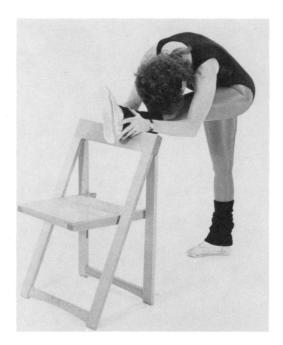

Stretch Exercise 5:
Hamstrings (standing)

In a standing position, place one leg on an object that is as high as your waist. Keep both legs straight. Try to grasp the ankle of the elevated leg and attempt to touch your forehead to the elevated knee. Hold for 10 seconds. Switch the positions of your legs; stretch. Repeat this sequence 10 times.

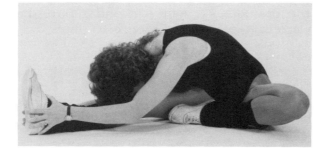

Stretch Exercise 6:
Hamstrings (sitting)

Sit down in the hurdler's position—with one leg extended forward and the other bent, with the foot's sole flat against the extended leg. Lean forward, attempting to grasp the ankle of the extended leg. Bring your forehead down to the knee of the straightened leg. Hold 15 to 20 seconds. Reverse the positions of your legs; stretch. Repeat this sequence 10 times.

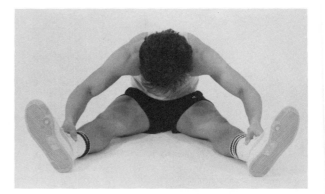

Stretch Exercise 7:
Groin and Hamstring

In a sitting position, with your legs extended and widely spread and your feet pulled back toward you, grasp your ankles and attempt to touch your forehead to the ground. Hold for 10 to 15 seconds. Repeat 10 times.

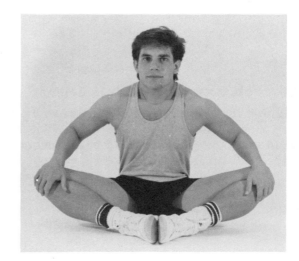

Stretch Exercise 8: Groin

In a sitting position, keep your back straight and bend your knees, with the soles of your feet together. Place your hands on your knees; push your knees toward the floor. Hold the stretch for 10 seconds. Repeat 10 times.

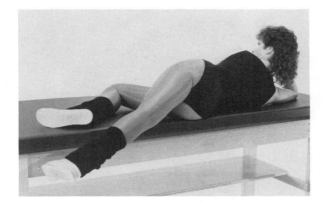

Stretch Exercise 9:
Iliotibial Band (lying)

Lie on a table with your unaffected side against the table and your affected side toward the ceiling. Allow your upper leg to hang over the edge of the table; allow gravity to assist the stretch. Hold for 15 to 20 seconds. Repeat five times.

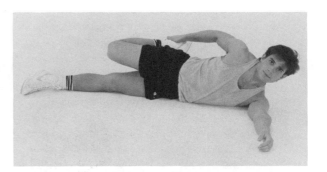

Stretch Exercise 11: Quadriceps

Lie on your side. Bring your foot up behind you; reach back with the arm on that same side and grab the ankle. Pull the leg toward you. Hold for 10 seconds. Repeat five times.

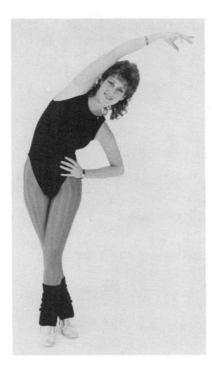

Stretch Exercise 12:
Lower Back and Hamstrings (standing)

Stand with your legs straight and your feet spread slightly. Bend at your waist and try to touch your toes. Hold for 5 to 10 seconds. Repeat 10 times.

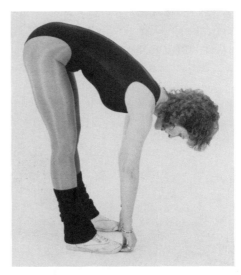

Stretch Exercise 10:
Iliotibial Band (standing)

"Windmill" stand with the affected leg crossed behind the other. Bending sideways at your waist, lean your upper body as far as possible toward the unaffected side, lifting the arm on the affected side over the top of your head. Hold for 15 to 20 seconds. Repeat five times.

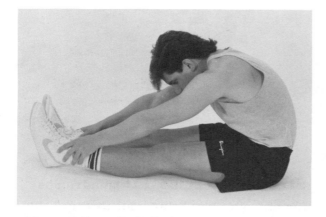

Stretch Exercise 13: Lower Back and Hamstrings (sitting—this is less strenuous for the athlete with back problems)

Sitting on the floor with your legs extended, reach forward as far as possible toward your feet; reach as far as is comfortable. Hold for 10 seconds. Repeat 10 times. (Gradually progress to reaching your toes.)

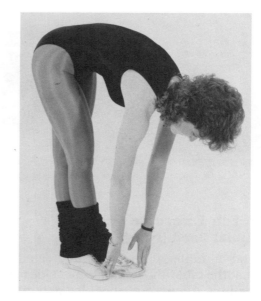

Stretch Exercise 15: Lower Back and Hamstrings

a. While standing, cross one leg in front of the other. Slowly bend forward from your waist and hips. Hang down, relax, and breathe regularly for 20 to 30 seconds. Stretch the other leg the same way. Repeat two times.

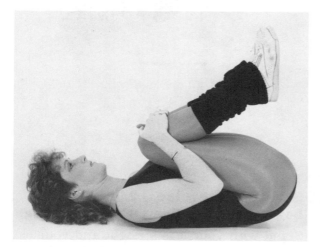

Stretch Exercise 14: Lower Back and Hip Extensor

Lying flat on the floor, bring both knees slowly toward your chest. Hold for 10 seconds. Lower your legs, then slowly bring one knee to your chest and hold for 10 seconds; lower this leg, then bring up the other knee. Repeat this entire sequence five times.

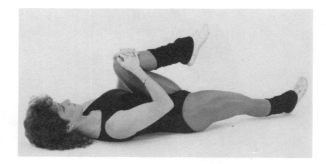

b. Lying flat on the floor, bring one knee slowly toward the chest. Hold for 10 seconds. Alternate knees. Repeat this sequence five times.

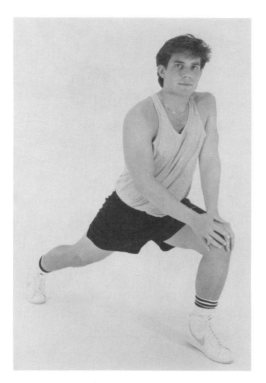

Stretch Exercise 16:
Starting Line Stretch for Psoas Muscle

Kneel as if you were about to take off from the starting line. Slowly rock forward and back (do not bounce). Continue for 10 to 30 seconds.

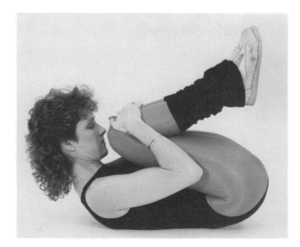

Stretch Exercise 17: Back

Lie flat on your back. Lift up your knees and raise your head; attempt to touch your knees to your chin. Hold for 5 to 10 seconds. Repeat five times.

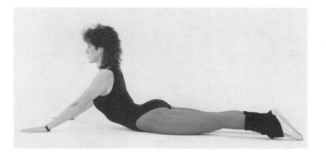

Stretch Exercise 18:
Back Extension

Lying on your stomach, use your hands and extended arms to lift your upper body, arching your back. Hold for 5 seconds. Repeat five times.

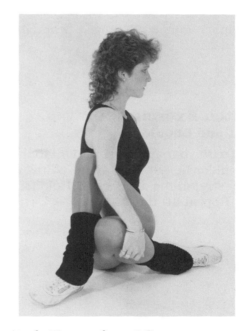

Stretch Exercise 19:
Spine and Trunk Rotators

Sit on the floor with your right knee bent and turned toward the left. Place your left leg over the right knee with the foot resting on the outside. Place your right elbow over your left knee and turn your head to the left, stretching your spine and trunk rotators. Hold for 5 to 10 seconds. Switch positions to the opposite side. Repeat this sequence three to five times.

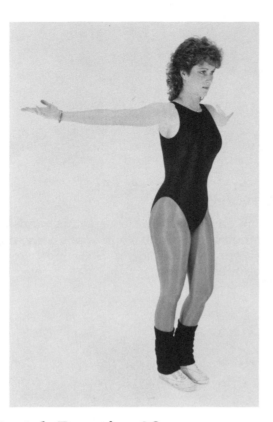

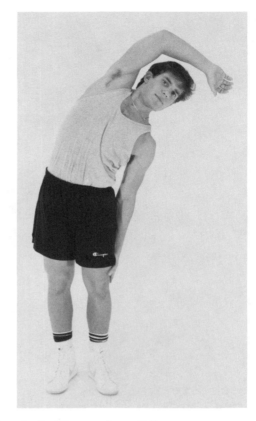

Stretch Exercise 20:
Chest and Shoulders

Stand with your arms out straight to the sides at shoulder height. Turn your palms up and gently stretch the arms back. Hold for 5 seconds. Repeat 10 times.

Stretch Exercise 21:
Side and Shoulders

Stand with your feet comfortably apart. Raise one arm over your head, reaching to the opposite side. Hold the stretch for 5 to 10 seconds. Do the same with the other arm. Repeat this sequence 10 times.

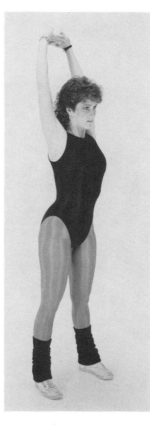

Stretch Exercise 22:
Shoulder and Wrist Flexors

Stand with your arms above your head, fingers interlocked and palms up. Keeping your arms straight, slowly pull your arms back. Hold for 10 seconds. Repeat 10 times.

Stretch Exercise 23:
Shoulder (triceps)

Stand with one arm raised behind your head as though you were trying to scratch your back. Grasp this elbow with the opposite hand; push down and away from the head. Hold for 5 to 10 seconds. Repeat with each arm 5 to 10 times.

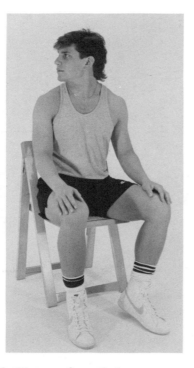

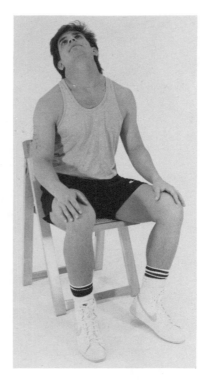

Stretch Exercise 24: Neck

(*Note.* The following two neck exercises are helpful for the athlete who works at a desk or a computer and is subject to neck and shoulder stress and muscle tension. These exercises can be done in a few minutes while you're sitting at your desk.)

Simply turn your head back and forth from left to right. Hold for 5 seconds at the limit of each motion. Repeat 10 times.

Stretch Exercise 25: Neck Roll

Sitting with your back straight, slowly roll your head in a circular motion (with only a partially backward motion, to avoid stressing the disks in your upper spine). Alternate the direction of the head roll.

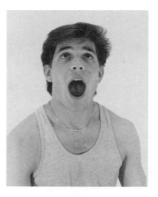

Stretch Exercise 26: Face Muscles

Sitting relaxed, raise your eyebrows and open your mouth as wide as possible. Hold for 5 seconds. Repeat 5 to 10 times.

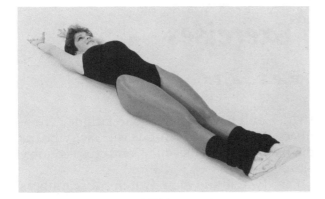

Stretch Exercise 27:
Total Body Stretch

Lie on your back with your arms outstretched over your head. Reach overhead with your arms while pointing the toes, gently stretching the entire body. Hold for 10 seconds. Repeat 5 to 10 times.

Strengthening Exercises

Katherine A. Braun, R.P.T., A.T.C.

Most sports require a combination of strength, speed, coordination, and endurance. Studies show that the stronger athlete experiences fewer and less severe injuries from overuse. Strengthening the muscles not only develops more forceful muscle contractions for kicking a ball farther or jumping higher but also reduces the stress on the joints. As the muscles develop in strength, they can better control the momentum of the torso and limbs, which experience tremendous forces and speeds while performing activities such as jumping, cutting patterns, and throwing. Muscle groups also need to be trained to fire in coordinated, synchronized patterns to prevent overstrain on any one muscle or tendon—the common overuse syndrome. Endurance training for muscles enables controlled motion, skill, and strength to be maintained over a prolonged period of time.

Developing a strength program for performance enhancement and injury prevention must focus on the demands of the athlete's sport. The basketball player needs lower extremity strength for jumping and sprinting, as well as good hand-eye coordination. The soccer player needs to pay extra attention to endurance and coordination. The best strength training programs include a combination of high resistance exercises (power training) and high repetitive exercises (endurance training).

Muscle Physiology

The human body has a tremendous ability to adapt to new stresses. In strength training, the muscles are expected to adapt to repeated stress and overload. Anatomically, muscles differ in structure both in muscle fiber alignment and in their neurophysiology (fast twitch and slow twitch). The fast twitch muscle fibers perform the explosive, fast contractile, high-tension, short-term, anaerobic activity. These muscle fibers produce the major forces in such activities as sprinting, jumping, and weight lifting. The slow twitch muscle fibers perform the slower contractile, low-tension, aerobic ac-

tivities and have resistance to fatigue. These fibers enable one to continue such activities as distance running, bicycling, and cross-country skiing.

Fast twitch and slow twitch muscle fibers both become larger (hypertrophy) in response to increased stress and demand. Fast twitch fibers exhibit a larger degree of hypertrophy in response to strength training, especially power training with high intensity and a low number of repetitions. The slow twitch fibers respond with a smaller degree of hypertrophy to endurance training (low intensity, high repetitions), but the muscles do increase in contractile strength and resistance to fatigue. Therefore, because different muscle fibers respond to different types of strength training, the athlete must develop an exercise program with balance.

Strength Training Programs

The basic methods of strength training can be grouped into three categories: isometrics, isotonics, and isokinetics. Isometrics requires contraction of a muscle against resistance without changing the length of the muscle or the angle of the joint. Isotonics requires a change in the length of a muscle and in the joint position as a resistance or weight is moved through an arc of motion (Figure 12.1). Isokinetics uses a constant speed with varied resistance through the arc of motion. Varied resistance means that the force against a muscle changes as the position of the joint changes. This is important because the strength of a muscle varies depending on the angle of the joint. By varying the resistance, the muscle is strengthened effectively in all joint positions.

In all three basic training methods, the optimal gains in muscular strength, power, and endurance occur through progression of weight training beyond current limits. Traditionally, the overload principle puts stress on the muscles through the increasing weight level and resistance. Remember, however,

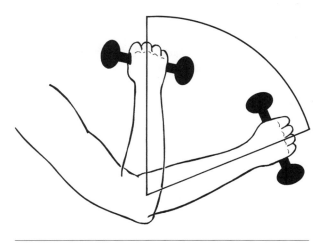

Figure 12.1 An arc of motion is formed by the movement at a joint by contraction of the muscles.

that muscles can also be stressed through varying sets and repetitions, duration of contraction, rate of movement, and rest intervals.

Isometric exercises create tension and resistance in the muscles without producing joint motion. These exercises often are useful for isolating specific muscles and in developing regions difficult to apply resistance to safely. Isometrics are especially helpful in strengthening muscles near joints that should not receive excessive resistance to movement. An example is in head and neck exercises (see Strength Exercise 1). Isometrics assists in producing increased tone in the muscles when initially recovering from an injury. This method's main disadvantage is that a muscle gains strength only in the one exercise position and not through its entire range.

Isotonic resistance exercises comprise most of the common strengthening programs. Isotonic resistance programs vary in design, although all center on the principle of overloading and stressing the muscles to develop new strength levels. Some of the various isotonic strength programs include progressive resistance exercise, the pyramid system, and power lifting.

The progressive resistance exercise (PRE) program, designed by DeLorme in the 1940s, is one of the most widely used training methods. It is an excellent program for both strength and endurance. Three sets of exercises are performed using a 5-second hold count, with 10 repetitions for each set. The first set is performed at 50 percent of the athlete's maximum resistance, the second set is

at 75 percent of maximum, and the third set is 100 percent of maximum. The maximum level and the entire program increases week by week. The graded progression of increasing resistance makes the system safer for new weight lifters and in medical rehabilitation.

The pyramid system for weight lifting progresses from light to heavy weights. The program starts with the athlete performing approximately 10 repetitions at a light weight, resting, increasing the weight level and performing 6 repetitions, resting, and finishing with 4 repetitions at the maximum resistance level. The pyramid system is often used by athletes desiring muscle mass and strength. Its main variations from the DeLorme PRE are that the weight range is higher and the weight is increased in larger increments.

The heavy to light weight system is sometimes called the *Oxford program* or *power-lifting program*. Some athletes who want power find the other methods too fatiguing and prefer to start at a maximal resistance level. The athlete starts with approximately 6 to 10 repetitions at his or her maximal resistance level. The weight level is decreased and another 10 repetitions are performed. The weight is decreased again and 10 repetitions are performed. This technique should be used only by the athlete with long-term weight lifting experience. It is very easy to strain muscles, tendons, and ligaments using this system, because minimal warm-up is used. The athlete must know from experience the maximal resistance level for the different exercises and his or her ability to progress to this maximal level.

Isotonic strength programs can be performed with dumbbells, ankle weights, home weight benches, Universal® gym systems, or Nautilus® equipment. All of the equipment systems use progressions to different weight levels. Isotonic resistance training is also one of the most accessible, effective, and least expensive techniques. Isotonic strengthening can be done with simple hand dumbbells at home or through joining a gym or health club.

Isokinetic strength training is one of the most effective and functional techniques for strengthening muscles. Isokinetics means that a constant speed is set and that resistance varies throughout the exercise motion. The athlete's effort and ability, rather than predetermined weights, influence the resistance levels. High speeds (for training quick muscle contraction and building endurance) and slow speeds (for strength and power) can be used in training. Most sportsmedicine and rehabilitative clinics utilize isokinetics extensively, because minimal strain is placed on injured joints and muscles.

Isokinetic exercises are usually performed on special equipment—such as Cybex®, Orthotron®, and Kincom®, which are principally found in sportsmedicine centers. However, some equipment manufacturers have recently produced machines that provide a similar function that use hydraulic systems and pneumatic resistance. Without expensive equipment, isokinetic training effects can be achieved by exercises performed with rubber tubing and resistance bands, or in a pool with water resistance controlling speed.

Weight Training Principles

A good, balanced conditioning program includes gentle warm-up exercises, flexibility stretches, strengthening exercises, and a cooldown. Simple calisthenics such as jumping rope, jogging in place, or jumping jacks are good warm-ups. Warm-ups also help you detect areas of stiffness and discomfort that need extra focus or caution in stretching and strengthening. Warm-up calisthenics and stretching increase the circulation to the heart and extremities, stimulate the joint receptors, and prepare muscle-tendon units for activity. Complete a simple stretching routine before and after weight lifting. You will perform better and have less chance of suffering muscle pulls.

A conditioning strength program should be performed at an intensity level sufficient to be strenuous and create muscle strain, but *never* to create pain. One of the worst adages to come from popular fitness lore is "No pain, no gain." Each muscle and tendon has limits to the degree of repetitive stress that can be tolerated. Never lift more than you can handle.

Allow muscles and tendons time to adapt to progressive increases in resistance. Increase the stress on a muscle adapting to a new weight level by increasing the repetitions or extending the hold time. If possible, allow the muscle to relax fully for 2 seconds between repetitions. Try to sequence the exercises to work your largest muscle groups, such as your thighs and legs, first. Also, try not to perform consecutive exercises with similar muscle groups; rather, stagger the exercises (e.g., bench press, bicep curls, then military press).

Lift weights and load a muscle in the comfortable ranges of motion for involved joints. Be careful not to overstretch any joint, especially while using heavy weights. Also, microtears to muscles and tendons can occur, which can create tendinitis problems as well as irritation of the bony joint surfaces.

Good technique also helps minimize injury and improve performance. Use slow, smooth movements that avoid any jerking forces. Lower the weight slowly to increase the eccentric work of muscles (contraction of muscle fibers as they are lengthening). Remember that proper breathing is essential to avoid strain and aids in the rhythm of the exercise. You should inhale before exertion, hold this breath while lifting, and exhale during completion of the lift. If possible, allow muscles to relax fully for two seconds between repetitions. The rest period between sets should be between 15 and 90 seconds. The shorter the rest period, the more the exercise becomes an endurance exercise, rather than a strength exercise alone.

A cool-down period should be allowed after each workout. Gentle stretching reduces muscle soreness after strenuous exercising. Stretching before and after exercising prevents a feeling of being muscle-bound and maintains joint flexibility.

In the ideal training schedule, maximum effect is achieved if you lift every other day, or three times per week. If you cannot get access to weights on the strengthening day, try to swim, bicycle, or jog. Strength building is related to intensity of exercise. Therefore, one can also work on strength in traditional endurance sports by performing sprints or fast, intense bouts of activity. Even with extensive strength training, there is no substitute for playing and practicing regularly—and not just through intensive weekend sports.

Planning days of rest from heavy lifting is important. Muscles need a 24-hour period to recuperate, or they may become overstrained. On rest days it is all right to engage in a low-level endurance activity.

When developing a strength program for performance enhancement or injury prevention for a specific sport, the exercises should focus on the muscles primarily used in the sport (see Tables 12.1 to 12.8, pp. 232-234). For example, if you are a baseball player, you need to concentrate on speed, hand-eye coordination, and endurance. Baseball requires shoulder movement patterns that involve a lot of rotation and diagonal motions of the shoulder and arm. The body needs neurological training of the muscles for strength, coordination, and endurance in these movement patterns. This is called *specificity of exercise.*

Cross-training is another form of conditioning that is very helpful in developing strength and endurance for a sport. This technique uses sports activities that are similar, but subtly different, to complement and work muscle groups other than those primarily used. Cross-training helps strengthen muscles that are not regularly conditioned, developing better muscle balance. The baseball player may add swimming and tennis to his regular activities. The runner may alternate regular running workouts with bicycling or cross-country skiing. Cross-training has been advocated by many top coaches and athletic trainers to minimize overuse injuries resulting from too much repetitive strain, coming when one activity or motion is overemphasized. A balanced combination of strength training with varied sports activities develops the best overall body conditioning.

Joint proprioception is the internal neurological feedback that monitors the spatial relationship of joint and body. It is the key to good balance and coordination. To translate strengthening into functional athletic performance, balance and coordination are critical. The athlete can develop better proprioception and balance by practicing a few drills. Standing and balancing on one foot for 25 to 60 seconds helps ankle proprioception. Using rocker boards is also very helpful for ankle strengthening, as well as proprioception. Continuous hopping in a side-to-side pattern, then in a forward and backward pattern, are helpful drills.

Exercise Equipment

For most persons desiring general strength and conditioning, a home system with simple dumbbell weights and Velcro® ankle cuff weights can be used. A compact, multifunctional home gym can also be purchased by the athlete desiring a more intensive strength program for developing muscle mass.

Such home gyms vary in design from simple elastic resistance bands and loose plate weights to elaborate pulley systems and multiuse hydraulic pistons.

Health clubs and gyms also provide equipment for strength training. Nautilus®, Kaiser®, Universal®, and Eagle® rigs, as well as numerous other types of equipment, all work on the principle of isolating a specific muscle group with each machine. Such equipment is helpful when the athlete has progressed to heavy weight levels.

Caution must be taken in using heavy weights on these units, especially at the extremes of ranges of motion. A prestretch is built into the ranges of motion of many units; however, maximum resistance should not be applied at the extreme ends of motion. When performing a power program, you should lift the weights through a comfortable range. You may need to block the motion and protect a joint by holding the motion bar or blocking the movement of the weights with the weight pins. This principle of protecting joints is especially important for the athlete with a history of tendinitis or joint strain. If there is any question about the use of the equipment, ask the attendant for guidance. Remember that a strengthening program should be strenuous, but never painful.

Conditioning Versus Rehabilitation

Isometric, isotonic, and isokinetic exercises are used in both conditioning strength programs and rehabilitative strengthening programs. The main difference is in the intensities of the exercise programs. In rehabilitative programs, more attention is given to the subtleties of the biomechanics of each exercise and to avoiding unnecessary stresses on the joints, ligaments, and tendon attachments. At a sportsmedicine center, a physical therapist can design a strengthening program to protect the injured region, with no irritation of the injured muscle or joint.

The athlete who has recently sustained an injury or strain should be very attentive to the problem. A period of rest and icing of the irritated region should be followed for 3 days to a few weeks. No exercise program should be painful to the body. Exertion, strain, and fatigue should be expected in a progressive strengthening program, but sharp pain and prolonged aching should not. Pain is the body's signal that it is doing more than it can structurally tolerate. The intensity of a painful workout should be decreased, or the program design altered.

(*Note*: The number of repetitions and sets of each exercise will vary, depending on your individual level of experience and conditioning. Review the introduction to strengthening exercises before starting to perform the following strength exercises.)

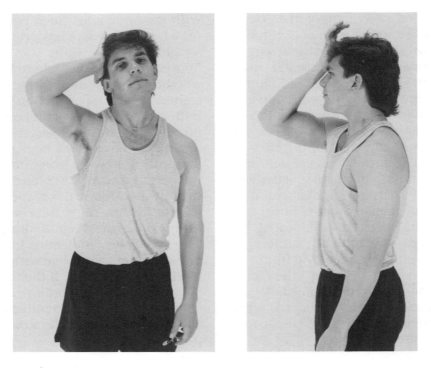

Strength Exercise 1: Neck Isometrics

Place a hand on the side of your head. Push your head into palm of your hand, with your hand resisting motion. Hold for 10 seconds. Do four patterns: to the right side, to the left side, forward, backward. Repeat 10 times for each side.

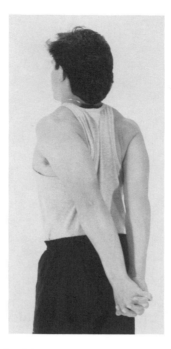

Strength Exercise 2: Rhomboid Isometrics

Standing or sitting, hold hands together behind your back with your elbows straight. Pull your shoulders back and squeeze your shoulder blades together. Hold for 10 seconds. Repeat 10 times. (This is a good postural exercise for people with desk jobs or secretarial or computer terminal work.)

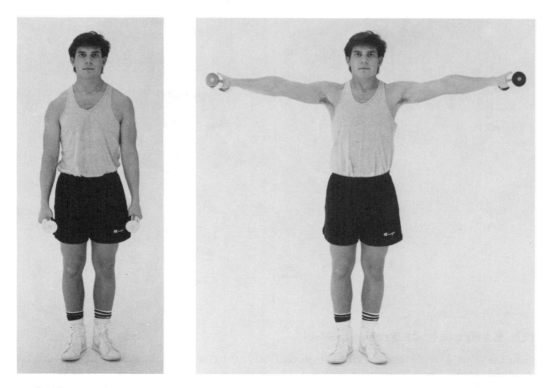

Strength Exercise 3: Deltoid (middle; posterior)

a. While standing, lift your arms to the side horizontal position. Hold for 5 seconds. Repeat.

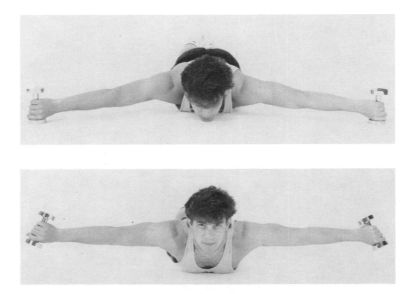

b. While lying on your stomach, position your arms perpendicular to your body, with your thumbs pointing down. Lift the arms from the shoulders, up and backward. Hold for 5 seconds. Repeat.

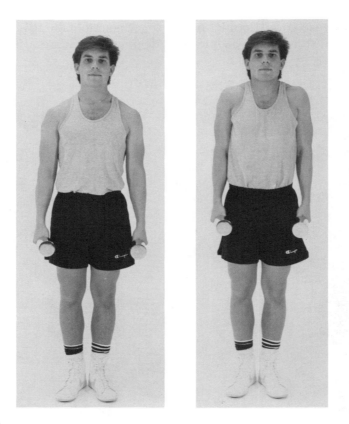

Strength Exercise 4: Trapezius

Standing, keep your arms straight next to your body, with a dumbbell weight in each hand. Lift your shoulders. Hold for 5 seconds. Repeat.

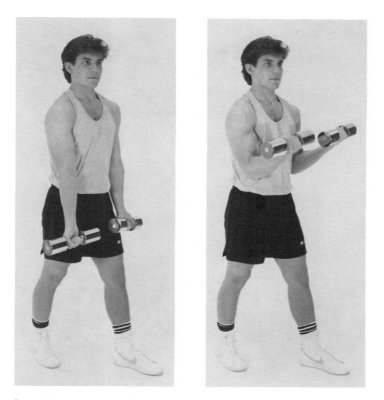

Strength Exercise 5: Biceps

Stand with one leg forward and one leg back, with your elbows in full extension next to your body. Lift the dumbbell with the palm facing upward and stop at a 100 degree angle at the elbow. Hold for 5 seconds. Repeat.

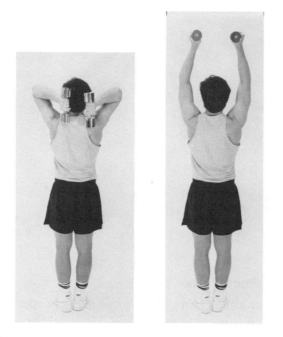

Strength Exercise 6: Triceps

a. Standing, lift a dumbbell weight overhead. Point your elbows toward the ceiling with your hands behind your head. Straighten your elbows while holding dumbbell weight overhead. Pause. Repeat slowly.

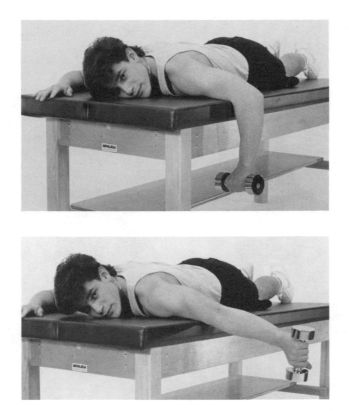

b. Lie on your stomach on a bed. Position your elbow at the edge of the bed, with your arm perpendicular to your body holding the dumbbell. Straighten your elbow to the horizontal. Hold for 5 seconds. Repeat.

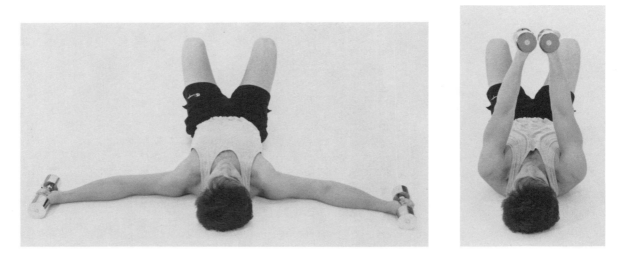

Strength Exercise 7: Pectoralis

a. Lie on your back with your knees bent. Place your arms perpendicular to your body. Lift the dumbbell overhead, keeping your elbows straight. Pause at the top, then slowly lower. Repeat.

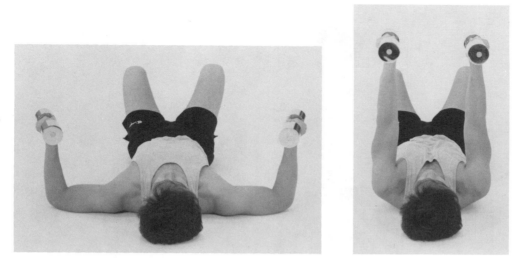

b. Lie on your back with your knees bent. Place your arms perpendicular to your body, with your elbows bent 90 degrees. Slowly lift the dumbbell overhead and straighten your elbows. Pause at the top, then slowly lower. Repeat.

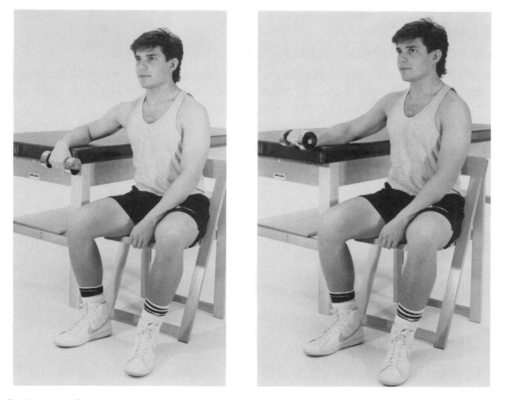

Strength Exercise 8: Wrist Extensors

Sitting next to a table, place your forearm on the table with your wrist at the edge. With your palm facing down, hold the dumbbell weight and cock your wrist up. Hold for 5 seconds. Lower slowly. Repeat.

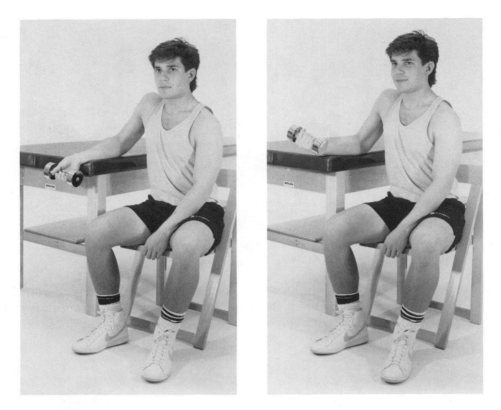

Strength Exercise 9: Wrist Flexors

Sitting next to a table, place your forearm on the table, with your wrist at the edge and your palm facing up. Holding the dumbbell, let your hand drop back over the edge. Lift and curl your wrist upward. Hold for 5 seconds. Lower slowly. Repeat.

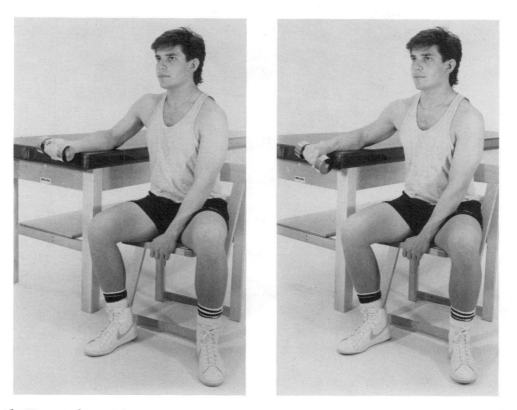

Strength Exercise 10: Forearm Pronators and Supinators

Sit next to a table with your forearm on the table and your elbow bent 90 degrees. Rotate your forearm with your wrist turning palm up, then palm down. Rotate slowly and keep the elbow position stationary.

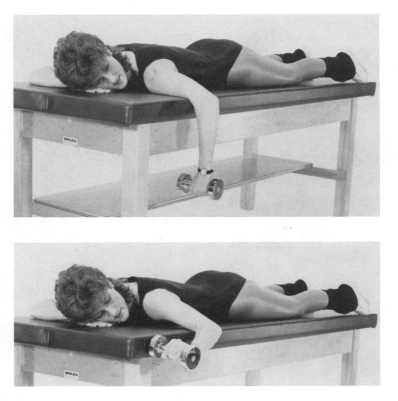

Strength Exercise 11: Shoulder External Rotators (rotator cuff)

Lie on your stomach on a bed. Position your elbow at the edge of the bed with your arm perpendicular to your body. Let your elbow bend at a 90 degree angle, with your forearm hanging over the edge. Holding the dumbbell, lift your forearm to the horizontal. Hold for 5 seconds. Repeat.

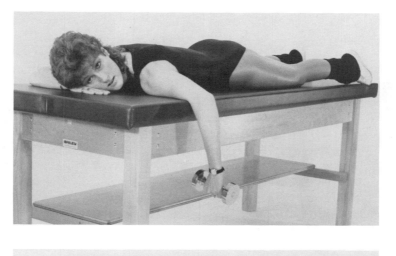

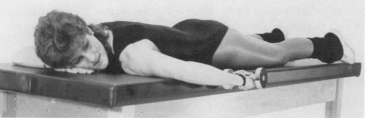

Strength Exercise 12: Shoulder Internal Rotators

Lie on your stomach on a bed. Position your elbow at the edge of the bed with your arm perpendicular to your body. Hold the dumbbell, and let your elbow bend at a 90 degree angle, with your forearm hanging over the edge. Lift your forearm backward with your palm facing up. Hold for 5 seconds. Repeat.

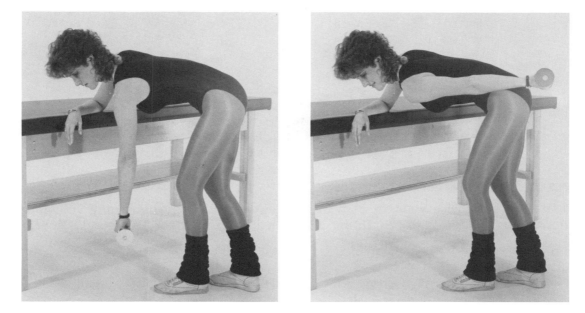

Strength Exercise 13: Latissimus Dorsi

a. Standing, lean forward from your waist to 80 degrees, supporting your trunk on one side. Your opposite arm hangs down, holding a dumbbell. Lift the dumbbell backward to the horizontal. Hold for 5 seconds. Repeat.

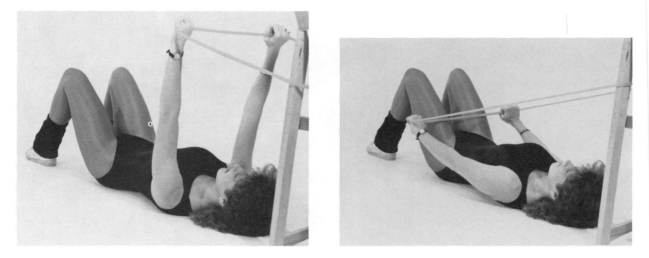

b. Lie on your back with your knees bent. Spread your arms 2 feet apart overhead; pull rubber tubing from overhead position toward your hips. Pull slowly and pause at the hips. Repeat.

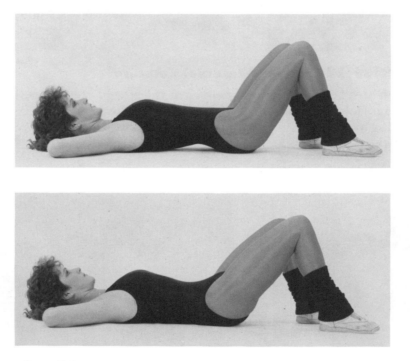

Strength Exercise 14: Abdominals

a. Lie on your back with your knees bent. Flatten your back by tightening your lower abdominal muscles and buttocks, tilting your pelvis back. Hold for 10 seconds. Repeat.

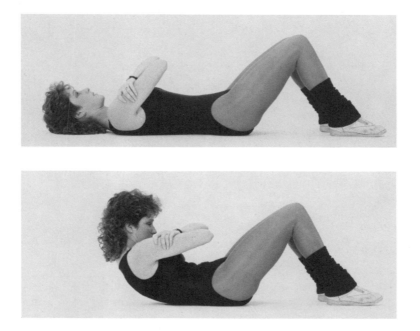

b. Lie on your back with your knees bent. Curl up your head and shoulders 30 degrees. Hold for 5 seconds. Repeat. Progress from your arms lying next to your body, to your arms across your chest, to your arms behind your head.

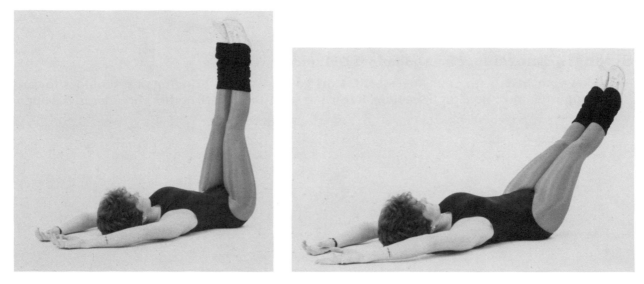

c. Lie on your back with your hips at 90 degrees and your legs vertical. Slowly lower your legs together. Stop at the position at which your lower back lifts off the floor. Do not lower your legs beyond 45 degrees. Hold for 5 seconds. Repeat.

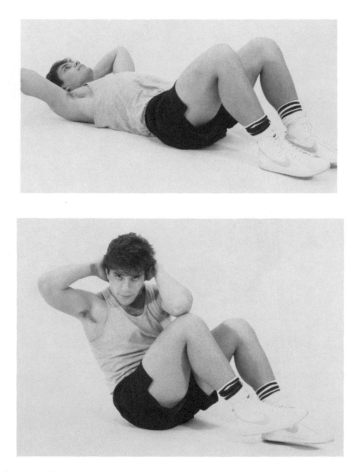

Strength Exercise 15: Abdominal Obliques

a. Lie on your back with your knees bent. Curl your trunk up, bringing one shoulder toward the opposite knee. Hold for 5 seconds. Return to start, then lift the other shoulder to the opposite knee. Repeat.

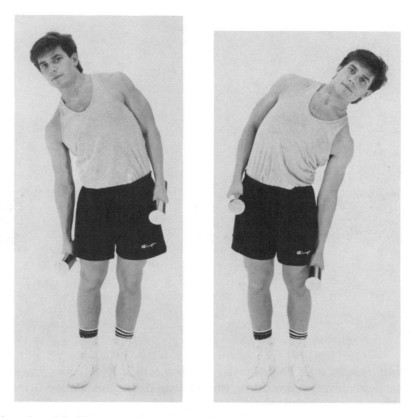

b. Standing with a dumbbell in each hand, side-bend your trunk. Pause, then slowly straighten your trunk to the upright position. Alternate with a side bend to the opposite side. Repeat.

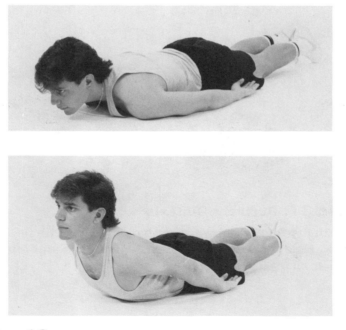

Strength Exercise 16: Back Paraspinals

a. Lie on your stomach, placing your arms next to your trunk. Lift your shoulders and upper chest; do not overextend your back. Hold for 5 seconds. Progress to letting your upper chest hang partially over the edge of a bed, lifting to the horizontal. Repeat.

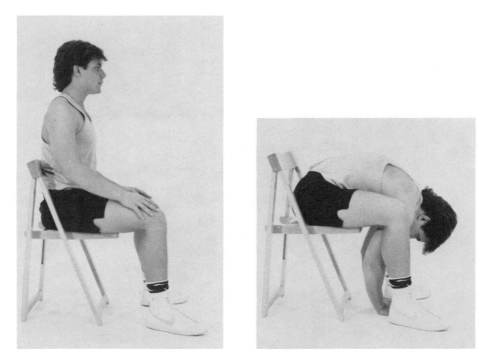

b. Sitting in a chair, slowly curl down between your legs and let your hands touch the floor. Concentrate on slow, controlled motion and curling the spine. Pause briefly, then slowly lift the back upright (do not use weights). Repeat.

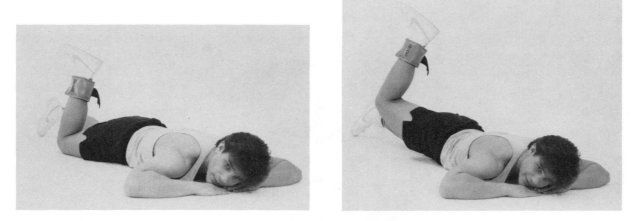

Strength Exercise 17: Buttocks/Gluteals

Lie on your stomach. Lift just slightly upward one weighted leg with its knee bent to 90 degrees; avoid arching the back. Hold for 5 seconds. Then, switch legs and repeat.

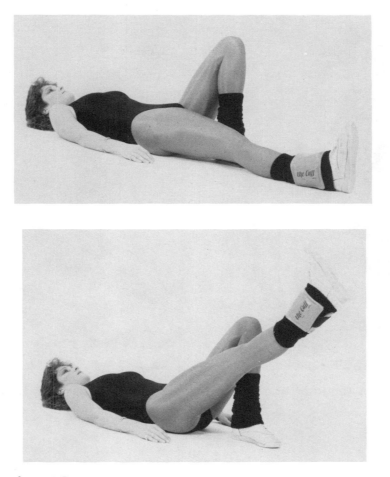

Strength Exercise 18: Quadriceps

a. Straight leg raise—lie on your back with one knee bent. Lift the opposite, weighted, straight leg 30 degrees off the floor. Hold for 5 seconds. Repeat. Progress from 2.5 to 15 pounds.

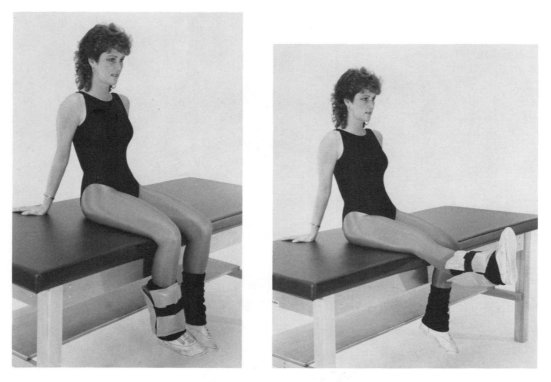

b. Sitting, straighten the knee of a weighted leg. Hold for 5 seconds. Repeat. Progress from 10 to 30 pounds.

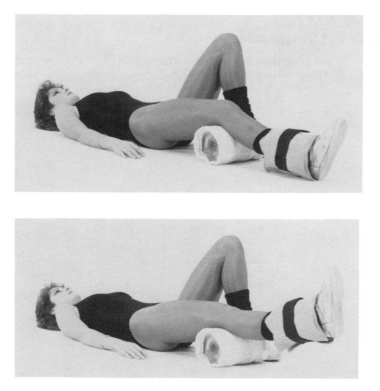

c. Terminal knee extension—lie on your back with one weighted knee over a padded coffee can or tightly rolled towel. Straighten the knee the last 45 to 30 degrees. Hold for 5 seconds. Repeat. Progress from 5 to 20 pounds.

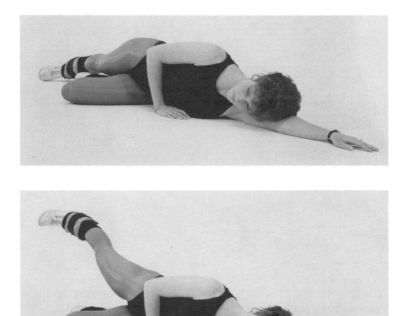

Strength Exercise 19: Abductor Group (tensor fascia latae, gluteus medius)

Lie on your side with your upper hip rolled slightly forward, the leg weighted. Lift 30 degrees above the horizontal. Hold for 5 seconds. Repeat. Progress from 2.5 to 10 pounds.

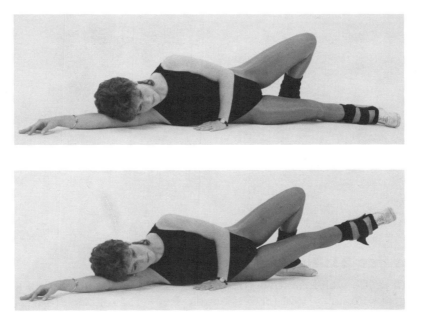

Strength Exercise 20: Adductor Group (adductor magnus, gracilis, pectineus)

a. Lie on your side and place your top leg behind your weighted, lower leg. Lift your lower leg 20 degrees. Hold for 5 seconds. Repeat. Progress from 2.5 to 10 pounds.

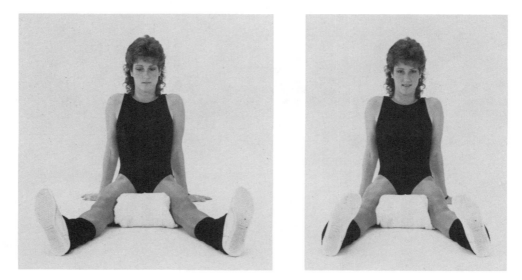

b. Sitting with your legs straight, place a large towel roll between and above your knees. Roll your knees and legs inward, squeezing them against the towel roll. Hold for 10 seconds. Repeat.

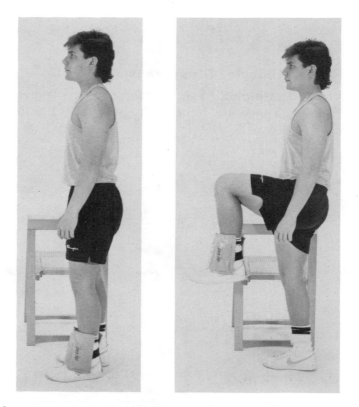

Strength Exercise 21: Hip Flexor

Standing, place an ankle weight above your ankle. Lift the corresponding knee to 90 degrees and hip to 90 degrees flexion. Hold for 5 seconds. Repeat. Progress from 5 to 15 pounds.

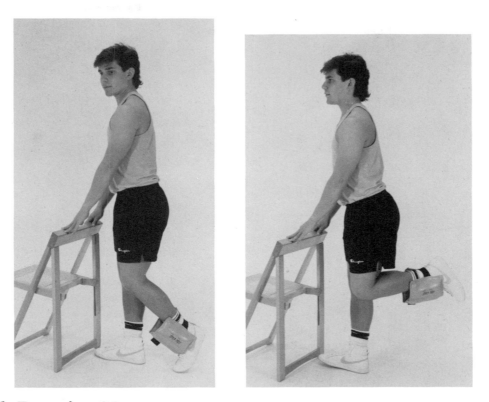

Strength Exercise 22: Hamstrings

Standing, place an ankle weight above your ankle. Lift the lower leg backward, with the knee bending to 90 degrees. Keep the upper thighs level in front. Hold for 5 seconds, then slowly lower. Repeat. Progress from 2.5 to 10 pounds.

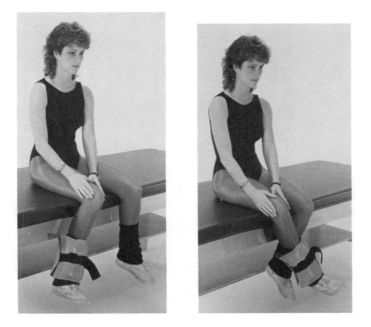

Strength Exercise 23: Hip Internal and External Rotators

Sitting on the edge of a bed, rotate your weighted lower leg outward to a 45 degree angle; prevent your knee from rolling inward too far. Hold for 5 seconds. Then rotate your lower leg inward to a 45 degree angle; prevent your knee from rolling outward. Hold for 5 seconds. Repeat. Progress from 5 to 10 pounds.

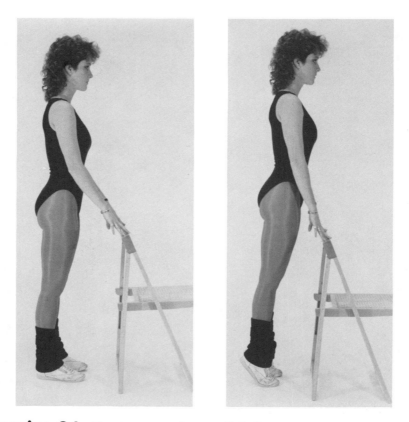

Strength Exercise 24: Gastrocnemius and Soleus

a. Standing, slowly stand on your toes. Hold for 10 seconds. Repeat.

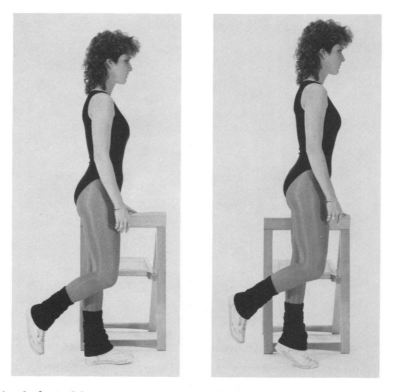

b. Progress from both feet, 20 repetitions, to one foot, 10 to 20 repetitions.

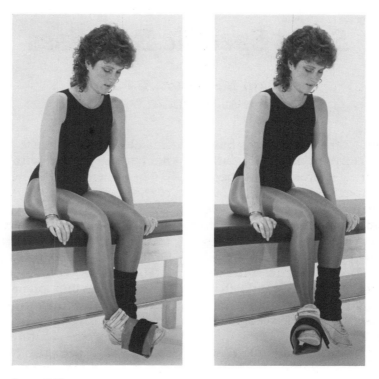

Strength Exercise 25: Ankle Dorsiflexors

Sitting on the edge of a bed, place an ankle weight on your forefoot. Lift the foot and toes upward. Hold for 5 seconds, then lower. Repeat. Next, lift the foot upward and inward. Repeat. Next, lift the foot upward and outward. Repeat. Progress from 5 to 10 pounds.

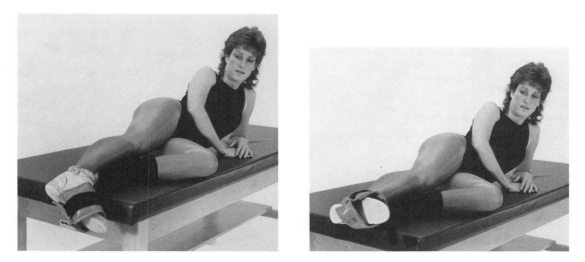

Strength Exercise 26: Peroneals

Lie on your side with one ankle hanging over the edge of the bed, with an ankle weight on your forefoot. Let gravity lower the forefoot slowly downward and inward. Pause. Lift the forefoot upward and twist the ankle outward. Hold for 5 seconds. Repeat. Progress from 2.5 to 10 pounds.

Sport-Specific Exercises

Paul M. Taylor, D.P.M.
Katherine A. Braun, R.P.T., A.T.C.

Stretching and strengthening exercises have been shown to be effective in preventing athletic injuries. Stretching exercises have been emphasized over the past several years. However, it is essential to maintain proper muscle balance, so combining strengthening exercises with stretching helps prevent injuries and may also enhance performance. Therefore, it is important for the athlete who participates in different sports to establish a stretching and strengthening program.

In a practical sense, it must be recognized that many casual athletes have a limited amount of time for such a program. Also, different sports stress different muscle groups. With these considerations, the following tables in this section offer a combination of stretching and strengthening exercises that are sport-specific. That is, the exercises emphasize the muscle groups that are most utilized or more likely to be injured within a particular sport.

These exercise routines can be done as part of the warm-up for the event, or they can be done at a different time of day. These exercises should be done on a daily basis. The specific techniques of how to do each exercise are described earlier in this chapter.

The athlete who has been injured and requires a rehabilitation program should refer to part II to review the recommendations for that specific injury.

The exercise routines recommended in Tables 12.1 through 12.8 should serve as general guidelines only. Persons vary in their individual needs to stretch or strengthen muscles. Anyone who suffers repeated injuries should obtain professional help for treatment and for recommendations for a rehabilitation program.

Table 12.1 Running

Stretch exercises	Strength exercises
2 or 4—calf	18a or 18c—quadriceps
5 or 6—hamstrings	22—hamstrings
11—quadriceps	25—ankle dorsiflexors
13—lower back and hamstrings	

Table 12.2 Tennis and Racquetball

Stretch exercises	Strength exercises
4—calf	3—deltoid
6—hamstrings	8, 9, and 10—forearm
8—groin	14b—abdomen
11—quadriceps	16a—back extension
13—lower back and hamstrings	18a or 18c—quadriceps
16—psoas	
20—chest and shoulders	
21—side and shoulders	
22 and 23—shoulders	

Table 12.3   Swimming

Stretch exercises	Strength exercises
20—chest and shoulders	2—rhomboid
22 and 23—shoulders	3—shoulder
21—side and shoulders	6a—triceps
24 and 25—neck	

Table 12.4   Basketball

Stretch exercises	Strength exercises
2 and 3—calf	16a and 16b—back
8—groin	18a, 18b, or 18c—quadriceps
11—quadriceps	24—gastrocnemius and soleus
13—lower back and hamstrings	
21—side and shoulders	
22—shoulders	

Table 12.5   Soccer

Stretch exercises	Strength exercises
4—calf	1—neck
6—hamstrings	18a or 18c—quadriceps
7—groin and hamstrings	20—adductors
8—groin	24, 25, and 26—ankle
11—quadriceps	
21—side and shoulders	
24 and 25—neck	

Table 12.6   Walking

Stretch exercises	Strength exercises
2 and 3—calf	17—gluteals
11—quadriceps	18a or 18c—quadriceps
12 or 13—lower back and hamstrings	22—hamstrings
14—lower back and hip extensor	24—gastrocnemius and soleus
	25—ankle dorsiflexors

Table 12.7   Aerobic Dance or Exercise

Stretch exercises	Strength exercises
1—plantar fascia	3—deltoid
2 and 3—calf	6—triceps
11—quadriceps	11—shoulder external rotators
18—back extension	18a or 18c—quadriceps
19—spine or trunk rotators	19—tensor fascia lata
21—side and shoulders	21—hip flexor
	24—gastrocnemius and soleus

Table 12.8   Cycling

Stretch exercises	Strength exercises
2 and 3—calf	18—quadriceps
9 or 10—iliotibial band	22—hamstrings
11—quadriceps	24—gastrocnemius and soleus
15—lower back and hamstrings	
24—neck	

PART III
Prevention of Overuse Injuries

Once the inevitability of athletic injury is accepted, it becomes easier to plan for the prevention of injury. Prevention of injury is not something that the athlete should consider only after suffering an injury. Successful prevention of injury requires developing the concept of incorporating prevention into the exercise program. This means that the athlete must be aware of physical changes within the body and the environment as well as mental changes. Prevention should also be extended beyond the exercise program into the athlete's complete lifestyle as well. This part offers guidelines for developing a program of injury prevention that considers many aspects of the athlete's life.

The basic three-step treatment plan for injury (from part II) is as follows:

1. Reduce or stop the stress causing the injury;
2. Reduce the inflammation and encourage the natural healing process; and
3. Correct any factors that will contribute to re-injury.

This treatment plan is expanded into a prevention plan in chaper 13, "How to Avoid Injury." The injured athlete should consider a conditioning program offering alternative fitness methods as detailed in "Maintaining Fitness in the Injured Athlete." Injury prevention includes physical dangers—such as cars and animals—as well as the effects of road surfaces or flooring and adverse weather and safety conditions when exercising. Such basic considerations as clothing and shoe and sock selection for injury prevention are also included in chapter 13.

A secure grasp of nutrition is also necessary for successful injury prevention. Diet factors such as cholesterol as well as special dietary conditions (anorexia and bulimia) are discussed in chapter 14. The athlete who is overweight or diabetic need not be severely limited, if guidelines are followed.

Bones, joints, and muscles, and the effects exercise has on them over a long period of time are discussed in chapter 15.

In chapter 16, the concerns of children as athletes are discussed. Injuries that are unique to children, such as growth center (epiphyseal) injuries and osteochondrosis, are reviewed.

First aid for minor injuries is included in chapter 17. The athlete needs to know how to treat and prevent minor injuries such as blisters, sprains, bruises, abrasions, and also to provide emergency care.

Prevention of injuries does not simply mean stretching for 10 minutes before exercising. A successful prevention program includes not only stretching and strengthening, but a mental awareness of what is happening to the body in order to recognize these changes and modify any negative behaviors before an injury occurs. This must include changes not only to your exercise program but also to your daily lifestyle.

CHAPTER 13

How to Avoid Injury

If you have been injured, prevention of future injuries should be considered during the treatment stage of the initial injury. Remember that the three steps of the basic treatment plan are:

1. Reduce or stop the stress causing the injury;
2. Reduce the inflammation and encourage the natural healing process; and
3. Correct any factors that will contribute to reinjury.

Prevention of injuries is a continuation of this final step of treatment. If an injury was due to a muscle imbalance and treated by a stretching and strengthening program, this program should be continued to avoid the recurrence of the muscle imbalance and a likely reinjury.

In fact, the wise athlete determines whether there is a potential muscle imbalance before an injury occurs and treats it appropriately. This can be done by using the stretching and strengthening exercises recommended in chapter 12 for use in conjunction with specific sports. By using these exercises on a routine basis, you can prevent muscle imbalance and possible injuries. Also, you can identify muscles that may be tight or weak and plan additional work for these muscles. If you find, while doing the stretching exercises, that there is extreme tightness in a particular muscle group, such as the calf or hamstrings, more time should be spent on this problem group. In a similar fashion, if there appears to be a weakness in a certain muscle group while you're doing the strengthening exercises, more time should be devoted to the exercises for this group.

Another method to avoid developing muscle imbalance is to cross-train. This requires that you participate in more than one sport, each emphasizing different muscle groups. By varying the activities, such as running, swimming, and biking, throughout the week, more muscle groups are involved and the potential for imbalance is reduced.

Muscle imbalance is one type of biomechanical variation. It reduces the efficiency of the body and makes the athlete more prone to injury. There are also structural biomechanical variations in the body that may cause similar problems. These variations may include a number of things, such as excessive pronation of the feet, bowlegs, curvature of the spine, or limitation of motion in the shoulder. Identifying any such problem early and treating it appropriately helps avoid injury.

Because there are so many of these variations that can occur in the body—and they can each occur in varying degrees—they are difficult to self-diagnose and treat. Therefore, if you suspect this type of problem, obtain professional help. Once the extent of the problem is determined, treatment can be initiated. This may include orthotic devices, braces, stretching and strengthening exercises, physical therapy, modifications in training techniques, and alternative exercises. A special program has to be established for each problem.

In addition to the structural biomechanical variations that can occur, there are also external biomechanical forces that may adversely affect the athlete. These are areas in which the athlete has more control and choice, such as training surfaces. A runner who always runs to one side of the road is affected by the banking of the road. Running along this slight incline for many miles places more stress on the lower extremities and increases the potential for injury. Prevention is effected simply by running on alternating sides of the road (where safe) or at least by changing the course to avoid always having the banking on the same side. An aerobic dancer who exercises on a solid floor, like a rug over concrete, is more prone to injury. Preventing injuries requires only changing to a floor that has more "give"; this reduces the adverse external biomechanical forces. Another commonly overlooked external biomechanical force comes from worn athletic shoes. As the heels wear or the midsole compresses, more stress is imposed on the feet and legs. Replacing shoes more frequently helps prevent this.

Each athlete may be able to identify other types of external biomechanical forces that may be encountered. This emphasizes the necessity to be mentally alert to changes occurring within our bodies and in the environment. Only by recognizing these changes early can we prevent injuries.

Suggested Reading for "How to Avoid Injury"

Canby (1981)

Crossen (1982)

Davis (1982)

Donaldson (1977)

Gaston (1983, March)

"How much pain . . ." (1984)

McGregor & Devereaux (1982)

Nirschl (1980)

Ottum (1982)

Pagliano & Jackson (1980)

Paulsen (1983)

Titus (1984)

Tropp et al. (1985)

Van der Meer (1984)

Wellemeyer (1983)

See reading list at the end of the book for a complete source listing.

Maintaining Fitness in the Injured Athlete

Walter R. Thompson, Ph.D.

Millions of people now enjoy the benefits of regular exercise. Many of them, unfortunately, also suffer from injuries that result from exercise. Recent statistics indicate that two out of every three runners are injured annually. Treatments vary as much as the injuries themselves—one of the least popular treatments being complete rest.

Scientific literature on the psychological aspects of sport has begun to identify an apparent "self-destruct" attitude in both amateur and professional competitors. It appears that many athletes literally run themselves into the ground, consciously or unconsciously, exacerbating injuries and creating much damage that could have been avoided. Popular literature often condones this behavior with such articles as "Running Through Your Injury."

Only after trying various self-prescribed home remedies do most injured athletes seek advice from doctors. Unfortunately, past attitudes of physicians have unintentionally encouraged such delays. Doctors' unsuccessful—and frequently unnecessary—prescriptions of time off to allow healing have discouraged many athletes from consulting medical professionals.

Correct Diagnosis

Identification of the injury and determination of its cause are the first and most important steps in the recuperative process. Is the injury a biomechanical defect or the result of a traumatic event? This is an important distinction in correct treatment. Also, is the athlete chronically aggravating an injury by overcompensation? What alternatives does the athlete have for maintaining his or her present level of fitness while giving the injury appropriate care? It is this last issue that requires creativity based on sound judgment, not only

from the physician or therapist but also from the injured athlete.

Decline of Fitness

Perhaps the most well-known (and often-quoted) study of de-training effects was reported by Bengt Saltin, Ph.D., and his colleagues in 1968. They demonstrated a 27 percent reduction in maximal oxygen consumption in athletes after 21 days of bed rest. (Maximal oxygen consumption is the product of cardiac output [heart rate times the amount of blood pumped with each beat] and the difference between oxygen content of arteries and veins. It is regarded by most scientists as the best indicator of endurance fitness.)

Saltin et al. demonstrated that the greatest portion of this decrease occurs within the central circulatory system; that is, cardiac output decreases by 27 percent after just 21 days of imposed bed rest. Because neither maximal heart rate nor oxygen difference in arteries and veins change during this time, stroke volume must be the limiting factor in response to maximal exercise endurance. Exercising muscles themselves still function as efficiently as they had prior to imposed bed rest.

Saltin and his co-workers inferred from this that if an athlete continues to train the central circulatory system while resting the injury, recovery can be achieved much more quickly than with complete bed rest. Thus, the way to maintain training effect during recovery from an injury (though not working the injured part) is to follow established training principles to maintain central cardiovascular fitness.

These basic training principles may be considered the minimal amount of activity for highly trained athletes. If you follow the three-times-a-week exercise program at 75 percent of maximum heart rate for 30 minutes nonstop, as the American College of Sports Medicine suggests, you can maintain a training effect.

Alternative Exercise Program

Studies show that an athlete's cardiovascular endurance decreases at almost the same rate (or more quickly!) as it was gained. Therefore, it is important to adopt an alternative exercise treatment program that allows you to maintain strength, flexibility, and cardiovascular fitness while resting the injured body site. If you do not maintain the preinjury level of central cardiovascular fitness, performance suffers upon return to participation, obviously.

Alternative forms of exercise include any activities involving large muscle groups that increase the heart rate and keep it at levels necessary to maintain the desired level of cardiovascular fitness. Activities such as swimming, running in a pool, bicycling, and bicycle ergometry (stationary bicycling) are acceptable. Swimming requires some skill and may not be the best alternative for some athletes (fear of water may be a consideration). Bicycling and bicycle ergometry require little skill and can be performed by most athletes.

Bicycle Ergometry

The best alternative is a combination of active arm and leg work. Some exercise bicycles provide both pedals for the legs and handlebars that move to provide exercise for the arms. This type of bike allows various combinations of exercises that can be used while resting an injured part.

This bicycle can be ridden as a normal bicycle ergometer, with active use of the legs and arms (as you pedal with your legs, the handlebars of the bike also move back and forth in a pedaling fashion, and vice versa). The practicality of this kind of ergometer rests in its flexibility. If you have a leg injury, all that is required is to rest the feet on the pedals and exercise with the arms. Range of motion is achieved by the legs, and cardiovascular benefits are derived from the arms. Conversely, if the injury is in the arm or shoulder region, active exercise can be performed by the legs while passive range-of-motion exercise is done with the arms.

As the rehabilitative process continues and the affected extremity becomes stronger, greater resistance may be forced upon the injured area. In other words, as the injured area becomes stronger, you can gradually increase resistance and move from a strictly passive exercise to one that requires full use of the injured area. This method allows for a rapid and complete return to regular activity.

Swimming

Swimming is another excellent exercise for the injured athlete. The buoyancy of water allows exercise without putting weight on the injury. In the beginning stages of rehabilitation, walking in the water, gradually progressing to swimming, is advised. (For leg and foot injuries, though, lower extremity activity should be kept to a minimum.)

If complete rest of the injury has been suggested, maintaining cardiovascular fitness becomes of paramount importance. Arm exercise, as in swimming without the use of the legs, allows the heart rate to increase enough to maintain the proper intensity. Because maximal heart rates for swimming often are not as high as running, for example, intensity should be kept at the lower end of the training range (75 percent of maximal heart rate).

Weighted Limbs

Another alternative, recently developed by Leonard Schwartz, M.D., is called *Heavyhands®*. Although Schwartz remarks that this technique is not designed for anyone with a "physical incapacity or illness," it does have the same advantages as most rehabilitative programs.

Heavyhands® is a technique of weighting the hands to increase intensity and duration of exercise. The athlete carries weights in the hands while performing some other type of activity (riding a stationary bicycle ergometer or walking, for example). Schwartz feels that by the athlete weighting the hands, the heart rate increases proportionately with the amount of weight carried. In an effort to maintain cardiovascular fitness in an injured athlete, this may prove to be ideal.

The Complete Cure

Total injury rehabilitation and maintenance of cardiovascular endurance during recovery from an injury are essential to any athlete. The self-destruct (training through injury) attitude often found in injured athletes should be of primary concern. Chance of reinjury or aggravation of an existing injury increases greatly if the athlete returns prematurely to regular workouts. A way of combating this is to stress the importance of alternative techniques in the maintenance of fitness.

Avoid the quick-cure attitude. Care for your injury properly without compromising the level of conditioning already achieved. Find enjoyable alternatives that are strenuous enough to maintain your preinjury level of fitness.

Avoiding Physical Hazards While Exercising

Susan Kalish, B.A.

The key to a safe workout is paying attention not only to your body but also to your environment. Since most people exercise for a healthy, long life, it is counterproductive to neglect your safety. You can choose to exercise in a safe environment; by this choice, you can enjoy your exercise program to its greatest advantage.

Plan ahead. There are a number of situations you can control that affect your safety. Choose a safe time and place to exercise; pay attention to who is around you. Tell someone where you are going and when you think you will be back. Better yet, exercise with a buddy so that you both can watch out for each other. Run or bike with your head up; a lowered head not only hinders breathing but also can reduce your field of vision.

Vehicle Hazards

Whereas feet were the most common mode of transportation 100 years ago, cars now outnumber pedestrians by a long shot. The ideal would be for cars to share the road with cyclists and runners. However, because cars are bigger and stronger, they should always be given the right-of-way. By using common sense and remembering what you were told years ago by the crossing guard, you will be able to safely exercise on the road. Avoid running on busy highways and interstates. Run on the shoulder of the road and face the traffic at all times, except when going around blind curves, when you should run on the outside. Frequently check behind you for cars coming from that direction.

However, remember—these precautions mean only that you can see cars better, not that motorists can see you. At dusk or at night, wear bright, reflective clothing. Put reflective tape on all your moving parts and try to use well-lighted, populated areas. Carry a flashlight, not so much in order to see the road as in order that others see you coming. Warn pedestrians and cyclists of your approach; shout "on the left" as you pass on that side.

When running or biking along the road in a group, go in single file. Obey all traffic signs and signals. Pedestrians do not have the right-of-way, except under certain conditions, such as in walkways when crossing at traffic signals. Slow down when you approach an intersection; when necessary, walk your bike across the street. Assume motorists do not see you. In fact, wave drivers through and try to get eye contact to be sure they really know you exist.

Avoid using roads when they are covered in snow. Cars have enough trouble avoiding each other in those weather conditions, and a cyclist or runner slipping and sliding along the road is an easy target for oncoming traffic. Also, streets banked with snow lend few escape routes for persons on them if a car should go into a skid.

Animal Hazards

They say dogs are man's best friend, but that is not necessarily the case when the man is a runner or cyclist. Many dogs instinctively chase, bark, or bite at moving objects. The best way to avoid getting attacked by a dog is to avoid the dog. Respect its territory; if possible, do not go through it. If you come across an aggressive dog, even with its owner, be careful. Never go between a dog and its owner, especially if the owner is a child. Even if the dog is on a leash, give it room, in case it lunges at you.

The best way to treat a barking dog is to act as if you are ignoring it. If you feign indifference, the dog may lose interest. Only *feign* indifference—actually, be alert. If a dog comes at you, face it. Usually you are bigger than the dog, and a smart dog knows this. If you act brave and forcefully yell "Go away!" most times dogs retreat. Do not turn your back on the dog; dogs like to attack from the rear. Stay alert, even when the dog leaves; it may come back.

If the dog comes at you, you have three choices: (a) try to make friends by talking softly, holding your hand out palm down, and praying; (b) assert your dominance by ordering the dog away, making threatening gestures, picking up a stick or stone (even an imaginary one could do the trick), and trying to be brave; and (c) become submissive by relaxing your muscles and glancing away, so that the dog thinks it has "won" (big dogs often respond to this and walk away).

These alternatives do not apply to packs of dogs. If more than one seemingly angry dog comes at you, run. Climb a tree or do whatever you can to get away. One mean dog is dangerous—two or more can be deadly.

It is a serious matter to be bitten by a dog. If your skin is broken, get medical help. Dogs transmit diseases through their saliva. If your skin is broken, you need at least a tetanus shot. Contact the dog's owner and your local police, animal society, or county health department. You need to know whether the dog has had its rabies shots lately. If the owner does not have written proof that the dog has had shots, contact the dog's veterinarian or the police.

Human Hazards

Because exercisers can by very vulnerable—that is, they often are alone, move through unpopulated areas, and are possibly tired—they are easy prey to muggers, rapists, and those bent on harassment. By being cautious, you can prevent many unhappy experiences. The key is to trust your intuition. If you feel uncomfortable in a situation, get out of it.

Plan your route carefully. Choose a time of day at which you know other people exercise in that area. Exercise in well-populated, well-lighted places. Avoid going near doorways, alleys, or dense shrubs. Have a variety of routes so that no one can assume you will pass their way at a certain time of day. Familiarize yourself with places along the route where you can get help, such as police or fire stations, 24-hour grocery stores, or other places of refuge. Be very familiar with the routes you use at night. Drive over them carefully in daylight. Save the safest areas for last, when you are the most tired. Reserve some energy for emergencies.

Act defensively. Carry mace or a whistle, look confident and strong. Ignore verbal harassment and use discretion in acknowledging strangers. If a driver or passerby asks for directions, answer from a distance. Anger is a good control weapon. When approached, spontaneous anger can intimidate, buy time, and give a potential attacker second thoughts.

Watch for cars turning off the road onto side streets. If you think a car is trailing you, turn and go the other direction. If you hear a car or footsteps, look behind you and assess the situation. Many attacks can be prevented if you act on your early intuition. Do not wait until you are attacked to scream. Attract as much attention as possible by blowing a whistle, yelling "fire," breaking a window, or doing anything else you can think of to call attention to the situation.

To avoid giving a thief or mugger ideas, do not wear conspicuous jewelry when you exercise. An incident that begins as theft may become something far worse. Carry only enough change for a phone call. If you are attacked by someone unarmed, try to escape. As a last resort, render quick, disabling blows and retreat. Attack the assailant's groin, eyes, and throat. This is more effective than scratching, punching, and kicking, which often can escalate the attacker's response. If you are attacked by someone who is armed, do not resist if all he or she wants is your property; your life is more important than your money. Make a mental note of the attacker's looks, mannerisms, and voice. Estimate the attacker's age, height, and weight by making comparisons with people you know.

Environmental Hazards

The quality of the air you exercise in affects not only your performance but also your health. There is a positive correlation between carbon monoxide exposure, which is found in air pollution, and a high incidence of cardiovascular disease. Because your breathing increases dramatically when you exercise, you breathe in a greater amount of harmful chemicals when exercising in a polluted environment than when you are still. In one study, runners had three times the concentration of harmful chemicals in their bloodstream after running in a polluted area than if they had just stood there for the same period. Such concentrations were equivalent to those of smoking 10 to 20 cigarettes that day.

Avoid running along highways and highly

congested roadways. Time your exercise to avoid peak traffic hours. Ozone levels increase soon after dawn and peak around midday. These levels usually drop again after rush hour or around 6:00 p.m.

Plan Ahead

Always carry some sort of identification when you exercise. A reflective ID tag is ideal. It should include your name, address, next of kin, and any pertinent medical information, such as your blood type, allergies, medications being taken, and special physical conditions.

By using common sense, you can enjoy a safe exercise program. The time of day you exercise, where you exercise, and the people around you contribute to your feeling of well-being. Be alert to these factors. A safe exercise program requires more than just proper training; it also requires a safe environment.

Suggested Reading for "Avoiding Physical Hazards While Exercising"

Pietschmann (1983)

See reading list at the end of the book for a complete source listing.

Avoiding Cold-Weather Injuries

Paul M. Taylor, D.P.M.

Prevention of cold-weather injuries requires attention to clothing, shoes, and the environment. The main consideration in coping with the cold is to maintain a safe balance between body temperature and air temperature. Exposed skin, wet clothes, and wind all influence the balance. By dressing properly, choosing your course well, and exercising common sense, the natural regulatory mechanisms of your body are adequate to deal with most temperature extremes.

You should be careful not to overdress for winter activities. Exercise generates body heat, which accumulates during exercise, so if you don't feel at least slightly chilled when you step out the door, you're already overdressed. After 5 to 10 minutes of activity, you usually find that your body's heating mechanism has warmed you sufficiently. If you wear enough clothing to be comfortably warm, clothing loose-fitting enough to allow for circulation of warm blood, and are prepared for temperature changes due to wind, snow, rain, or the setting sun, you can step out with confidence. Just follow the basic principles of dressing for the cold.

Several layers of lightweight garments work better than one bulky layer in trapping air, a natural insulator, close to the body to keep it warm. It is most important to keep your torso warm. Start with something light and absorbent, like a cotton T-shirt. Next, protect your arms and neck area and insulate your torso with a long-sleeved turtleneck. The ideal top layer is wind and water resistant; nylon windbreakers, down vests, sweatshirts, and wool sweaters are the most popular. Winter gear made of new materials such as Gortex® that allow air to circulate but keep out moisture makes it much easier to exercise in very cold climates. Their main disadvantage is their cost, and they may be too warm for climates that get only occasional cold weather.

Much body heat can be lost through improper protection of the hands, feet, legs, and head. In fact, over 40 percent of your body heat can be lost through an uncovered head. In cold weather, protecting the head is essential. Watch caps are popular because they also protect the ears; hoods don't get lost and are quickly adjusted. To protect the face against extreme wind, many athletes wear ski masks; others smear Vaseline® on their skin. Scarves are another means of facial protection. Don't forget to protect your hands. Mittens are more effective than gloves. Football players need warmth but also must be able to grip the football; leather gloves may be effective for this purpose.

As for the feet, under most conditions they should stay fairly warm. Wool socks retain heat. Treads or waffle-soled shoes help provide traction; when the activity surface is wet, you can spray shoes with a silicone compound to repel some of the moisture. For field events the length of cleats needs to be changed, depending on conditions.

Legs are usually comfortable with just one layer of clothing. Dance tights, sweatpants, pantyhose, or long underwear worn underneath runnning shorts can provide warmth without a lot of bulk. Males should give serious consideration to additional insulation in very cold weather, with extra shorts underneath the long coverings.

Good preparation for winter exercise isn't just a matter of knowing the weather forecast and dressing warmly. You should be participating in activities consistently while the weather turns colder, in order to acclimate yourself to the colder temperatures. Also, be sure to warm up thoroughly indoors before you step outside. Your muscles won't loosen as quickly as they do in the summer's warmth, and you need to stretch them carefully. You also want to build up body heat and step up your circulation before you go out into the cold. When you start to exercise, begin slowly to let your body warm up gradually. If you tax yourself suddenly, you may overheat and find yourself slowing down midway into your workout and becoming too chilled and tired to continue. After exercising, be sure to get out of wet clothes immediately to avoid getting a chill.

The thermometer tells only part of the cold weather story; the windchill factor is even more important. Windchill indicates the effects of temperature combined with wind velocity. Be aware of temperature and wind changes.

Although in most cases running shoes with treads or field shoes with cleats provide adequate traction, temperatures below 30 degrees Fahrenheit call for caution. Whenever possible, avoid ice. When running on a tricky surface, try to stay relaxed and maintain an even, rhythmical running stride. Run carefully to avoid falls, twisted ankles, and sprains. If you do pull something, don't be afraid to skip a day or so of activity. You can cause further damage to the injured area by forcing yourself to limp on treacherous surfaces.

Frozen lungs are not a danger to athletes. Cold air can't damage your lungs, because the air you breathe is warmed adequately in your mouth and throat before it ever reaches your lungs. Although cold, dry air can irritate your throat, only under unusually extreme conditions are normal body mechanisms insufficient to adequately warm the air going down your windpipe.

Anyone who spends time outdoors in cold weather should be aware of frostbite, usually a result of prolonged exposure to low temperature. The skin temperature drops below 32 degrees, causing the formation of ice crystals in the skin or tissues underneath. Frostbite can be further promoted by exhaustion, fatigue, wet clothing, or insufficient circulation. Fingers, toes, ears, nose, and cheeks are the most frequently affected areas; athletes who go out for long periods of time should take care to protect these areas. The skin of the affected area first turns ruddy and may burn and sting. As the initial redness fades, the skin becomes pale and grayish-yellow and feels numb or cold, but with no pain.

The threat of frostbite can be met through physical action such as wiggling fingers and toes, making faces, and otherwise working the muscles to increase the supply of warm blood to the area. Also, you should avoid becoming overheated, because moisture and perspiration can help promote frostbite. Again, proper dress is critical. If you suspect frostbite, make the affected area warm and dry. Seek the attention of a physician as soon as possible.

Hypothermia is a drop of one or more degrees in the internal body temperature, usually caused by prolonged exposure to cold air or water. Hypothermia can occur even in temperatures as seemingly mild as 30 to 50 degrees Fahrenheit. As the skin and related tissues cool rapidly, the body reduces the circulation of blood from the extremities to try to keep the core of the body warm. When the body begins to lose heat faster than it produces heat, hypothermia becomes a threat.

Symptoms include intense shivering, slurred speech, loss of coordination, stumbling, and mental deterioration. Hypothermia is a life-threatening condition. Concentrate warming efforts on the core of the body. Immediately seek shelter from the wind and the cold; get out of all wet clothes. Take in warm (not hot) food and drink, and rest the body in a warm environment. Dressing properly for the cold and knowing how to react to symptoms of hypothermia are important in any outdoor winter activity.

Properly prepared and outfitted, the athlete can continue to exercise or to play sports throughout the coldest winter months.

Suggested Reading for "Avoiding Cold-Weather Injuries"

Kent (1983)

See reading list at the end of the book for a complete source listing.

Avoiding Heat Injuries

Paul M. Taylor, D.P.M.

Extremes of temperature, both heat and cold, present potential injuries for the athlete. Exercise in extreme heat requires careful preventive techniques because, as Dr. George Sheehan says, "Heat is the only thing that can kill a healthy athlete."

Heat dissipation is crucial for the body at work. In order for body tissues to function efficiently and not become damaged, the body core temperature must remain relatively stable. At racing speeds, working muscles produce much more heat than at rest. Therefore, the body must disperse this heat while exercising. The primary method of reducing heat buildup in the body is through perspiration. The sweat on the skin evaporates, creating a cooling effect; in essence, this mechanism is the body's radiator. If anything within the body or any external factors interfere with the cooling, a heat injury may result. A temperature increase of only a few degrees can injure the more fragile body tissues, such as the brain, liver, or kidneys. The brain is particularly susceptible to heat injury, which is why people frequently become disoriented with heat injuries (see Table 13.1).

The three principal types of heat injuries are heat cramps, heat exhaustion, and heatstroke. Heat cramps, or muscle cramps, are due to a loss of fluid and a lowering of the essential minerals needed for proper muscle function. Treatment for muscle cramps requires stopping the activity, resting in the shade or a cool area, and drinking water or a weak electrolyte/sugar fluid replacement.

Heat exhaustion is a condition that comes on gradually. It is primarily a cardiovascular problem and is due to the gradually decreasing level of fluids in the body. The symptoms may include weakness, malaise, faintness, and the skin becoming cold and clammy. A low blood pressure may develop, for which the heart may try to compensate by developing a rapid, weak pulse. Because heat exhaustion usually develops gradually over a period of a few days, as soon as the symptoms are recognized, treatment with rest and fluid replacement should be started.

Table 13.1   Heat Index/Heat Disorders

Heat index*	Possible heat disorders for people in higher risk groups
130° or higher	Heatstroke/sunstroke highly likely with continued exposure
105°–130°	Sunstroke, heat cramps, or heat exhaustion likely, and heatstroke possible with prolonged exposure and/or physical activity
90°–105°	Sunstroke, heat cramps, and heat exhaustion possible with prolonged exposure and/or physical activity
80°–90°	Fatigue possible with prolonged exposure and/or physical activity

*See Table 13.2.

Heatstroke is a serious and potentially fatal condition. This is a situation in which the body core temperature rises so high that the body is unable to maintain its normal temperature through regulating mechanisms. This results in a sudden increase in the tissue temperature, with serious complications. An athlete experiencing heatstroke develops blurred vision, dizziness, and nausea. This progresses to a very high temperature with hot, dry skin. The body's cooling mechanisms break down, and the person stops sweating. The person becomes irritable or delirious, the pulse rate and blood pressure increase, and, ultimately, loss of consciousness may occur.

Emergency medical care must be summoned, but treatment to cool the body must be started immediately. The victim should be kept in a cool area, the body fanned and doused with water or packed in ice. If conscious, the victim should be given fluids. Medical care, including intravenous fluids, should be started as soon as possible. Heatstroke may cause serious damage to such vital body organs as the brain, heart, liver, or kidneys. Careful medical follow-up care is essential.

The first step in the prevention of heat-related injuries is recognizing the conditions that may predispose the athlete to heat injuries. Although high temperatures alone contribute to exercise-related injuries, a combination of high temperature and high humidity is even more dangerous. The "Heat Index Chart" from the U.S. Department of Commerce provides a guide to identify which conditions may become hazardous (Table 13.2). If the table is not available, the rule of 150 may be applied. Add together the temperature in degrees Fahrenheit and the relative humidity percentage; if their sum exceeds 150, caution must be used in exercising. Again, be aware that as the temperature and humidity rise, there is a significant danger of heat injury. These precautions are especially important in activities in which heat problems are compounded by heavy padding and clothing, such as summer football practice.

During summer exercise, the following preventive measures should be taken:

- Gradually adjust to the increasing temperatures. Allow time for your body to become acclimated to the warmer weather. Do not try to increase the duration or intensity of your activity while the weather is getting hotter.
- Adjust your training schedule according to the weather. If the temperature and humidity are high, do not do a hard workout, even if it is in your schedule.
- Wear lightweight clothing. Wear running shorts and a loose singlet or T-shirt. Light-colored clothing is also better, reflecting more of the sun's radiation than dark clothing.
- DO NOT wear sweat suits or rubber suits in an attempt to increase sweating to lose weight. This is extremely dangerous and can easily cause excessive heat buildup in the body, with resultant heatstroke.
- Drink plenty of fluids. Water, fruit juice, or dilute electrolyte solution should be taken before, and regularly during the activity. Drink a pint of fluid before the activity and continue drinking 6 to 8 ounces every 15 to 20 minutes. These are just guidelines; they vary depending on the particular person's level of fitness, the temperature and humidity, and the intensity of the exercise.
- DO NOT take salt tablets. Intake of salt tablets was once commonly done while exercising in hot weather. However, most experts have recently advised against using them. It is felt that salt causes a retention of fluid in the stomach and is unable to circulate to other tissues, where it is needed.
- Wear comfortable, well-padded shoes. In hot weather, the activity surface temperature can become excessively hot. This causes higher body temperatures and also increases the potential for developing blisters and other injuries. Socks should be worn to help "wick" the perspiration away from the body and to help cooling.
- Eat a diet that replenishes minerals such as magnesium and potassium. These are found in such foods as cantaloupes, watermelons, tomatoes, carrots, and cucumbers.
- Exercise when the temperature is coolest. Exercising in the early morning or late evening reduces the chance of heat injuries.
- Splash water over your body during exercise to help the body's cooling mechanisms.
- Exercise with a partner. Thus, if any problems develop, help is immediately available. Also, someone else may recognize the signs of heat injury even before you do.
- Know the signs and symptoms of heatstroke and heat exhaustion. Don't try to exercise through these symptoms; this may push the body to the point at which you become disoriented and unaware of what is happening.
- Apply a sun block or lotion to areas that may burn. However, do not apply it excessively, because this may interfere with sweating and cooling.
- Extra caution should be taken by children. They generate more heat but perspire less than adults, so they are more prone to heat injury.

It is not necessary to discontinue exercising during hot weather. It is necessary to take certain precautions. In some climates, the temperature and humidity reach the danger zone.

Table 13.2   Heat Index Chart

Air Temperature and Relative Humidity Versus Apparent Temperature

Air temperature (°F)	Relative humidity (%)																				
	0	5	10	15	20	25	30	35	40	45	50	55	60	65	70	75	80	85	90	95	100
140	125																				
135	120	128																			
130	117	122	131																		
125	111	116	123	131	141																
120	107	111	116	123	130	139	148														
115	103	107	111	115	120	127	135	143	151												
110	99	102	105	108	112	117	123	130	137	143	150										
105	95	97	100	102	105	109	113	118	123	129	135	142	149								
100	91	93	95	97	99	101	104	107	110	115	120	126	132	138	144						
95	87	88	90	91	93	94	96	98	101	104	107	110	114	119	124	130	136				
90	83	84	85	86	87	88	90	91	93	95	96	98	100	102	106	109	113	117	122		
85	78	79	80	81	82	83	84	85	86	87	88	89	90	91	93	95	97	99	102	105	108
80	73	74	75	76	77	78	78	79	79	80	81	81	82	83	85	86	86	87	88	89	91
75	69	69	70	71	72	72	73	73	74	74	75	75	76	76	77	77	78	78	79	79	80
70	64	64	65	65	66	66	67	67	68	68	69	69	70	70	70	70	71	71	71	71	72

Heat index (or apparent temperature)

Note. From "Heat Wave: A Major Summer Killer" by the U.S. Department of Commerce and the National Oceanic and Atmospheric Administration, 1985, NOAA/PA 85001.

In such environments it may be wise to change to a different activity, such as swimming or exercising in air conditioning. Being aware of changes in your body, listening to those signs, and applying common sense allow for safe exercising throughout summer.

Shoe Selection for Prevention of Injuries

Paul M. Taylor, D.P.M.

Proper shoe selection can aid in the prevention of sports injuries. Shoes should be selected for the specific sport and for your individual characteristics.

Current advances in the development of athletic shoes provide improved performance and protection against injury. Sport-specific shoes are now available for almost every sport. Each sport places unique stresses on the lower extremity and imposes unique demands pertaining to directional stability, traction, and shock absorption. Because shoes are designed to meet specific needs, you should wear the shoes that are best suited for whatever sport in which you participate. The days of having one pair of sneakers for all sports activity should be over. Running shoes are designed to stabilize the foot and provide maximum shock absorption in a unidirectional fashion. Tennis shoes are designed for the rapid changes in direction that the sport requires. Different outer sole or tread designs are also available for different court surfaces. Sports such as basketball and volleyball require shoes that provide protection not only for running and rapid changes of direction but also for jumping. Wearing shoes that are sport-specific helps to reduce injuries. The dedicated athlete should take advantage of the new shoes that are available.

In certain sports in which there is a demand for a large number of shoes, manufacturers have been able to provide shoes that are not only sport-specific but also specific for the demands of the individual. This includes shoes for specializing in certain events as well as shoes designed for certain body types or foot types.

Running shoes have evolved into both racing "flats" and training shoes. There are different shoes for sprinters and long-distance runners. There are shoes designed for each event in track and field. These shoes can be further modified by changing the spikes. The biggest variety can be found in running shoes. However, as participation in other sports continues to increase, a wider variety of shoes should be available for other sports, also.

Running shoes have been customized for particular body types or foot types. Shoes are advertised as providing maximum pronation or supination control. There are shoes especially suited for the heavy runner. Running shoes can be further individualized to suit the runner by modifying the shoe through a series of plugs, wedges, or small apertures that can be filled with shoe sole repair material.

Finding well-fitted shoes that are ideally suited for an activity certainly helps provide injury protection, but it can also provide a lot of confusion. With such a large selection of shoes available, it becomes difficult to choose the correct ones. However, there are a number of things that you can do to select the best shoes without having to buy several pairs. The main criteria in selecting shoes is to be sure that they fit properly. The best designed shoes are not going to help if they don't fit correctly. Frequently, because shoe retailers are limited in their inventories, stores may not stock the shoe style you want in your size. If this is the case, either order the shoe in the right size or make another selection. Use the following as a guide when purchasing new shoes:

- Try the shoes on with the same type of socks that you wear during the activity the shoes are intended for.

- If you wear orthotic devices, bring them with you to try them on in the shoes.

- Do not assume that you always wear the same size shoe. Sizes vary between manufacturers, and your foot size changes occasionally, also.

- Tie the laces and stand in the shoes. There should be a space about the width of your thumb between the end of the shoe and your longest toe.

- Walk or jog around the store in the shoes. They should be comfortable, without any pinching, rubbing, or slipping at the heel. If your heels slip but the toeroom is correct, do not go to shorter shoes to keep the heels from slipping. Ask for shoes that come in a narrower size or are made on narrow lasts; different brands of shoes have different widths.

- Wear the shoes around the house for 1 or 2 hours before running in them. If they become uncomfortable in the house, return them and start over.

The fit is the most important consideration in buying shoes, but it is always difficult to decide on a particular brand or style. If you have been running in the same style of shoes for a long time without any problems, it is probably better to stay with that style, even if there are shoes with higher ratings. If you do need a different style or brand, check the running magazines. They regularly provide shoe surveys that can be used as guides in selecting proper shoes. Talking to other runners who may have similar problems also helps. Furthermore, shopping at a store that specializes in athletic shoes should help, because they should have a better selection and should be better able to determine the best type of shoes for your needs. If you have been treated by a podiatrist, consulting with him about the shoes that may be best for your foot type may help, also.

Finding the best shoes is critical to an exercise program. This is true of all sports. The above guidelines can be used in choosing shoes for any sport. Finding the right shoes for your activity, in regard to fit and function, is a big step in preventing injuries.

Sock Selection for Prevention of Injuries

Paul M. Taylor, D.P.M.

Recent developments in athletic socks help provide more protection to the athlete's feet. Much attention has been directed to athletic shoes over the past several years; however, socks may be equally important. Socks help provide cushioning, shock absorption, shear reduction, cooling, and wicking. (Wicking is the ability to draw moisture away from the skin. Shear reduction helps to reduce blisters and callus formation.)

More consideration than usual should be given to sock selection, because socks provide a vital interface between the shoes and the feet. Better quality socks provide more comfort during sports participation. Just as with sport shoes, special socks are now available for individual sports. Socks have been designed to meet the specific needs of running, tennis, basketball, golf, skiing, and other sports. Taking advantage of these better quality socks is to your benefit.

Natural fibers such as cotton and wool have been traditionally rcommended for athletic socks. However, recent developments have made socks designed with synthetic materials just as acceptable. This provides you the opportunity to choose which type of sock is best for you. Because the cost of some of the best socks is only 5 or 6 dollars a pair, you can try different types to see which works best.

Socks are part of athletic equipment and they should be carefully selected and properly cared for. Because socks vary in thickness, the socks that are worn in sports should be worn when the athlete tries on new shoes. All footwear should be considered part of a system, this system being made up of shoes, socks, and, in some cases, an orthotic device. It is important to balance this system in order to get the most out of each part. Taking the time to properly select each part of this system helps prevent injuries to the foot and possibly to the entire lower extremity.

Once the socks have been purchased, they should be properly cared for, as is any other piece of athletic equipment. Manufacturers' washing recommendations should be followed. Socks should be washed after each use, because washing restores their fibers and helps to maintain their protective features.

Customer surveys have shown that people give little consideration to why they purchase particular socks. This should not be true of the athlete; he or she should give careful consideration to which type of socks is best and purchase high-quality products. It is attention to details such as these that contributes to injury prevention.

Orthotic Devices

Paul M. Taylor, D.P.M.

Orthoses, or orthotic devices, are braces or supports used to straighten or maintain any deformed part of the body. Due to the recent emphasis on using orthotic devices to control foot function in the athlete, the terms frequently refer to these types of foot-aiding appliances in particular.

The athlete should understand that there is a large variation in the types of orthotic devices available, providing various degrees of protection. These can range from simple shoe inserts or wedges to complex, custom-made orthotic devices. Knowing the potential benefits and limitations of each appliance helps the athlete determine which type of device is needed.

Soft Shoe Insoles

Shoe insoles are soft, flat sheets of material that provide additional cushioning for feet. Insoles are designed to absorb shock and reduce shear forces. Many athletic shoes have insoles built into them. Otherwise, insoles can be purchased separately and inserted into shoes. Soft insoles provide extra shock absorption, can prevent calluses or blisters, and are useful as fillers in shoes that are a little too wide. Such insoles are usually available for under 10 dollars. They provide a minimal amount of protection, without any motion control, but they are useful to cushion minor calluses and to increase shock absorption somewhat.

Heel Cups

Heel cups protect heels through increased cushioning and by providing contact areas that more closely follow the contours of heels than the inside of most shoes do. These devices are helpful for heel spurs, heel bursitis, heel neuromas, and even for reducing the calluses, dry skin, and fissuring of skin that sometimes occur around the edges of the heels. Heel cups are made of various materials; some have ripple designs on the bottom to increase shock-absorbing capabilities. Heel cups cost between 3 and 10 dollars. They are somewhat limited in use because they are available in only one or two sizes.

Molded Shoe Insole

Molded shoe insoles, made of soft materials, can provide contoured heel and medial arch support and occasionally feature metatarsal pads. Molded insoles are frequently placed in shoes by the manufacturer, or they can be purchased separately and added to the shoe. Some models have pronation pads that include wedges in the heels or varying densities of material, which keep the heel in a slightly inverted position to prevent excessive pronation. These devices generally cost under 15 dollars. They are intended to provide arch support but are limited in success. This is because corrections and padding must be minimal, because each type of mass-manufactured correction must fit everyone who wears that size of shoe. Because foot construction varies considerably among people, changes in the insoles are not always beneficial for each wearer.

Individually Made Over-the-Counter (OTC) Orthotic Devices

The limitations of the previously mentioned devices are primarily due to the fact that one size fits all. This may be adequate for cushioning, shock absorption, and mild pronation control. However, when more motion control is needed, an individually made device may be required. Several companies offer these devices through the mail. The athlete receives a package containing instructions on making neutral impressions or tracings of the feet. These are then returned to the lab for custom fabrication of the devices. This type of individually made appliance should provide the best correction of all OTC orthotic devices.

However, there can be some problems with these devices, also. Their use requires the athlete to make a diagnosis of the foot problem and to decide if this type of device constitutes appropriate treatment. Due to the complexities of foot biomechanics, this is not a simple task. Also, the critical factor in making an accurate orthosis is to have a proper cast. This is not easy for someone with no previous experience. Inexperience can prove costly: These mail-order orthotic devices cost 60 to 90 dollars. Because of the difficulty in obtaining proper casts and in providing accurate corrections on the devices without examining the patient, these devices are not as accurate as doctor-prescribed devices.

Prescription Orthotic Devices

For serious foot problems or when the devices mentioned previously fail to provide relief, prescription orthoses may be necessary. Such devices are prescribed by a doctor following a complete evaluation. This careful evaluation determines whether the orthotic device is the most appropriate treatment.

There are several steps involved in obtaining these devices. Initially, a history is obtained from the athlete. This may include reviews of the chief complaint, how the injury occurred, any other injuries, self-treatment, shoes, level of activity, and any other information that may relate to the problem.

An examination of the lower extremity is then done. This determines any biomechanical problems that may be present. The alignment of the joints and the amount of motion within the joints is determined. X-rays may also be obtained to more accurately assess the relationships of the bones and joints. A gait evaluation of the extremity in motion may also be done at this time.

After it is confirmed that an orthotic device is the best treatment, casts of the feet are obtained. This must be done carefully, in order to capture the contours of the feet and to maintain the neutral positions of the feet (these are positions in which the feet are neither pronated nor supinated). The casts are then sent to a laboratory, where models of the feet are constructed. The orthotic devices, including any corrections or modifications that may have been requested by the doctor, are fabricated on these models.

After the orthosis is dispensed to the patient, a gradual break-in period is needed. During this time, additional minor corrections may be done on the orthotic device to "fine-tune" it for the patient.

It should be remembered that an orthosis is not the final answer for treatment or prevention of injuries. It may only be part of an overall treatment plan, which may include such other modalities as medication, physical therapy, surgery, rehabilitation, and training modification. The main disadvantages of prescription orthotic devices are their high cost (300 to 400 dollars) and the fact that they may not always work. Yet, if the evaluation is done properly and the orthotic devices are used as indicated, there is a very high success rate.

The injured athlete faces a dilemma in trying to choose which type of orthotic device is most helpful. If the injury is minor, and the athlete has a sense of where the problem may be, trying a simple device may be enough to resolve the problem. However, if the injury becomes more severe or recurs, professional help should be obtained. It is also important to realize that a visit to a sports podiatrist or physician should not be considered only to obtain an orthosis. The doctor should also provide more information about the injury and should offer alternatives and suggestions about simpler types of devices.

Shoe Modifications

Paul M. Taylor, D.P.M.

Foot difficulties are frequent and recurring problems for runners and other athletes. Many foot troubles are of a mild nature and frequently can be self-treated with shoe modifications or inserts. These modifications can balance mild structural abnormalities of the foot and protect areas of tenderness. To make such changes it is necessary only to obtain some readily available materials, to identify where on the foot the pain is located, and to be prepared to spend a little time on trial and error until the corrections are comfortable.

Either felt or sheet cork material can be used for the corrections. These materials are available with or without adhesive backing and come in thicknesses of ⅟₁₆, ⅛, or ¼ inches. They can be obtained from medical and surgical supply stores and sometimes from shoe repair stores. If these materials cannot be located, thick moleskin in double or triple layers can be substituted. This can usually be obtained from drugstores.

When the correction is under a weight-bearing area of the foot, any sharp edge becomes uncomfortable. Therefore, it is necessary to use beveling or tapering techniques while cutting the edges of the correction. One way to bevel the edges of the material is to hold the scissors at an angle (Figure 13.1). For materials of ¼-inch thickness, it is necessary

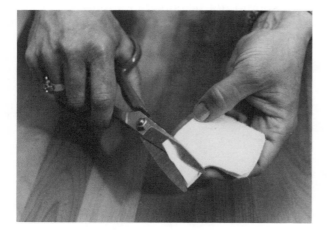

Figure 13.1   The edges of the pad can be beveled by holding the scissors at an angle.

to skive (pare) the edges. This is done with a sharp knife and with the felt flat on a cutting board. Start about 1 inch from the edge; angle the cut so the thickness tapers to almost nothing at the edge (Figure 13.2). Once the corrections are made, they can be placed inside the shoe.

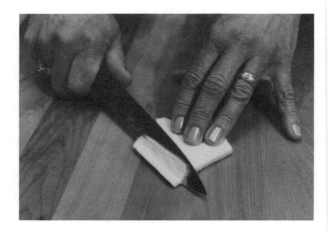

Figure 13.2   A more gradual feather edge can be obtained by using a sharp knife to skive (pare) the pad.

It is even more effective to use the removable insoles that come in many running shoes. If a pair of shoes does not have these insoles, they can be obtained at most athletic shoe stores. They are available both as flat insole material and as molded insoles that contour to the arch and heel. When an insole is used, it is better to place the padding on its bottom.

Padding for Specific Problems of the Foot

The following illustrations (see Figures 13.3 to 13.7) show how to pad for different problems. The general idea is to pad around a painful or tender area, to take the pressure off that spot. The initial correction should not be more than ⅛ inch; it can be increased later as needed. To get the proper positioning of the padding, use a felt pen to draw the correction on the bottom of your foot and then stand in the shoe. The pressure will transfer the mark to the insole. Then the insole can be removed and the correction trimmed and glued in the proper position.

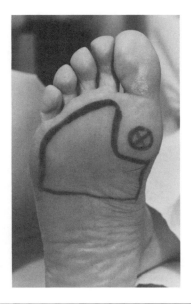

Figure 13.3 In order to properly position the pad, first draw an outline of the pad on the foot. The X marks the painful area on the foot.

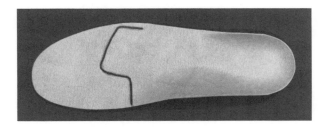

Figure 13.4 Transfer the mark to the insole by placing the insole in the shoe, putting the shoe on the foot, and standing. The marking for the position of the pad is now on the top of the insole.

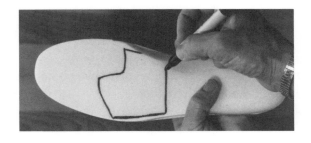

Figure 13.5 Transfer the markings to the bottom of the insole.

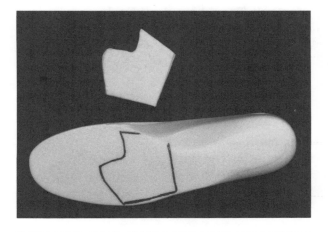

Figure 13.6 Cut the pad to the shape of the outline. Bevel the weight-bearing edges.

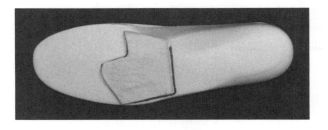

Figure 13.7 Glue the pad in place on the undersurface of the insole.

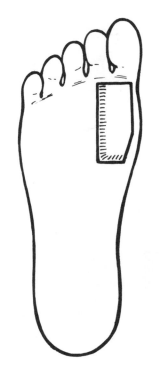

Figure 13.8 Padding for Morton's toe. The short lines indicate the edges of the pad that should be beveled.

Morton's Toe (Short First Toe)

When the first toe (actually the first meta-tarsal) is short, it does not bear weight as it should, and the medial or inside of the foot is unstable. Simply placing a pad under the first metatarsal helps to stabilize the foot (see Figure 13.8).

Sesamoid Pain (Pain Under the Ball of the Foot)

The ball of the foot is commonly injured in sports that require jumping and rapid changes in direction. A pad for this is frequently called a "dancer's pad" (see Figure 13.9).

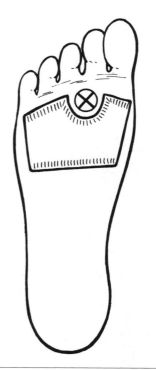

Figure 13.10   Padding for lesser metatarsal pain under one metatarsal.

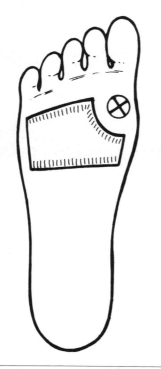

Figure 13.9   Padding for sesamoid pain (dancer's pad).

Metatarsal Pain (Metatarsalgia)

If any of the lesser metatarsals are injured, padding can be used to take the pressure off the area. The cutout portion of the pad should be under the painful metatarsal or metatarsals (see Figure 13.10). If the pain involves more than one or two metatarsals, a standard meta-tarsal pad can be used (see Figure 13.11).

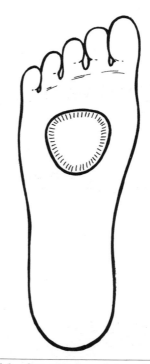

Figure 13.11   Standard metatarsal pad for metatarsalgia. The pad should be placed behind the area of greatest sensitivity.

Arch Pain

An arch support is used for pronation control and may also help protect a plantar fasciitis (see Figure 13.12).

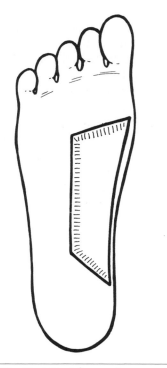

Figure 13.12 Padding for arch support. If the arch pad is placed under the insole, the edge on the inside of the foot should extend to the edge of the insole.

Heel Pain

An aperture heel pad helps protect any pain on the bottom of the heel (see Figure 13.13).

Heel Raise

A heel raise can be used to compensate for a leg length discrepancy or for Achilles tendinitis. The heel raise should be of material at least ¼-inch thick (see Figure 13.14).

Aperture Pad for Any Bony Prominence

Because of the many bones and joints in the foot, it is common to have an area where one of the bones may be more prominent; this can cause irritation from the shoe. A "donut"

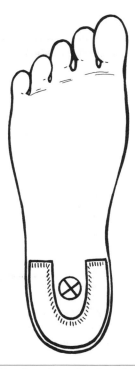

Figure 13.13 Aperture heel pad. The area of greatest sensitivity, X, should not be covered by the pad. The area marked with the small lines should be beveled.

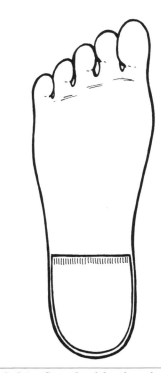

Figure 13.14 Standard heel pad.

pad can be placed around such an area to prevent chronic irritation. This type of pad may be available precut from drugstores (see Figure 13.15).

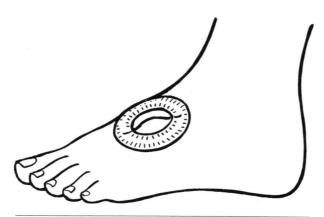

Figure 13.15 Aperture pad to protect any prominence. The pad should encircle the bump and be beveled on all sides.

Summary

The different corrections described above can be used in combination, as well as singly. For example, a person with a Morton's toe usually tends to pronate. Therefore, a Morton's pad and an arch pad could be used in combination.

The use of shoe modifications frequently helps relieve some of the common minor injuries that befall the athlete. However, if the corrections in the shoe do not provide relief or if they make the pain worse, the use of the pads should be discontinued; a consultation with a podiatrist should be obtained. If various shoe modifications have been tried unsuccessfully, and a visit to a podiatrist becomes necessary, the pads that were tried should be taken to the doctor; this may help with the diagnosis of the problem.

CHAPTER 14

Nutritional Factors Affecting Exercise

Every machine requires high-quality fuel to function at its peak level—and the human machine is no exception. When the quality of dietary input is poor, the body's performance suffers. What's worse, very harmful conditions may arise from long-term misuse of food. Awareness of these problems, which are discussed in this chapter, should be of the utmost importance to the conscientious athlete.

Cholesterol: Re-Tarnishing a Bad Reputation

Rebecca Riales, Ph.D.

Textbooks written on the development of atherosclerotic disease (hardening) of the arteries are laden with complicated theories of blood vessel injury, monocyte migration, and smooth-muscle-cell proliferation. More easily understood, however, is the role played by various aspects of our everyday lives in our probability of developing heart disease. These are called *risk factors*, and each one makes a contribution—small, moderate, or large—to our overall risk. If you are middle-aged or older, if you have a blood relative who developed heart disease in middle age or younger, if you are male, or any combination of the above, you are at a certain degree of risk of developing atherosclerotic disease. Although this is unfortunate, you can hardly alter these facts of your life.

The list of risk factors over which you do have control, fortunately, is longer. Are you a slender, nonsmoking, physically active person whose blood pressure, stress level, and sleep habits are in good shape? Good for you! You are already taking care of most of the remaining risk factors—those that are largely under your control and, thus, can be weighted in your favor.

Perhaps the most discussed modifiable risk factor in heart disease is blood cholesterol, if only because it seems to be so firmly and dismayingly linked to the eating of rich (and in the opinion of most people, delicious) foods. Not all of the body's cholesterol comes from the diet, though. The largest portion, in fact, is synthesized by the body to meet bona fide physiological needs. A white crystalline substance found in all animal tissues, cholesterol is essential for normal nervous system function and is used in the production of cortisone and sex hormones. Cholesterol in the body in excess of what is required to meet these physiological needs is, however, due to dietary excesses.

Cholesterol is a type of lipid, or fat, and therefore does not dissolve in blood, which is water-based. To circulate through the body, cholesterol must attach to a microscopic lipoprotein (lipid-plus-protein) globule that can be suspended in, and travel through, the blood. These lipoproteins come in three main types:

- HDL-cholesterol—High-density lipoprotein cholesterol, the "good" cholesterol, whose levels are inversely correlated with heart disease.
- LDL-cholesterol—Low-density lipoprotein cholesterol, the "bad" cholesterol, whose levels are directly correlated with heart disease.
- VLDL-cholesterol—Very-low-density lipoprotein cholesterol, a fraction (or portion) of total cholesterol that appears to be neutral with respect to its heart disease prognostic value.

The sum of these three types equals total blood cholesterol.

There is an important difference between HDL- and LDL-cholesterol. LDL-cholesterol is delivered by the blood to cells, where it is taken up by them. HDL particles, on the other hand, pick up excess cholesterol, possibly even removing it from the cells, and deliver it back to the liver, where it is reprocessed or excreted in the bile.

This process continues in the bloodstream day in and day out. In certain susceptible persons, cholesterol builds up in artery walls. In fact, the inside artery walls may become so narrowed by plaque (rich in cholesterol, platelets, smooth muscle cells, and large white blood cells called *macrophages*) that sufficient blood does not flow through them. In the case of an artery feeding the heart, this can result in a heart attack from the heart muscle not receiving enough oxygen from the blood to function properly.

Truly safe and healthful levels of total cholesterol (LDL plus HDL) in the blood are believed to range between 130 and 150 milligrams of cholesterol per deciliter of blood (mg/dl). However, in our culture, in which diets typically contain 40 to 45 percent of their calories as fat (plus dietary cholesterol associated with fat from animal sources), average total serum cholesterol concentrations range from 230 to 250 mg/dl—100 milligrams too high.

Experts say that to have low serum cholesterol levels, we each must eat only about half as much fat as the average American consumes. How sure are they, though, that if we agree to make these sacrifices, healthier arteries will result? How firm is the evidence for the so-called diet-heart theory that lower dietary fat and cholesterol lead to lower serum cholesterol levels, which result in lower risk of heart disease?

New Findings

For many years medical scientists had to content themselves with two major types of evidence in support of the diet-heart hypothesis: (a) studies of large groups of people and their diets that revealed a strong statistical association, but did not prove a causal link, between occurrence of heart disease and high intakes of fat; and (b) experimental work on laboratory animals, including nonhuman primates, that proved that high-fat diets did lead to high levels of cholesterol in the blood that lead to atherosclerosis.

The crucial third type of evidence was not forthcoming for many years—namely, use by humans of experimental diets, drugs, or a combination of the two, which caused not only lower levels of circulating cholesterol, but also less subsequent heart disease. Many large clinical studies yielded results that strongly hinted in this direction but fell short of what medical science considered proof.

We now have conclusive evidence of this long-suspected link. Results of a study, published in the January 20, 1984, *Journal of the American Medical Association*, have generated excitement throughout the United States and around the world. Funded by the National Heart, Lung, and Blood Institute, the study cost more than $150 million, took more than 10 years, involved 17 research sites, and studied over 3,800 men at increased risk of heart disease due to elevated levels of cholesterol. Subjects took a cholesterol-lowering

drug—cholestyramine—or a placebo or both, and ate a cholesterol-lowering diet. Various serum lipids were measured in the laboratory, and angiographic (x-ray) studies were carried out, allowing three independent teams of radiologists to visualize atherosclerotic disease processes in coronary arteries as they occurred over time.

When all the data were compiled and analyzed, it was found that the combined drug and diet regimen had caused significant improvement in serum lipid levels when compared to the placebo treatment, and the patients with the greatest decreases in the "bad" cholesterol and the greatest increases in the "good" cholesterol had the least disease progression. In fact, the patients with the greatest decrease in their ratio of bad cholesterol to good cholesterol had less than 1/3 of the amount of disease progression seen in the group with the smallest change in the ratio: 15 percent versus 47 percent. The bottom line is that *if total cholesterol levels of Americans were decreased by 25 percent, the risk of heart disease would be lowered by 50 percent.*

LDL-Cholesterol-Lowering Strategies

What tactics are available to the motivated, health-conscious person for lowering his or her LDL-cholesterol level? The premier strategy continues to be a low-fat/high-carbohydrate diet. If blood cholesterol levels are extremely high, drugs may be warranted. Drugs are expensive, though ($150 for a one-month supply of cholestyramine), and may have unfavorable side effects. They are not considered the treatment of choice, except for a small minority of patients.

A diet that derives at least half of its calories from complex carbohydrate foods is an optimal approach. The most popular complex carbohydrate sources are whole grains, beans and peas (legumes), garden vegetables, potatoes, corn, oats, rice, and pasta. These foods result in less fat in your blood, and probably less fat in your silhouette as well. Dietary fiber that accompanies many of these foods can be a cholesterol-lowering bonus. In particular, the gelling and mucilaginous fibers associated with legumes and certain vegetables and grains (but not wheat bran) may have a cholesterol-lowering effect.

Animal fat has a cholesterol-raising effect; therefore, animal protein foods selected should be as low in fat content as possible. In general, Americans can eat less animal protein because so much protein is provided by complex-carbohydrate foods. If only 25 percent of your daily calories are derived from fat, and you use these calories judiciously, your diet can still be very tasty.

HDL-Cholesterol-Raising Strategies

Can the above dietary strategy increase your HDL-cholesterol level, though? Probably not. Studies to date have failed to show a strong link between diet and concentrations of this good cholesterol in the blood. The best means of raising the HDL-cholesterol level seems to be a program of vigorous aerobic exercise. (A less-than-vigorous exercise regimen may improve your physical fitness but be insufficient to improve your serum lipids.) Alcohol may have a beneficial effect on HDL-cholesterol levels, but researchers hesitate to promote its use because abuse poses an additional set of risks to a portion of the population. Cessation of cigarette smoking and reduction of obesity have also been reported to be associated with raising HDL-cholesterol concentrations, particularly if levels were below average initially.

The Whole Picture

Before we become totally engrossed in this examination of the trees (blood cholesterol levels), may we take three paces back to look once again at the forest (risk of heart disease)? Although no one can quarrel with the desirability of lowering LDL-cholesterol, let us not assume that if everyone's LDL-cholesterol levels were ideal, there would be no atherosclerotic heart disease. This serum lipid is only one factor in the large puzzle that leads to cardiovascular disease. For maximal decreases in your risk of having a myocardial infarction, it is necessary to pay responsible attention to all the factors known to put you at less risk, including low blood pressure, not smoking, weight control, stress management, and regular exercise.

Both common sense and experimental evidence indicate that the lower your LDL-cholesterol/HDL-cholesterol ratio, the smaller your risk for heart disease, as far as the cholesterol risk factor is concerned. Twenty percent of American men have a heart attack by age 60. The average ratio of LDL to HDL cholesterol associated with this rate is as follows:

$$\frac{\text{LDL of 160 mg/dl}}{\text{HDL of 45 mg/dl}} = \text{ratio of 3.55}$$

A half-average risk ratio is 1.00, a twice-average risk ratio is 6.25.

Until recently, researchers and physicians relied on total cholesterol levels to determine heart disease risk. It now appears, however, that the relative proportions of cholesterols is more significant.

Suggested Reading for "Cholesterol: Re-Tarnishing a Bad Reputation"

Hagan et al. (1983)

Penny et al. (1982)

Rotkis et al. (1981)

Sady et al. (1984)

See reading list at the end of the book for a complete source listing.

Diet and Ulcers

Gabe Mirkin, M.D.

One American in 10 develops an ulcer in his or her lifetime. Although medical research has not yet determined the exact cause of ulcers, it has shown that eating certain foods can make them worse.

Location

Ulcers can occur in any area exposed to stomach juices, but they are formed mainly in two sections of the gastrointestinal tract. Duodenal ulcers, the most common type, appear in the first 11 inches of the small intestine, the duodenum. Less common are gastric ulcers, which occur in the stomach.

Description

Ulcers are small erosions of the surface lining of the gastrointestinal tract, generally ⅛ to ¾ of an inch in diameter. They look like small craters, similar to canker sores in the mouth. They arise from the failure of the mucosal lining of the stomach or duodenum to protect itself from its own gastric juices. If left untreated, ulcers may eat through (perforate) stomach or duodenum walls, leaking stomach acid to surrounding areas. Perforation may lead to serious internal bleeding.

Symptoms

Ulcer symptoms include a steady, often burning, pain in the abdomen between the breastbone and the navel occurring when the stomach is empty. Pain caused by contact of the ulcer by stomach acid usually is felt several hours after a meal—after the stomach empties—and again early in the morning, 6 to 10 hours after dinner. Pain from gastric ulcers often intensifies with eating because of direct irritation to the ulcer by food churning in the stomach.

Causes

Stomach acid is necessary for ulcers to occur. Hyperacidity frequently accompanies the onset of an ulcer, but patients often do not show signs of excess acid. Other factors—such as smoking, which inhibits the flow of a neutralizing juice from the pancreas; a family history of ulcers; type O blood; hormonal abnormalities; liver, lung, and kidney disease; and a lack of resistance in stomach and duodenal walls to the hydrochloric acid secreted by the stomach—are potential contributors to ulcer formation. Many medications, including aspirin, almost all antiarthritis drugs, and cortisone-type drugs, increase your chances of developing ulcers because they increase stomach acidity.

Doctors regard personality as a factor in producing or prolonging duodenal ulcers. Tense people often are viewed as more likely to get them; nevertheless, there are just as many examples of high-strung persons who never get ulcers as there are placid people who do.

Beverages to Avoid

Of all beverages, beer and milk cause the greatest increase in stomach acid; not far behind are coffee and carbonated drinks. All forms of alcohol—wine, beer, and hard liquor—stimulate the secretion of hydrochloric acid in the stomach, producing a higher level of acidity than nonalcoholic beverages. Milk, once recommended as a remedy for ulcer patients, is no longer prescribed. Its alkaline quality neutralizes stomach acid, and the stomach responds by markedly increasing its acid output.

Caffeine, once thought to aggravate ulcers, is no longer believed to do so. Recent studies show that the stomach responds with the same acid output to regular coffee, decaffeinated coffee, and carbonated beverages. Also, it appears to make no difference whether or not the carbonated drinks contain caffeine.

Treatment

There is no single best ulcer diet recommended for the healing phase, averaging 40 days but taking anywhere from 13 to 230 days. The best treatment includes medications that control or lower the concentration of acid in gastric juices as well as the avoidance of acid-producing drinks.

In addition to avoiding acid-producing foods, frequent small meals are recommended. Six meals evenly spaced throughout the day keep the stomach full. If antacids are used, they should be taken 1 or 2 hours after a meal, when the stomach is emptying. There is no good evidence that spicy or hot foods cause discomfort. If they bother you, do not eat them. If they do not, go ahead.

Ulcer medications limit acid secretion and neutralize acid after it has been secreted. Two drugs, cimetidine and ranitidine, effectively limit stomach acid production. Many over-the-counter antacids are also available to neutralize stomach acid.

Exercise

You can also use exercise as part of your ulcer treatment, as long as you exercise for more than 10 minutes. During exercise, the acidity of your stomach usually remains the same as before. However, for several hours after exercise, stomach acid is markedly reduced. Try running, cycling, swimming, or any other continuous exercise as part of your self-treatment.

Warning Signs

Because hyperacidity often precedes and accompanies an ulcer, modify your diet accordingly. If you notice a burning in your abdomen or chest that feels better after you eat, if you experience frequent belching with a sour taste, find a white coating on your tongue, or have a persistent sore throat, check with your doctor. If you do have hyperacidity or an ulcer, you may benefit by restricting your intake of coffee, carbonated drinks, alcohol, and other acid-producing substances.

Anorexia Nervosa and Bulimia

Diane K. Taylor, B.A.

Anorexia nervosa and bulimia are two serious eating disorders characterized by a need for strict control over body image and size. Although these disorders manifest a polarity in symptoms, there are similar psychological traits that predispose the development of each. A high percentage of the victims of these disorders are female. They are generally self-effacing, hard-working, goal-oriented high achievers who are uncomfortable with anger. They can become obsessed with being thin and, therefore, with food.

In anorexia the victim perceives herself as fat and begins to diet; as the condition progresses, the anorexic cannot seem to stop dieting, because the ultimate thinness is never reached. The anorexic sees a fat body no matter how thin it really is, and becomes in danger of starving to death. In an intense effort to remain small and thin (and, perhaps, perpetually childlike, not grown up), the anorexic severely limits caloric intake and exercises compulsively in order to burn off more weight. Weight loss becomes a competitive sport, and the anorexic "wins" with each pound lost.

For the victim of bulimia, eating huge amounts of food in short periods of time is controlled by vomiting after eating or by overuse of laxatives. The bulimic forms a binge-purge cycle that becomes addictive. Whereas the anorexic becomes painfully thin and can then be diagnosed and treated, the bulimic is often average or slightly above average weight and is much more difficult to recognize and treat.

The common denominator of both these eating disorders is control of both body and food. Either disorder signals a person out of touch with her own body, both in feeling: not listening to body signals; and in image: not seeing the body as it really is. There is a possibility that the anorexia victim may develop symptoms of bulimia during treatment, but there is rarely a crossover from bulimia to anorexia.

Although no studies have been done definitively linking athletics to either of these disorders, there are some behavior patterns that the athlete can fall into, signaling a potential progression to either disorder. To the athlete, a lean body means enhanced performance—the less body fat, the more efficient the exercise. If the athlete is in a competitive situation, a drop in body weight often increases performance. In training for a specific event, the athlete may begin to increase the amount of time in activity, and in the process lose weight and feel better about the resulting condition.

The difference between the healthy, lean, well-trained athlete and the anorexic seems to be in the self-perception of the athlete. If the goal is better performance, neither training nor eating are obsessive. In the anorexic, the training and exercise are used to get thinner; the satisfaction is not in the exercise itself, but in its contribution to being thin.

In many sports, body weight is a large part of the training goal. For example, wrestling has weight limitations for each classification. In ballet and gymnastics, a light, supple body is necessary for grace and mobility. In many instances, the day of the performance is weighing-in day. Under these circumstances, some athletes eat as if in training, then vomit before weighing in. This can start the binge-purge pattern of bulimia. The athlete who is accustomed to large amounts of food during training can find in the off-season that eating is hard to control except by improper eating habits.

The most telling factors in the development of these disorders are behavior changes that may signal a serious problem. If you begin to value body image obsessively or need to control body image with exercise, you may be thinking along the wrong lines. It is natural for those who exercise regularly to miss that exercise if they must stop for any reason. Yet, sudden increase in activity or inability to stop activity is not a healthy attitude, especially if the reason for exercise is to control body size.

Because victims are very secretive, these disorders are often difficult to diagnose. In bulimia, there are some signals: scars on the knuckles from inserting the fingers down the throat to force vomiting, dental problems from stomach acids damaging teeth, stomach problems, and a noticeable large ingestion of food without weight gain. Anorexia is more difficult to diagnose, but excessive concentration on exercise and thinness are certainly signals.

These disorders need professional help. They cannot be self-treated; they do not go away spontaneously. Many sportsmedicine centers now have a specialist in eating disorders on staff. If this is not available, a local mental health clinic should be able to refer you to a treatment center.

Suggested Reading for "Anorexia Nervosa and Bulimia"

"Anorexia nervosa and bulimia" (1986)

Blumenthal et al. (1984)

Braisted et al. (1985)

Goldfarb & Plante (1984)

Katz (1986)

Malony (1983)

Szmukler et al. (1985)

Weeda-Mannak & Drop (1985)

Yates et al. (1983)

Zucker (1985)

See reading list at the end of the book for a complete source listing.

The Overweight Athlete

Paul M. Taylor, D.P.M.

Being overweight means different things to different athletes. To the long-distance runner, whose percentage of body fat averages 5 percent for males and 10 percent for females, any additional fat may be considered overweight. For the 6-foot male runner, average weight would be 150 to 160 pounds. For the football player of 6 feet, though, the average weight is 190 to 210 pounds. Therefore, in considering the overweight athlete, the sport, level of activity, and family history determine what the weight should be.

Different athletes have different concerns about being overweight. For the fitness athlete who exercises for health, maintaining a proper weight is one aspect of a total fitness program. For a wrestler, being overweight would mean having to compete in a different weight class.

Whatever the reason for wanting to lose weight, there are certain principles related to weight loss of which the athlete should be aware. The percentage of body fat is frequently used to monitor unnecessary weight. Body fat percentage varies depending on the athletic activity and the level of participation. For males, body fat may be as low as 3 percent for the distance runner or up to 13 or 14 percent for the football or baseball player. A similar range occurs in the female athlete, with a 10 to 12 percent minimum for the distance runner and 20 to 25 percent for participants in sports such as swimming and tennis. The woman with body fat below 13 percent, it should be noted, may experience amenorrhea (see chapter 10, "Irregular Periods").

Measurements of body fat are usually obtained through one of two techniques. Underwater weighing with measurement of lung residual volume is an accurate method, but not very convenient. The most common method is through skinfold measurements using a skinfold caliper. Measurements are taken at three different parts of the body; from the sum of these measurements, the approximate percentage of body fat can be determined. Determination of body fat is helpful in establishing a weight training program for the athlete.

For example, two football players both weigh 210 pounds and are 6 feet tall. They may initially appear equal, but the body fat of one is 14 percent and the other is 25 percent. Because the player at 25 percent has a greater percentage of fat, he has less muscle bulk; this could indicate that he is not in proper condition.

If the athlete is found to be overweight or, more accurately, overfat, a weight loss or weight training program may be necessary. In a weight loss program by diet only, there is a loss of muscle, as well as fat. Weight loss through exercise alone is very slow, because it requires burning 3,500 calories to lose one pound. Based on the amount of calories that are used up with different exercises, an individual would have to run for 4 hours or walk for 17 hours to lose one pound.

To achieve weight loss, a combined program of exercise and dieting is much better than exercise alone. The setpoint theory offers an explanation of why exercise alone helps with some weight loss, though. This theory suggests that the body has a certain setpoint percentage of body fat that it tries to maintain, much as the way a thermostat regulates temperature. Persons with a low setpoint appear to have a higher metabolic rate; they can consume more calories without gaining weight. Those with a high setpoint usually do not metabolize the calories as rapidly and tend to gain weight. It is now thought that regular exercise lowers the setpoint, resulting in more effective weight loss. This is consistent with the findings that the body continues to burn calories at a higher rate even after exercise.

The person beginning an exercise program primarily for weight loss should be aware of the following guidelines:

1. Consult with your doctor before beginning an exercise program.
2. Maintain an appropriate diet during the exercise program. A well-balanced diet, with selections from each of the four food groups, should be continued.

3. Your calorie intake level should be reduced to allow a loss of 2 or 3 pounds per week. Consult with your doctor or a nutritionist to determine the best diet.
4. Maintain a normal fluid intake at all times.
5. Begin the exercise program gradually.
6. Wear proper shoes to help prevent injury. If you are overweight, this places more stress on your lower extremities. Overuse injuries are very common when persons start exercise programs.
7. DO NOT use rubber suits or other methods to lose weight that cause dehydration.
8. Start with an exercise that looks like fun. It's easier to continue a program if it's enjoyable.
9. Exercise with a friend. Work with someone at a similar level of fitness.
10. Don't set unrealistic goals; this only leads to frustration and giving up the exercise program.

Weight loss or weight training is a complex situation that involves a lot of theory and varies from one person to the next. It appears that a combination of diet and exercise is best. The person who has chronic weight problems or is obese should consult with a professional on the best combined program.

Running With Diabetes

Jeffrey L. Young
Michael O'Shea
Charles M. Peterson

What do Bobby Clarke, Bill Talbert, and Ron Santo have in common? They are all professional athletes who enjoyed successful careers in their respective sports—and they all have diabetes. During their professional athletic careers, they were considered unusually courageous because they dared to stay active in spite of their health problem. Today, they serve as examples that with proper care, people with diabetes can exercise as much, as hard, and as safely as nondiabetics.

Diabetes mellitus is a metabolic disorder in which the body has problems transporting and utilizing its fuel sources, most notably glucose (sugar). This can result from the body's failure to produce insulin, the hormone necessary for carrying glucose into the cells; or it may result from a decreased sensitivity to this hormone, despite its presence in normal or supranormal levels. In either case, the end product is hyperglycemia, an elevated concentration of glucose circulating in the bloodstream. If prolonged hyperglycemia is left uncorrected, it may lead to degeneration of nervous and muscle tissue, disorders of the eyes and kidneys, and increased risk of developing cardiovascular disease.

A person whose pancreas does not produce insulin has Type I diabetes and must inject insulin into his or her body. A person whose pancreas still produces insulin but who, for some reason (e.g., obesity or being overfat), still exhibits excessively high blood sugars (normally, blood glucose is between 60 and 140 milligrams per deciliter) has Type II diabetes. These people take insulin, oral medications, or, in some cases, nothing extra at all to keep their blood glucose levels in the normal range.

It has been shown that with good blood glucose control, the disease process leading to secondary complications of diabetes may be reversed and the chances of developing these complications may be reduced. Good control is achieved by taking the right amount of insulin, eating appropriate types and amounts of food, and regular exercise.

The best regular exercise program for the diabetic is, for the most part, the same as one that promotes fitness in the nondiabetic person. It should include flexibility exercises to increase range of motion of joints and decrease the possibility of muscle strains and tears, strength training to increase muscle size and tone, and 20 to 30 minutes of aerobic exercise at the appropriate intensity to stimulate the cardiovascular system.

Some restrictions are placed, though, on the diabetic with uncontrolled hypertension, coronary disease, or certain eye conditions (e.g., retinopathy), in which great changes in blood pressure could damage already weakened blood vessels. This person should refrain from weight lifting or isometric activities that, potentially, could cause body systolic and diastolic pressure to increase too much. Walking, stationary bicycling, stretching, and mild calisthenics performed at the appropriate intensity would be permitted.

The person with diabetes can enjoy the same beneficial effects of regular exercise as his or her nondiabetic friends: decreased heart rate and blood pressure responses to physical work and emotional stress; a lower resting heart rate; and enhanced ability to transport oxygen to, and use oxygen in, working muscles. The combination of glucose control, strength training, and aerobic conditioning also increases the amount of glycogen (packaged carbohydrate) stored in the muscles and liver, offering more "reserve fuel" for emergency situations or when the blood sugar is dropping too low.

Metabolic Response

Most of the concern the diabetic has about exercise, however, has not been with whether there are the same long-term effects of conditioning as for the nondiabetic person, but rather with the unpredictability of his or her own metabolic responses to exercise on a day-to-day basis.

When the nondiabetic exercises, the blood glucose level stays remarkably stable. Uptake of glucose by working muscles is matched by availability of glucose from digested food and through breakdown of stored glycogen into simpler sugar. Since exercise augments the rate at which glucose is removed from the bloodstream, the pancreas virtually shuts off, letting out only tiny amounts of insulin, helping to maintain normoglycemia.

The situation with the diabetic becomes more complex. He or she does not have the luxury of a pancreas that changes its insulin output to adjust glucose levels. The amount of insulin present in the system varies according to when the last insulin injection was given and the type and volume of insulin administered. In general, if there is some "extra" insulin circulating when the diabetic person exercises, his or her blood glucose level does not remain stable, but falls. This is of great use for the diabetic person when the glucose level is a bit high. Without taking an additional injection of insulin, he or she can lower and normalize blood sugar levels.

However, glucose levels are not always the same going into every exercise session. A potential problem arises when the preexercise glucose level is in the lower end of the normal range. Here, even a 2-mile jog could make the blood glucose level uncomfortably low, unless a snack to prevent hypoglycemia is taken before the exercise session. On the other hand, if the preexercise sugar level is too high (greater than 250 milligrams per deciliter), the glucose level may go up even more.

Finally, not all types of exercise have the same effect on blood glucose. Calisthenics, yoga, and stretching do not lower glucose levels appreciably. Weight lifting generally has little effect, occasionally even raising glucose levels if the workout is too stressful. Jogging, bicycling, cross-country skiing, race-walking, and racquetball generally make glucose levels drop considerably.

Impact of Exercise

It is apparent, then, that the runner who has diabetes must be a bit more clever than his or her nondiabetic running friend. The diabetic runner has to be able to predict how glucose levels will respond to a run. The best way for anyone with diabetes to know how individual metabolism is influenced by exercise (or by insulin—or by a given food, for that matter) is to measure its changes. Sugar level of the blood (not urine!) should always be sampled before and after the session. It is a good idea to measure blood glucose in the middle of a session as well—particularly as the runner with diabetes aspires to greater distances, like a 10K run.

Lightweight, portable reagent strips that indicate the glucose concentration of sampled blood are available commercially. Using this method, the uncertainty is removed, hypoglycemic events may be prevented, and appropriate adjustments may be made so training may continue on a regular basis. Most athletes with diabetes find they not only need less insulin coverage going into an exercise session, but throughout the rest of the day as well.

Eventually some athletes want to attempt 15K, 20K, and even marathon runs. This is well within the grasp of the runner with diabetes if he or she takes proper care during training and on the day of the race. As training distances increase, it is wise to increase the number of times blood sugar is sampled until the runner gets a relatively clear picture of new glucose trends. It is also a good idea to get in a habit of carrying snacks in a pocket while running, in case glucose levels fall too much. Raisin-and-nut mixtures, for instance, are good. As the marathon approaches, the runner should experiment by running under conditions similar to those on the day of the race. This way, final adjustments based on the time of the day the race will be run, how much insulin will be in the system, and how long it will take to run the 26 miles may be made.

Race-Day Regimen

On the day of the race, if the diabetic is on an NPH/regular or lente/regular insulin schedule (schedules that combine a short-acting insulin with an intermediate-acting insulin), the short-acting insulin (regular) should be omitted from the morning injection. A small breakfast may be eaten, but it should be low in carbohydrates because there will be no insulin to compensate for the increase in glucose from the meal. The longer-acting dose of insulin should be cut at least in half, because the event itself may last from 3 to 5 hours. If the race is in the morning, and the runner is on an insulin schedule in which he or she takes a longer-acting insulin the night before, the morning injection may be omitted entirely.

During the race the runner should be sure to replenish liquids at least every 10 to 15 minutes. The fluid probably should have a little sugar in the solution, but not too much or it will slow the rate at which water leaves the stomach. The person with diabetes should have verified the effects of these solutions on blood glucose during training.

Last but not least, the diabetic marathoner should have people waiting at the finish line to offer congratulations and to help measure his or her blood sugar.

The importance of the person with diabetes getting blood glucose levels under control can-

not be overemphasized. Such control is not an easy task. It takes much time and effort to learn how to adjust insulin and to understand the composition of different foods and their effects on blood glucose levels. However, the diabetic owes it to him- or herself to get it done. Ultimately, gaining control offers greater freedom to enjoy not only exercise, but all of life as well.

Suggested Reading for "Running With Diabetes"

Jones & Johnson (1981)

See reading list at the end of the book for a complete source listing.

CHAPTER 15

Bone and Joint Factors Affecting Exercise

Bones and their joints, though the hardest elements of the body, are not impervious to assault from trauma, overuse, or other problems that can reduce or destroy their usefulness in certain activities. This chapter examines a few conditions that can adversely affect the bones and joints of the athlete.

Osteoarthritis in Athletes

Paul M. Taylor, D.P.M.

Osteoarthritis is a disorder of the joints that is characterized by a deterioration of the cartilage, and the formation of new bone, at the joint surfaces and around the periphery of the joint. Although this condition is generally associated with the aging process, it can sometimes develop earlier in a joint that has been subjected to acute trauma or repeated stress. Because athletics increase the likelihood of acute injury to a joint, and because there is repeated stress on the joints of the athlete, there is concern that there may be an increased potential for osteoarthritis in the athlete. Studies have shown that a joint that has been injured may develop arthritis. However, it also appears that the normal stresses of athletics—particularly running—do not increase the risk of osteoarthritis.

In a normal joint, there are smooth linings of articular cartilage covering the meeting ends of the bones, allowing for the smooth, gliding motion of the joint. The joint space is also filled with fluid that helps to lubricate the joint (Figure 15.1).

There are a number of synonyms for *osteoarthritis*, including hypertrophic osteoarthritis, degenerative joint disease, old age arthritis, wear and tear arthritis, and osteoarthrosis.

Although the mechanism for the development of osteoarthritis is poorly understood, there are certain chemical and cellular changes that occur within the joint. These lead to a softening and eventual breakdown of the normal cartilage. Defects develop within the cartilage, and thickening of bone and development of bone spurs occur below the joint surface and around the joint (Figure 15.2).

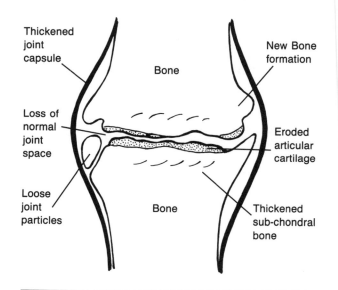

Figure 15.2 Osteoarthritis disrupts the normal, smooth gliding surfaces of a joint and produces irregular bone formation around the joint.

As osteoarthritis continues, physical changes occur, including pain, swelling, crepitus (a grating sound or feeling in the joint), and restriction of motion. Such changes within a joint obviously adversely affect the performance of an athlete.

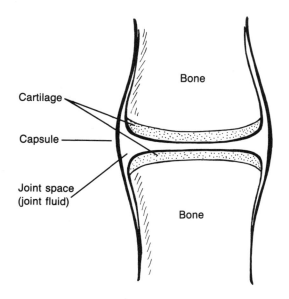

Figure 15.1 Normal configuration of a joint.

Participation in certain sports causes an increased risk of osteoarthritis in certain joints of the athlete. The soccer player is at risk of osteoarthritic changes in the feet and ankles; football players, in the knees and neck; pitchers, in the elbows; and ballet dancers, the big toes.

Osteoarthritis in the athlete sometimes appears to be primarily due to an acute trauma to a joint. This would occur from the knee being injured during football or from repeated injuries to the feet and ankles during soccer. Whenever there has been injury to a joint, internal damage may occur, including damage to the surface of the cartilage; fracture of bone; rupture of ligaments; and, in knee injuries, tearing of the meniscus. When damage occurs, there may be uneven distribution of weight on certain areas of the joint. This results in focal areas of increased stress and eventual development of osteoarthritis. Whenever a joint is subjected to uneven stress, there is increased potential for cartilage damage and osteoarthritis.

This uneven stress can be caused by biomechanical problems, as well as by trauma. Biomechanical imbalance can include such things as a knock-knee problem; this places excessive stress on one side of the knee, with softening of the cartilage and subsequent fraying and gradual osteoarthritic changes. If the kneecap does not track properly over the femur, similar changes can occur. Any joint may be subject to these changes if there is a biomechanical imbalance placing stress upon it.

Normal joints are able to withstand the stresses of athletics because the body has a number of protective mechanisms for them. First, there is a passive mechanism, such as the absorption of shock by the soft tissue in the heel pads and of stress by the bones and ligaments. Second, there is a major shock absorbing mechanism in the active, reflex-controlled stretching of the muscles. As joints move, the related muscles stretch under the slight tension; this helps to relieve the joint of the stress.

Because the body has a number of mechanisms to protect the joints from the normal, repetitive stresses of athletics, it would seem that the primary causes of osteoarthritis in the athlete are trauma and biomechanical imbalances. Situations in which the joint is placed under rapid loading—when the muscles' protective mechanisms are not able to function fast enough—also tend to increase the potential for osteoarthritis. This would seem to indicate that the athlete in a contact sport, in which injury and trauma are likely, has the highest risk for osteoarthritis in particular joints. Sports such as running, in which the shock-absorbing mechanisms are effective, would pose a minimal risk, as long as the athlete has not had a previous injury or a biomechanical imbalance. This does in fact appear to be true; a number of reports have concluded that running or jogging, as long as there is a normal musculoskeletal system, do not cause osteoarthritis.

If the athlete does develop an osteoarthritic joint, treatment should initially include the development of an understanding of the problem and how it affects activity. An appropriate period of rest may be needed to allow the changes within the joint to subside, before subjecting it to additional stress. Any factors that are causing excessive stress on the joint should be corrected. A period of physical therapy and rehabilitation may be necessary. The extent of treatment, including rest, therapy, and rehabilitation, depends on which joint is affected and the degree of involvement. Modifying the type and extent of athletic activity may also be necessary.

In severe cases, medication—either through oral anti-inflammatories or, occasionally, injection of a painful joint—may be needed. If severe osteoarthritis develops, surgical correction is sometimes required. The objectives of short-term treatment should be the relief of pain and of localized stiffness. Long-term goals should be the continued relief of pain and stiffness and the prevention of permanent stiffness or deformity.

Prevention of osteoarthritis in athletes requires careful preparation in order to avoid injury. This includes appropriate training schedules and stretching and strengthening programs. Early and appropriate treatment of any joint injury is essential, as is trying to correct or compensate for any biomechanical imbalances that may impose excess stress on a joint. It is also necessary to avoid stressing an already injured joint. Do not participate when fatigued; fatigued muscles cannot provide enough protection to joints.

Given the increased incidence of osteoarthritis with aging, the athlete who participates a long time in a sport is subject to developing this problem. However, with early recognition and appropriate treatment, it is possible to minimize the adverse effects of osteoarthritis in the athlete.

Suggested Reading for "Osteoarthritis in Athletes"

Hellman et al. (1985)

Hollander (1974)

Lane et al. (1986)

McDermott & Freyne (1983)

Meisel & Bullough (1984)

Panush et al. (1986)

Raskin & Rebecca (1983)

Roy & Irvin (1983)

Sohn & Micheli (1985)

Stulberg (1980)

Yale (1984)

See reading list at the end of the book for a complete source listing.

Fractures and Dislocations

Paul M. Taylor, D.P.M.

Fractures and dislocations are acute injuries that are due to physical trauma. A *fracture* is a break in the continuity of a bone; it may be either an open or closed fracture. In a closed fracture, the skin remains intact; in an open fracture, the skin has been broken. A *dislocation* is an injury of a joint in which the normal alignment of the joint has been disrupted. It is possible to sustain a fracture-dislocation, where there is a fracture of a bone as well as the dislocation of an adjacent joint (Figures 15.3, 15.4, and 15.5).

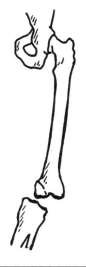

Figure 15.5 This bone is fractured at the end, with a dislocation of the joint.

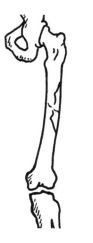

Figure 15.3 This bone is fractured at the mid-point, without displacement.

With a fracture or a dislocation, the athlete has pain and is unable to move the injured area. In some cases, the body has a protective mechanism in which there is minimal pain immediately after the injury; but the pain begins to increase gradually. Swelling and bruising also increase after the injury. With some mild, nondisplaced fractures, the athlete can move the injured area. Therefore, it should not be assumed that an injury has not resulted in a fracture just because the athlete still has movement.

With any suspected fracture or dislocation, emergency medical help should be summoned and first aid provided. Do not move the patient. Control any bleeding and dress the wounds. If emergency medical help is expected shortly, it is best just to keep the individual still and comfortable until the help arrives. If help is going to be delayed, or if the person must be moved, immobilize the affected area. The injured area can be splinted with wood, cardboard, or even rolled-up magazines, supported with ties of cloth. Avoid moving any area that is suspected of being fractured or dislocated.

Once the patient reaches the hospital, x-rays determine the extent of the injury. If there is

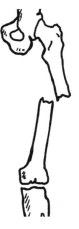

Figure 15.4 This bone is fractured with displacement.

no displacement, the area can be protected with a cast. If displaced, the fracture has to be realigned through manipulation, then set with a cast. On some occasions, these measures do not provide adequate correction; surgery to reposition and internally fixate the bone fragments may be necessary.

Any broken bone or dislocation is a serious injury. Any injury in which there is a suspected fracture or dislocation should receive immediate medical attention.

Suggested Reading for "Fractures and Dislocations"

Shonds & Raney (1967)

See reading list at the end of the book for a complete source listing.

Osteochondral Fractures

Paul M. Taylor, D.P.M.

An osteochondral fracture is an injury to a joint resulting in a break or fracture through the articular cartilage and a portion of the bone (*osteo*, bone; *chondral*, cartilage). Articular cartilage is the smooth lining over the end of a bone forming part of the joint. An osteochondral fracture is usually caused by an acute injury to a joint, such as twisting a knee or spraining an ankle. The sudden force on the joint can cause a bone fracture that can extend into the cartilage. As another mechanism of injury, a pulling on the cartilage can cause it to tear and pull away a portion of the bone, causing a fracture (Figure 15.6).

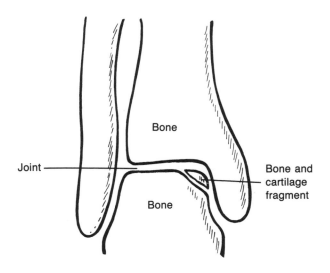

Figure 15.6 An osteochondral fracture may leave a fragment of bone in the joint.

Because of the force needed to create this injury, the symptoms make the seriousness of the injury immediately apparent. There is immediate pain and inability to bear weight or move the injured part. Bleeding into the joint and swelling around the joint develop quickly. X-rays after the injury may show the fracture to the bone; however, cartilage does not show on x-rays, so sometimes the extent of the injury is not immediately apparent.

When this injury is recognized early, the treatment depends on the joint involved and the extent of the fracture. If a bone or cartilage fragment is evident in a large joint, such as the hip or knee, surgery may be necessary to pin the fragment in place. If there is only a small fragment, but it is loose in the joint, the fragment is removed. If the fracture fragments are in good alignment, or if a smaller joint is involved, treatment with a non-weight-bearing cast may be used.

In some injuries, the osteochondral fracture is not evident on x-rays because cartilage does not show and the fracture of the bone may be hidden by other parts of the joint. In cases where the nature of the injury and the symptoms indicate a fracture may be present, additional tests—including special x-ray views, arthrograms (injecting dye into the joint to give better detail on x-rays), bone scans, and, possibly, arthroscopic surgery—are needed to identify the fracture. (Arthroscopy involves inserting fiber-optic lenses via a needle to see the inside of a joint.) If fragments are found during this time, it is possible to remove some of them using special surgical techniques.

Despite the various diagnostic techniques, occasionally an osteochondral fracture is not identified. This omission can happen with an injury to any joint. It presents problems later because if the fracture does not heal properly, it can cause irritation or rubbing inside the joint, which can lead to arthritis. This type of injury should be suspected when the athlete continues to have pain and swelling in a joint after an injury for a much longer than normal time. If the athlete has suffered an ankle sprain or twisted knee and continues to have pain and swelling for more than 2 or 3 months, an osteochondral fracture should be suspected, and the testing—including the arthrogram, bone scan, computerized axial tomography, and arthroscopy—should be repeated.

Treatment for an osteochondral fracture that is diagnosed late includes rest, modifying the level of activity, physical therapy, oral and injectable anti-inflammatories, immobilization, and, if the joint does not improve, surgical repair.

Osteochondral fractures are generally acute injuries and require immediate treatment. However, in a few cases, the injury is not recognized early, and later problems or continued pain may occur. With either scenario, there may be permanent injury in the joint, with some loss of function. This can be minimized by early diagnosis, appropriate treatment, and adequate physical therapy and rehabilitation.

Suggested Reading for "Osteochondral Fractures"

Hopkinson et al. (1985)

Irvin et al. (1985)

Israeli et al. (1981)

Naumetz & Schweisel (1980)

Thompson & Loomer (1984)

See reading list at the end of the book for a complete source listing.

Myositis Ossificans

Paul M. Taylor, D.P.M.

Myositis ossificans is a rare condition in which calcification develops in a muscle following an injury. The mechanism of the injury is that the athlete sustains an initial injury to a muscle, such as a muscle pull or a direct blow to the muscle. This causes bleeding within the muscle belly and development of a hematoma (a blood clot within the muscle). The normal physiological response of the body would be gradual absorption of the hematoma and repair of the muscle. Unfortunately, in a few cases, the body responds abnormally: The clot is gradually replaced with calcified, or bony, tissue. This bony formation within the muscle (myositis ossificans) interferes with the normal function and motion of the muscle and may be painful with activity.

The best prevention of myositis ossificans is early and appropriate treatment of any muscle injury. If the problem does develop, treatment requires rest until the ossification process has been completed, which can be determined only by x-rays. This process may take several months to over a year. Once the ossification has matured, if it continues to be painful or to interfere with normal function, surgical removal of the ossification may be necessary.

Fortunately, myositis ossificans is not a common problem. It can usually be avoided by proper treatment of muscle injuries. When it does occur, though, medical care with careful follow-up is necessary.

Suggested Reading for "Myositis Ossificans"

Nicholas & Reilly (1985)
Shonds & Raney (1967)

See reading list at the end of the book for a complete source listing.

CHAPTER 16

———

Developmental Factors Affecting Children's Exercise

Many adults have recognized the benefits of exercise. Should children be encouraged to develop similar exercise habits? Do children receive enough exercise through normal play, school physical education, and organized sports?

According to the National Children and Youth Fitness Study, sponsored by the U.S. Department of Health and Human Services: "approximately half of the American children and youth in grades 5 through 12 do not perform the minimum weekly requirement of vigorous physical activity needed to maintain an effectively functioning cardiorespiratory system" (Ross, Dotson, & Gilbert, 1985, p. 85). The activity level considered the minimum in this study was defined as "exercise which involves large muscle groups in dynamic movement for periods of 20 minutes or longer, three or more times a week, and which is performed at an intensity requiring 60 percent or greater of an individual's cardiorespiratory capacity" (Ross et al., 1985, p. 83).

Accepting the premise that "appropriate physical activity may be a valuable tool in therapeutic regimens for control and amelioration (rehabilitation) of obesity, coronary heart disease, hypertension, diabetes, musculoskeletal problems, respiratory diseases, stress, and depression and anxiety" (Ross et al., 1985, p. 82), should efforts be made to increase the level of exercise among children? It would appear that more children should be encouraged to exercise and to develop appropriate lifetime physical activities. These activities should also be continued on a year-round basis.

These activities are available to children through a number of sources. These would include free play, physical education classes, community programs, and the family. The benefit of free play in fitness is difficult to determine, because of the variation of the levels of physical exercise among different children at play. Physical education classes may not always provide enough time or their activities may not provide adequate cardiorespiratory stimulus. However, this time can be used to teach appropriate techniques and to emphasize the importance of lifetime physical activity. Community programs—particularly in organized sports that provide activity that maintains an effectively functioning cardiorespiratory system—help meet these fitness goals if the programs are performed frequently enough. The family should also consider opportunities to provide additional exercise. This may include any number of physical activities, such as walking, hiking, jogging, biking, or any other activity that can be included in the family routine.

By using a variety of these sources, a much greater percentage of children can become involved in appropriate physical activity.

It does appear that increasing the exercise levels among children is beneficial. However, certain precautions should be taken. Children are not adults, and they should not be expected to perform at an adult level. Children exercise at a level closer to their maximum capacity and may not be as aware of fatigue as adults are. They are also more prone to heat injury because of their higher proportion of skin surface area to body volume when compared to adults. They also have different levels of endurance and are subject to injuries unique to children, such as epiphyseal fractures and osteochondrosis. Any of these problems can be avoided through adequate supervision.

The little league syndrome should also be avoided. This occurs when adults over-emphasize winning and encourage children to compete at a level for which they are not emotionally or physically prepared. In reference to organized sports, Dr. J.J. Gugenheim (1985) has suggested,

> We must establish sports programs that are appropriate for the physical and psychological levels of development. From age 6 to 10, we should foster an emphasis on awakening interest in sports, having fun, learning basic skills, and socialization. There should be reinforcement of positive results with compliments and rewards, not comparing performance between children. From 11 to 14 years, the emphasis should be on developing versatility, proper techniques, and tolerance for increased training. Highly organized sports before age 12 retard spontaneity and probably lead to early burnout. During age 15 to 18, we should emphasize an increased training such as strength and/or endurance or individual sports and begin extensive competition. (p. 5)

Through play, physical education classes, community activities and the family, children should be encouraged to develop lifetime physical activities. However, children should be properly supervised in exercise. Also, they should not be so forced into exercise that it becomes a negative, rather than a positive, experience.

Suggested Reading for "Developmental Factors Affecting Children's Exercise"

Gugenheim (1985)

See reading list at the end of the book for a complete source listing.

Endurance and Pubertal Development

Alan Rogol, M.D., Ph.D.

The child is not a scaled-down adult. Thinking of one as such would make medical science easier and pediatrics obsolete, but it is just not the case. In fact, the child is much different in almost every way from the grown-up. He or she is at, or near, the beginning of a developmental period that will take his or her mind and body through tremendous changes, eventually landing on the far side of puberty as an adult.

If the child is different from the adult, the adolescent is *very* different. It is during puberty that the child grows most rapidly, at a rate second only to the first 2 years of life. Normal growth averages between 2 and 3 inches per year from age 2 to the beginning of puberty, which usually begins between 8 and 13. However, during puberty, which usually lasts 5 or so years from its onset, the adolescent may grow anywhere from 2 to 6 inches per year.

Puberty is also the beginning of organized athletic activity for many children. The middle-school- or junior-high-aged child becomes involved for the first time in such often intense sports competition as running, swimming, soccer, gymnastics, and any number of other aerobic activities. Recent studies have shown that intense participation in these endurance-type activities before or during puberty may interfere with pubertal development in girls as well as boys. Although the evidence is certainly not all in, it appears that this disturbance, if there is any at all, has little or no long-term effects on the adolescent-turned-adult.

Normal Growth

One important measure of pubertal development is statural growth, or height measurement. The rate of growth, or growth velocity, is a much more important measure of normal growth during puberty than height at any certain age. In fact, there is no specific entity called "normal growth," but rather a statistically defined range that is considered normal for any child. Some children may begin puberty at 9, others at 12; once begun, though, it is a relatively orderly process. Only deviations from this orderly rate of growth are considered abnormal.

The child's growth pattern is the result of a complex interaction of genetic potential, nutritional and psychological factors, and the presence of specific diseases that may hinder the process. Only after all these factors are taken into account can an explanation of a specific growth pattern be made.

Normal growth rate after puberty has begun is 2.5 inches per year. Growth over 6, or under 2, inches per year is considered abnormal. Minimum normal growth between 2 and 12 is usually accepted as 2 inches per year. After puberty, from the beginning of adulthood onward, little or no change in height is experienced.

Adolescent Sexual Development

The most common method of observing adolescent sexual development is to keep a close watch on growth of pubic hair. Once puberty has begun, this growth continues uninterrupted in the normal child.

Five stages of pubic hair growth have been identified by James Tanner, M.D.: (a) prepubertal—no pubic hair; (b) sparse growth of long, slightly pigmented hair; (c) further darkening and coarsening of hair, with spreading over the pubic area; (d) pubic hair adult in character, but not in distribution—it has not yet spread to the inner thighs; and (e) adult pubic hair, with growth extending to the inner thighs.

Along with pubic hair growth, Tanner and his associates have also plotted breast development in girls and testicular development in boys. Although these three factors develop independently of the others, several rules of thumb help identify normal growth. For example, normal testicular enlargement in boys usually begins any time between 9.5 and 13.5 years of age. With girls, breast budding—

the first elevation of the breast area—normally begins between the ages of 8 and 13. Both of these are the first outward indications of the beginning of puberty.

These structural changes are the visible signs of rising levels of sex hormones in developing children. Some of these indications, such as growth spurts and beginning of menstruation, may seem to occur at abnormal times; in fact, they are perfectly normal. The growth spurt in boys happens relatively later in puberty than it does in girls, and most girls have their first menstrual period late in puberty, well after their greatest growth rate.

Exercise and Pubertal Development

Irregularities in reproductive system function and growth due to intense exercise may occur in either boys or girls, and the best indication is a slowing down of the normal pubertal development process. This is usually noticed as an unusually long time for a child to pass through height, genital, breast, or pubic hair developmental stages.

Preliminary studies show that boys who reduce their intake of calories in weight-related sports, such as wrestling, experience reduced growth during the competitive season. None of these studies shows any slowing of sexual maturation during this time, however. During the off-season, when boys once again eat normally, growth resumes—sometimes more rapidly than normal, seemingly to make up for lost time. The long-term effects of reduced eating during puberty among boys on ultimate height development is not known but are probably minimal, in light of the many weight-class participants who continue with competition into adulthood.

Determining the effects of exercise on development in boys is difficult because most male sports require strength and speed—normally attained only well into puberty and beyond. Because of this, most boys begin strenuous activity after they enter adolescence. Effects of exercise on girls are easier to study because pubertal development does not confer an advantage in many sports. In fact, sports such as gymnastics and ballet often necessitate a lean and flexible prepubertal body configuration.

Developmental Studies

In a study published in the early 1970s, it was shown that female track athletes had later first periods (menarche) than a more sedentary control group, and that Olympic women athletes experienced menarche later than high school or college athletes. These observations must be taken with caution, however. The obvious conclusion is that training and competition caused a later onset of menarche, but it may also be true that the athletic physiques of the women runners, not the training itself, predisposed them to later first periods.

The reason for delayed puberty and slower growth among women athletes during competition is currently being debated in the medical community. Dr. Rose Frisch of Harvard University has cited low body weight and a low percentage of body fat as the main reason for reproductive system dysfunction in women. A similar case has been presented for reduced numbers of periods or lack of periods in adult women involved in intense aerobic exercise.

It is now apparent that the body weight/body fat hypothesis is not the sole reason for menstrual system irregularities. In two well-documented studies, most long-distance runners who had fewer menstrual periods than normal women were above Dr. Frisch's critical weight or body fat percentages, but they simply did not menstruate regularly.

Michelle Warren, M.D., assistant professor in the Department of Obstetrics and Gynecology, St. Luke's Roosevelt Hospital, New York City, recently studied a number of ballet dancers who had either never menstruated or menstruated at irregular, prolonged intervals. Although most remained below the critical weight or body fat level necessary according to the Frisch hypothesis, they began to menstruate at the same low body weight if they stopped their high intensity aerobic activity. The reason for this is not known, but it seems to hint that intensity of activity, or energy drain, and not just body fat and weight, plays a major role in menstrual irregularities.

Although the long-term consequences of such intense exercise loads are not precisely known, a large number of dancers and runners have borne children either during or following a major decrease in the quantity and quality of their exercise. Dr. Warren has also shown that young women dancers rapidly progress through puberty or have their first periods when forced to stop exercising (usually due to an injury)—again, without change in body weight or body fat.

Dr. Frisch also studied women swimmers and runners who trained intensively before puberty and found they had delayed onset of puberty when compared to women who began training after puberty. She noted a 0.4-year delay in menarche for every year of prepubertal training. The implication here is that puberty was delayed because of the early onset of training, but again, these young swimmers and runners may have already been predisposed to late puberty.

Many women athletes who succcessfully pass through menarche may notice irregularities in menstrual bleeding patterns—either amenorrhea (lack of periods) or oligomenorrhea (fewer than six periods in 12 months). These may be due to the amount of training each week, the intensity of the training, or both, although there is no conclusive evidence to pinpoint any cause.

Endurance-type exercise is only one, but a major, factor that places stress on the developing and mature female reproductive system. Although the result is often oligomenorrhea or amenorrhea, the underlying causes are still not known. In addition to energy drain, length of exercise, body weight, and body fat, other factors—such as diet, nutrition, and the physiological effects of stress from training or other sources—must be considered. The more young women we see, the more we realize that menstrual system dysfunction and pubertal development irregularities may have a variety of causes.

Suggestions

Any developmental irregularities in the child should be referred to a medical professional. Parents who notice delayed development in their child and who can find no reason for it other than involvement in sports should feel assured that the condition is most likely reversible.

The first step in reestablishing normal development is to reduce the amount of exercise. With boys, the off-season normally takes care of any catching up they have to do. The amount of exercise a girl's system can tolerate while still developing normally varies widely. Some can maintain 50-mile training weeks and develop regularly; others may need to stop exercising entirely. Only experimentation can determine the correct amount of exercise.

"Should my child exercise at all?" is a question often asked. The answer is an overwhelming yes, under one condition—that he or she must want to. The child has an amazing capacity to do what he or she can and then stop when rest is needed. It is the parents, more often than not, who interfere with this natural process of stress and rest. There is still no better example of the perfect animal than the nine-year-old at play who runs, then plays under a tree for a while, then eats until full, then goes to bed for a good night's sleep—and he or she doesn't even call it exercise!

Epiphyseal Injuries

Wayne B. Leadbetter, M.D.

The epiphysis is a growth center of a bone. As such, only growing persons have epiphyses. Because different bones cease growing at different ages, a child may have some bones that have reached maturity and some that have not. There are technically two types of growth centers: epiphyses, which are found at the ends of bones and are responsible for longitudinal growth of the bone, especially in the legs; and apophyses, which are found at the attachments of muscles and do not contribute to longitudinal growth, but accommodate that growth and allow for the muscle and tendon attachments to keep up with growth. Both epiphyses and apophyses cease to grow upon maturity, which occurs normally at 16 in girls and 18 in boys.

There has been much attention focused on the risks to the growth centers of children playing sports, primarily because of the attention attracted by the phenomenon of little league elbow. Although it is possible to have injuries due to repetitive loading and trauma to growth centers in the legs from running or in the arms from throwing, these are not serious or prevalent.

On the other hand, some of the most dramatic and serious injuries in children do involve growth centers. These centers are affected by the strong pull of growing and enlarging muscles and by the great forces applied there when the child's growth is rapid. This rapid growth causes dynamic changes in leverage on arms and legs. The growth centers also receive stress when children play competitive sports.

The most common epiphyseal injury seen is the broken wrist, which typically involves the displacement of the epiphysis of the radius (forearm bone) from a blow or fall. Repetitive activities, such as throwing, have been shown in rare cases to produce an actual stretching of the growth center, especially in the upper arm, near the shoulder. This can actually lead to a slightly longer throwing arm upon maturity if childhood activity was intense. Professional baseball players and tennis players often have this characteristic, which has never been shown to be detrimental.

Running has not been shown to be of great harm to growth centers in the legs, but this remains a subject of research. There have been no studies confirming stunting of growth because of running activity. The significance of injury to the epiphysis is that whereas the vast majority of growth centers can be treated effectively, a small proportion are complicated by alterations or cessation in growth, resulting in disturbance in the eventual length of the bone. This is notoriously true of the knee and hip, where injuries can result in a leg length discrepancy that may have to be corrected as the child grows older.

Injuries to growth centers also produce potential angulation deformities, especially about the elbow and ankle, which result in either noticeable cosmetic deformity or alterations in function, requiring later correction. For these reasons, epiphyseal injuries are carefully treated and any trauma to a child resulting in persistent pain, swelling, or inability to play should necessitate an x-ray.

Apophyses are more often injured by repetitive stress activities, such as throwing or running, in which muscle attachments are stressed so much that they can pull apart from the bone (the classic example is Osgood Schlatter's condition of the knee). These injuries about the heel, knee, hip, and elbow in the young athlete cause pain and tenderness to palpation as well as a change in function. X-rays reveal a widening or stretching apart of the attachment of the tendon to the bone and signal a necessity for protection or rest for recovery and healing. Occasionally, the apophysis is pulled completely off and requires reattachment, but, fortunately, this is rare. The "growing pains" of children are often due to the pain of apophyseal injury.

Pads and arch supports for the heel, braces and strengthening for the knee, and conditioning programs for the upper extremity are useful, along with local icing and alterations in intensity of play. These should control the apophyseal complaints and allow for the child's successful participation in sports. As the child's growth slows down or ceases, apophyseal pains and problems disappear.

Studies have revealed that the incidence of serious epiphyseal injury is low, and the occurrence of serious apophyseal injuries is also rare. Therefore, concern for growth center damage should not be an inhibition to children's participation in sports.

Suggested Reading for "Epiphyseal Injuries"

Caine & Linder (1985)

Gregg & Das (1982)

Harvey (1982, 1983)

Smith & Reischl (1986)

Tursz & Crost (1986)

See reading list at the end of the book for a complete source listing.

Osteochondrosis
(Osteochondritis Dissecans; Apophysitis)

Mark E. Julsrud, D.P.M.

Osteochondrosis is a disease of the growth, or ossification, centers of bones in children. It begins as a degeneration or necrosis (areas of dead bone), followed by repair through regeneration and recalcification. It is theorized that some degree of trauma is needed to initiate the bone compaction, destruction, and changed architecture seen on x-rays in osteochondrosis. The fact that the spine and lower limbs are chiefly affected indicates the importance of trauma during the transmission of minor stress and weight bearing.

In growing bone, the development of the epiphysis, or growth center, is mainly cartilaginous and, therefore, most susceptible to the osteochondrotic process. The bony epiphysis grows rapidly; thus, the cells are also vulnerable to generalized hormonal or nutritional changes. When there are added mechanical pressures applied to the growing bone, the changes of osteochondrosis may occur. These changes are even more likely to occur when there is a delayed appearance of ossification centers—as often seen in Köhler's disease, in which the relatively fragile navicular bone of the foot appears late and is at risk between the normally developing talus and cuneiforms.

Most osteochondroses occur in early childhood around the so-called midgrowth spurt. Others, such as Osgood-Schlatter's disease, occur during puberty, the time of the adolescent growth spurt.

With the exception of Freiberg's disease, which affects the metatarsal heads, osteochondrosis is far more common in boys than girls. This fundamental constitutional difference between the sexes probably stems from the delayed appearance and maturation of secondary growth centers in males. In addition, boys' bodies are probably subjected to more trauma and stress in early childhood. Many affected persons are below average in height and relatively undersized at the end of skeletal growth.

It was not until the turn of the century that osteochondrosis was described as a discrete entity. Probably the earliest such descriptions were those of Osgood, an American orthopedist, and Schlatter, a Swiss surgeon; in 1903, these two doctors independently published articles on osteochondrosis of the tibial tubercle (knee). Listed in Table 16.1 are the eponyms and the anatomical areas of the most common osteochondroses.

Many of the osteochondroses seen in the adolescent are referred to as *apophysitis* or *nonarticular osteochondrosis*, meaning that, rather than a joint being involved, the traumatic component mainly appears to be traction at a tendon or ligament insertion into bone. Fragmentation or avulsion (separation) of cartilage at the point of attachment, disruption of cartilage production, attempts at repair by forming new bone, and thickening of fibrous tissue account for the changes seen on x-ray. Clinical signs of pain, tenderness, and swelling are usually well localized to the involved area.

A decrease of the normal pressure or traction on the apophysis may result in slowing of bone growth, whereas excessive forces may result in disorderly growth. Trauma, coupled with poorly understood constitutional factors that make some youngsters more vulnerable than others, appears to play a large role in the apophyseal osteochondrosis. Mechanical disruption of the normal bone growth may be evident as microfractures that do not heal, stemming from repeated trauma, calcification at tendon and ligament attachments, and the irregularity, fragmentation, mottling, and enlargement seen on x-rays.

Treatment generally requires only a reduced level of activity until symptoms subside. Ice massage to the affected area relieves pain and swelling. Oral anti-inflammatories may occasionally be needed. In severe cases, complete rest and, occasionally, cast immobilization are necessary. The condition is self-limiting, with full healing at the completion of the growth period. In some cases, there may be residual

Table 16.1 Location of Common Osteochondrosis and the Person for Whom They Are Named (Eponyms)

Eponym	Location
Blount	Tibia, proximal
Brailsford	Radius, head
Buchman	Iliac crest
Burns	Ulna, distal
Buschke	Cuneiform
Calvé	Spine, vertebral body
Diaz	Talus (astragalus)
Felix	Femur, lesser trochanter
Freiberg	Second metatarsal head
Friedrich	Clavicle
Froehlich	Humeral condyles
Haglund	Tarsal navicular, accessory
Hass	Humeral head
Iselin	Fifth metatarsal base
Kienboeck	Carpal lunate (semilunar)
Köhler	Patellar center, primary
Köhler's second	Tarsal navicular (scaphoid)
Legg	Humeral epicondyle, internal
Legg-Calvé-Perthes	Femoral capital epiphysis
Lewin	Tibia, distal
Mandl-Buchman	Femur, greater trochanter
Mauclaire	Metacarpal head
Monde-Felix	Femur, lesser trochanter
Mouchet	Talus (astragalus)
Oldberg	Ischiopubic junction
Osgood-Schlatter	Tibial tuberosity
Panner	Humeral head
Perthes	Femoral capital epiphysis
Pierson	Symphysis pubis
Preiser	Carpal scaphoid
Ritter	Fibular head
Schaefer	Radius, proximal
Scheuermann	Spine, marginal
Schlatter	Tibial tuberosity
Sever	Calcaneal apophysis
Sinding-Larsen-Johansson	Patellar center, second
Thiemann	Phalanges
Treves	Sesamoids
Valtancoli	Ischial tuberosity
Van Neck	Ischiopubic junction
Waldenstroem	Femoral capital epiphysis

irregularity and prominence of the bone, which does not, however, interfere with joint or muscle function or influence the growth and length of the bone itself.

Osteochondrosis can affect any of the bone growth centers in the body. The treatment is basically the same; however, certain areas require special limitations of activity and modifications in the level of activity, as well as specific strengthening exercises. When osteochondrosis does not respond to initial treatment, a sportsmedicine specialist should be consulted.

Suggested Reading for "Osteochondrosis (Osteochondritis Dissecans; Apophysitis)"

Gregg & Das (1982)

Harvey (1982, 1983)

Julsrud (1985)

Kujala et al. (1985)

Orava & Virtanen (1982)

Orava et al. (1982)

Tursz & Crost (1986)

See reading list at the end of the book for a complete source listing.

CHAPTER 17

First Aid

Anyone who participates in sports is going to receive minor injuries. These may include such things as blisters, sprains, bruises, and lacerations. The athlete should be prepared to apply first aid to these minor injuries. This section deals with how to prepare for and help prevent these injuries. Detailed description about how to treat each injury is covered in the injuries chapters (part II).

First aid consists of being prepared to provide emergency care when an injury or sudden illness occurs. The purpose of first aid is to protect the injured person until professional help can be obtained. In some cases of minor injuries, first aid may be the definitive treatment. In life-threatening emergencies such as heatstroke or heart attack, first aid involves stabilizing the condition of the person and keeping him or her alive until professional help arrives.

Cardiopulmonary resuscitation (CPR) and the Heimlich maneuver are emergency techniques with which everyone should be familiar. CPR is used to maintain blood flow and breathing in a person who has suffered a cardiac or respiratory arrest. The Heimlich maneuver is used to dislodge an obstruction in the airway of a choking victim. Learning CPR and staying current through refresher courses may help you save the life of a fellow athlete or a family member from a heart attack or an injury-provoked cardiac or respiratory arrest.

Cardiac arrest and choking are life-threatening situations for which immediate treatment is necessary; there is not enough time to wait for medical assistance. It is essential that everyone becomes familiar with these two techniques. It is not possible to teach either of these methods in this book—they must be

demonstrated and practiced. The routine of administering CPR should be learned in a course, allowing for supervised practice. Anyone who is active in athletics should complete the basic life support course. Almost every community offers this course through the local heart association, Red Cross chapter, or fire department.

In order to be prepared to provide first aid when these injuries occur, you should keep a first aid kit at home; also, a smaller kit is helpful for travel or for taking to your athletic events. The materials in both kits should be checked periodically and replaced as they become outdated.

The American Medical Association's *Handbook of First Aid and Emergency Care* recommends that the following items be kept available in the home:

- Roll of gauze bandage
- Sterile gauze pads
- Band-Aids®
- Butterfly bandages
- Roll of adhesive tape (1-inch)
- Scissors
- 3-inch elastic bandage
- Cotton-tipped swabs
- Absorbent cotton
- Aspirin
- Children's aspirin*
- Oral and rectal thermometers
- Petroleum jelly (for use with rectal thermometer)
- Syrup of ipecac (to induce vomiting)
- Tweezers

---

*Recent studies have linked aspirin taken by children to Reye's syndrome, so check with your pediatrician before giving aspirin to children.

- Safety pins
- Hydrogen peroxide (3% solution)
- Calamine lotion
- Bar of plain soap
- Flashlight
- Snakebite kit (especially for camping)

The athlete may also add moleskin, antibiotic ointment, a paper clip (see chapter 4 on "Black Toenails"), alcohol swabs (prepackaged), and an ice bag.

Because the above items would fill a large box, which would be rather cumbersome to carry, a smaller travel first aid kit should be prepared. The following list of items should fit in a small shaving kit and cover most first aid needs during traveling:

- Roll of gauze bandage
- Sterile gauze pads (individually wrapped)
- Band-aids®
- Adhesive tape (1-inch)
- Small scissors
- 3-inch elastic bandage
- Tweezers
- Safety pins
- Moleskin
- Tube of triple antibiotic ointment
- Paper clip
- Alcohol swabs (individually wrapped)
- 25 cents (to make a call in an emergency)

These suggested kits should be modified to meet your individual needs or the needs of any member of your family.

Certain preventive measures should also be taken by the athlete who runs or participates in sports away from home. One simple measure is to always carry identification. At least carry an ID card that gives your name, address, and the phone number to reach in an emergency. This can be carried in a pocket or in an ID pouch attached to the shoe. This would allow emergency medical personnel to contact your family in case of an injury. If you have any medical problems, you should carry an emergency medical ID. In fact, you should carry this with you all the time. This can provide any important medical history, including allergies, present illnesses, contact lens use, medications, and blood type.

Most people feel that injuries happen only to someone else, but sports activity increases the risk for minor injuries and, in some cases, serious injuries. These injuries can best be handled by your being prepared ahead of time to treat them. Having a first aid kit available and always having identification are two simple ways of preparing for any injury. Anyone who is involved in athletics should have a basic understanding of first aid. The best way to develop this knowledge is through completion of certified basic first aid courses. These are generally offered in the community through various organizations, such as the American Red Cross. It is recommended that everyone complete such a course and continue with recertification courses, in order to be prepared when first aid skills are needed.

Suggested Reading for "First Aid"

American Medical Association (1980)

Good Housekeeping (1980)

Kunz (1982)

See reading list at the end of the book for a complete source listing.

Minor Wound Care
(Cuts; Abrasions; Splinters)

Paul M. Taylor, D.P.M.

Frequently during athletic participation, minor wounds occur. These may involve various cuts, abrasions, and splinters. When these wounds are of a minor nature, appropriate local treatment should allow rapid healing.

Proper wound care requires controlling any initial bleeding, followed with a dressing. When a cut in the skin occurs, apply a clean dressing and light pressure until the bleeding stops. The best dressing is a sterile gauze pad; if this is not available, use a clean handkerchief or small towel. If you cannot control the bleeding within several minutes, or if the cut exposes the fatty layer under the skin, immediate medical attention is needed, because suturing of the wound (stitches) may be necessary. If the bleeding is controlled, and the wound does not appear to be deep, clean the area around the cut with soap and water, without rubbing over the wound. Apply a dry dressing. Do not apply topical antibiotics when initially treating the wound.

For an abrasion—the top layer of the skin is scraped off by rubbing against a rough surface—the treatment is the same as for minor wounds. If there is dirt in the abrasion, you can remove it by lightly brushing off the area, but do not attempt to remove deeply imbedded foreign material. Again, clean the area around the wound and apply a dry dressing.

Remove such foreign bodies in the superficial layers of skin as splinters with a needle or tweezers that has been cleansed in alcohol. Clean the area and cover it with a dry dressing. When a foreign body penetrates below the skin, apply a dressing and obtain medical help.

Deep puncture wounds, such as from stepping on a nail, require special attention. This type of wound may appear to be minor because of the small hole and minimal bleeding. However, because dirt and bacteria may have been pushed into the deeper tissue layers, a potentially serious infection could develop. If there is any question at all that an object may be under the skin, medical treatment should be obtained.

With any wound, especially puncture wounds, there is potential for tetanus infection. Keep immunizations against this problem current. If there is any doubt, obtain information related to the need for additional boosters from the family physician.

Most minor wounds heal well following self-treatment. However, if there is any question that a foreign object may remain in the wound, or if any signs of infection (pain, redness, swelling, drainage) develop, medical attention is necessary. With any type of wound, if there is increasing pain, redness, swelling, continued bleeding, or any drainage, immediate medical attention is needed.

Sunburn

Gabe Mirkin, M.D.

Beware of excessive exposure to sunlight when you exercise. A single exposure can cause your skin to burn. Repeated exposures can cause aging, wrinkling—and even cancer.

Even on hazy days, you can be exposed to significant amounts of sunlight. The sun's rays are reflected off clouds, buildings, trees, and even the ground.

When you exercise, try to protect your skin from direct exposure to sunlight. White clothing reflects the sun's rays more effectively than dark clothing and tends to be more effective in preventing overheating. However, when it comes to blocking the sun's rays, the weave of the cloth is far more important than color. A porous weave can permit more than 50 percent of the sun's rays to pass through. On the other hand, a tight weave can block all of the sun's rays.

Most of the sunscreens on the market contain the chemical PABA, which does not block all of the sun's rays. However, a combination of PABA and zinc oxide *does* block all of the sun's rays and has the added advantage of not being washed off by perspiration.

Don't depend on pain to tell when to get out of the sun. You won't even find out that you have a sunburn until after your skin has already been burned. The pain from a sunburn is caused by the delayed release of certain chemicals called *prostaglandins* by the damaged cells. Because aspirin and other anti-arthritis drugs prevent the formation of prostaglandins, they are effective in stopping the pain of sunburn. If you are uncomfortable from a sunburn, you can take three adult aspirin tablets; repeat this dosage in 6 hours. However, people who have excessive stomach acidity (as evidenced by belching, a burning pain in the stomach that is alleviated by eating, a sour taste in the mouth, mouth odor, or a white coating on the tongue) and those who are allergic to aspirin should avoid this medication.

Here are some tips to help prevent sun damage:

Avoid exercising outdoors on hot summer days between 10 a.m. and 2 p.m. Sunlight is most intense when the sun is directly overhead. This occurs around noon.

If you have lightly pigmented skin, try to cover your face and the back of your hands when you go out in the sun. People who have light-colored skin are the ones who are most susceptible to developing aging and skin cancer upon exposure to sunlight. The areas that are most likely to be damaged are the face, top of the ears, and the backs of the hands. So, wear a hat and use PABA-containing sunscreens on your hands and face.

Skin Infections
(Pyoderma; Folliculitis; Boils; Carbuncles)

Gabe Mirkin, M.D.

If you develop crusted areas on your skin or small blisters filled with a yellow fluid, check with your doctor. You probably have an infection that can be cured easily by taking the appropriate antibiotic. Such skin infections (pyoderma) develop when there is a break in the skin and bacteria invade the tissues. These areas may itch; by your scratching, the infection can be spread to wider areas of the skin. Hair follicles may become infected (folliculitis); if the infection advances deep into the hair follicle, a furuncle (boil) may develop. If not treated properly, this infection may extend to other hair follicles, causing multiple drainage sites of infection—a carbuncle.

If you develop recurrent skin infections, ask your doctor to do a nasal culture for bacteria. The chances are that you are carrying a *Staph aureus* germ there, even though you may have no nasal symptoms whatsoever. Years ago, it was almost impossible to clear this germ from the nose. Now, such infections can be cured by taking a combination of two prescription medications, rifampin and cephalosporin.

Skin infections can be prevented by careful hygiene and proper care of any minor wounds or insect bites. If any break in the skin shows increasing redness, itching, or drainage, you should see your doctor.

The Human Skeleton

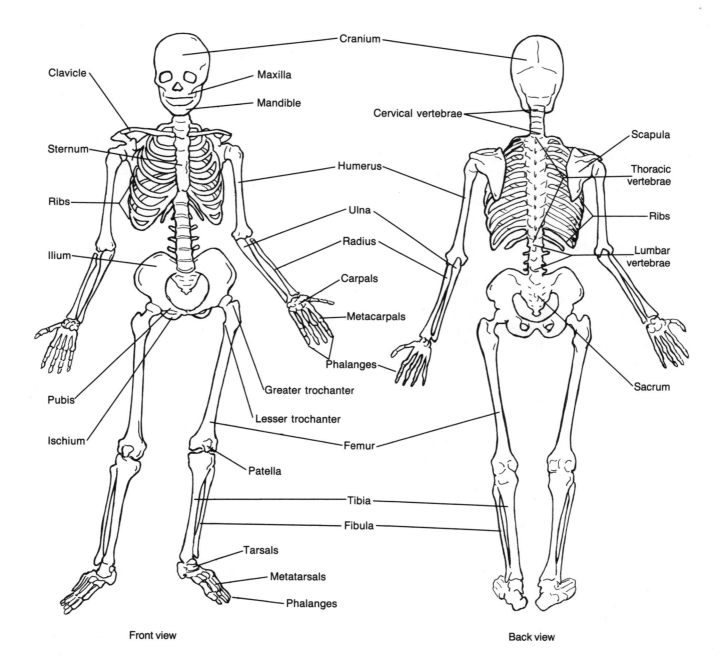

Front view

Back view

APPENDIX B

Body Plane and Movement Terms

Standardized terms of reference to body planes and movements describe positions and motions of the body and its parts. This system starts with the body in the *standard anatomical position*. The body is erect with the palms of the hands facing forward, three planes can be visualized as dividing lines. The *sagittal*, or *median*, plane runs from the front to the back of the body, dividing the body into left and right halves. The *coronal*, or *frontal*, divides the body from side to side into back and front halves. The *transverse*, or *horizontal*, plane divides the body into top and bottom halves.

Portions of the body near the sagittal plane are said to be *medial* (in, or toward the middle); structures farther away from the sagittal plane are *lateral* (to the side). Portions of the body in front of the coronal plane are *anterior*; behind the coronal plane, *posterior*. Viewed relative to the transverse plane, structures close to the head are *superior*; those farther from the head, *inferior*.

Additional terms define the positions of structures anatomically. *Superficial* refers to structures near to the surface of the body; *deep*, those more internal. Also, in the hand, the palm is the *palmar* surface; the back of the hand, the *dorsal* surface. The top of the foot is also called the *dorsal* surface, but the sole is called the *plantar* surface.

Limbs require terms to describe their positions in reference to the body. The parts of a limb far from the trunk are *distal*; those closer to the trunk, *proximal*.

Not only do these body plane terms describe the absolute and relative positions of parts of the body but they also help describe the various movements the body and its parts can perform. Movement of the trunk or neck in the coronal plane (from side to side) is *lateral flexion*. In the sagittal plane, forward bending is *flexion*, backward bending, *extension*. *Rotation* is any movement around the long axis where the sagittal and coronal planes intersect.

Regarding movement, as well as position, limbs require additional terminology. However, the use of the planes and similar principles still apply. Limb movement in the sagittal plane is *flexion* or *extension*. Flexion is when a bending occurs at a joint. For example, bending the forearm forward (from the standard, palm-up, anatomical position) at the elbow is flexion. Extension is the reverse of flexion or straightening the elbow. Movement of a limb in the coronal plane is *abduction* when it carries the limb farther away from the sagittal plane; *adduction*, closer. For example, raising the arm away from the side of the body is abduction; returning it to the side is adduction. Rotation can also occur in the limbs. When the rotation turns the lateral side of the limb anteriorly, or inward, this is *medial rotation*. The opposite motion is *lateral rotation*.

Pronation and supination are complex motions that occur in the hands and feet. In the hand, *supination* makes the hand face anteriorly (palm up); *pronation*, posteriorly. In the foot, supination and pronation each occurs in all three body planes at one time. In *supination*, the foot is moved in plantar flexion, inversion (being turned inward), and adduction. In *pronation*, the foot is moved in dorsiflexion, eversion, and abduction. In the foot, *plantarflexion* is movement toward the sole, and *dorsiflexion* is movement upward toward the front of the leg.

Although references to body planes and movements may initially seem complex, you can see how this standardization of terms allows for a clearer verbal understanding of how different parts of the body move and of their relationships to one another (see Figure 1).

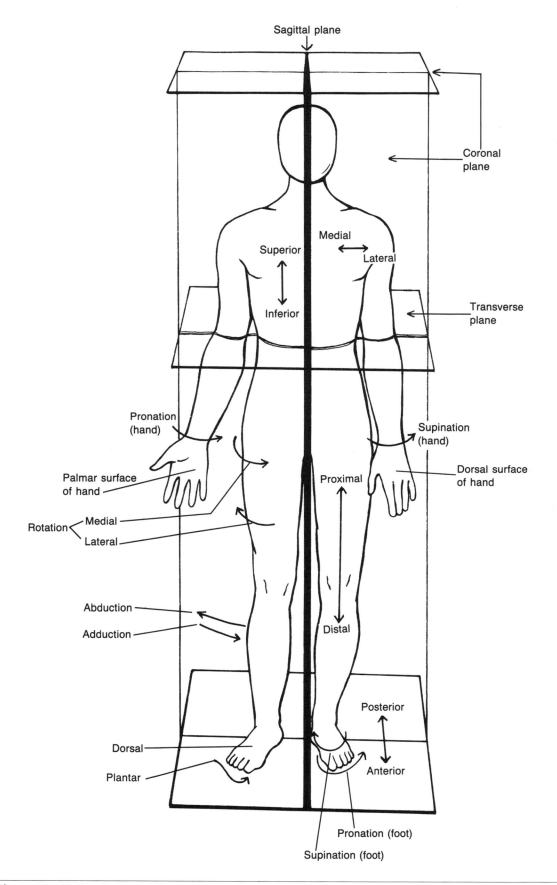

Figure 1 Body planes and movement terms.

Glossary

abduction Turning outward, away from the axis of the body.

abscess A localized collection of pus in a cavity formed by the disintegration of tissues.

acetaminophen A nonprescription pain and fever medication. It does not contain aspirin, nor is it anti-inflammatory.

acute A sudden, short, rather severe course of injury or disease, as opposed to *chronic*.

Achilles tendon (tendo calcaneus Achillis) The powerful tendon at the back of the heel.

adduction Turning inward, toward the axis of the body.

adipose Fat.

aerobic Pertaining to a process or activity that uses oxygen, as aerobic exercise.

amenorrhea The absence or abnormal cessation of menses.

anaerobic In exercise, activity that creates an oxygen debt—literally without oxygen.

aneurysm A sac, filled with blood, formed by the dilation of the walls of an artery or vein.

anorexia Loss of appetite.

anorexia nervosa A serious condition in which a person systematically reduces food intake to the point of emaciation.

antibiotic An agent that kills bacteria.

antiemetic Anything that relieves nausea and/or vomiting.

antiseptic An agent that inhibits the growth of microorganisms on animate surfaces (e.g., on skin).

apophysitis An outgrowth or swelling disease of the growth center of a bone (apophysis).

arteriosclerosis A condition marked by loss of elasticity, and a thickening and hardening, of the arteries.

arthritis Inflammation of a joint.

arthrograph An x-ray of a joint.

arthroscope A device used to examine the interior of a joint.

articular cartilage Fibrous tissue lining of a joint.

aspirin (acetylsalicylic acid) A nonprescription pain, fever, and anti-inflammatory medication.

athlete's foot (tinea pedis) A chronic superficial (skin) fungal infection of the foot, especially between the toes and on the soles. Symptoms are cracking and scaling of the skin, with intense itching.

atrium The portion of the heart, in two sections, left and right, which receives blood and passes it to the ventricles.

avascular Not supplied with blood cells.

axis of motion A line about which a revolving body turns.

bacteria A microorganism, the presence of which indicates infection.

biomechanics The use of mechanical laws applied to living things, especially the locomotor system of the human body.

bone scan A process by which a radioactive "tag" is injected into the body and appears in the bone to be examined by special equipment.

bunion (hallux valgus) A swelling of the bursa of the ball of the big toe.

bursa A fluid-filled sac, found throughout the body, which provides protection by cushioning and reducing friction.

bursitis Inflammation of a bursa.

callus Of skin: a circumscribed thickening due to friction, pressure, or other irritation; of bone: an unorganized meshwork of woven bone over a fracture.

candida A yeastlike fungus.

capsule   A membranous structure surrounding another structure.

chondromalacia   An unnatural softening of cartilage.

chronic   Persisting over a long period of time, as opposed to *acute*.

contrast baths   A physical therapy technique alternating hot and cold baths.

contusion   A wound that does not break the skin.

cortisone   A carbohydrate-regulating adrenal hormone. Synthetic cortisone is used for treating inflammation.

crepitus   The crackling sound produced by the rubbing together of fragments of fractured bone or the movement of an inflamed tendon.

diabetes   A condition wherein the body cannot properly process sugar or produce insulin.

diaphysis   The long shaft of a bone.

diaphragm   The muscular membrane that separates the thoracic (chest) and abdominal cavities.

diathermy   The generation of heat in the body tissues by electricity.

disinfectant   An agent that inhibits the growth of microorganisms on inanimate surfaces.

disk   A rounded plate or organ, here referring to a spinal vertebra.

dislocate   To displace a bone or joint.

distal   Remote; farther from a point of reference.

diuretic   An agent that increases the output of urine.

dorsiflexion   Backward bending, as of a hand or foot.

dysmenorrhea   Painful menses.

eczema   An inflammatory skin disease with symptoms of watery lesions forming scales and crusts. It is often attended by fever, restlessness, itching, and burning.

electrical stimulation   A form of physical therapy using electrical impulses to stimulate a muscle or nerve.

electrocardiogram   (EKG, ECG)   A graphically plotted measurement of the electrical impulses of the heart.

electrolyte   A fluid containing mineral elements and an electrical potential, the balance of which are important to normal body function.

electromyograph   (EMG)   An instrument that records the changes in the electrical potential of a muscle.

epiphysis   The end of a long bone, wider than the shaft; the growth center.

evert   To turn outward.

exostosis   A bony growth extending from a bone.

extension   The straightening of a joint; the opposite of flexion.

flexion   The inward bending of a joint, as in curling a limb; the opposite of extension.

fracture   A break, as of a bone. Simple fracture: unbroken skin; compound fracture: broken skin.

fungus   A type of growth, nonbacterial, on the body.

gait cycle   (a) The motions that occur during walking. (b) The time period from one point to the return to that same point.

gastrointestinal   Referring to the stomach and bowel.

gout   A condition wherein the purine metabolism is disturbed, forming excess uric acid in the blood, which causes chalky deposits in the joints and, therefore, severe arthritic attacks. Treated with diet and medication.

granulation tissue   The small, rounded, fleshy masses formed around wounds.

groin   The lowest part of the abdominal wall near its junction with the thigh.

hallux limitus   Limitation of motion of the great toe.

hallux rigidus   Absence of motion in the great toe.

hallux valgus   (bunion)   A lateral deviation of the great toe.

hammer toes   A contraction deformity of the toes.

hamstrings   A group of muscles in the back of the thigh.

heel spur   An abnormal projection of bone from the heel bone.

hematuria   The presence of blood in the urine.

Hydrocollator®   A physical therapy method using heated gel-filled packs to apply heat to specific body areas.

hydrotherapy   The application of water to treat disease or injury.

hyperextension   Extreme or excessive straightening of a limb or other body part.

hypermobile Excessively or abnormally mobile or flexible.

hyperpronation Excessive pronation.

hypertension High blood pressure.

hyperuremia (polyuria) Excessive urination.

hypothermia Abnormally low body temperature.

ibuprofen A nonprescription, nonaspirin, pain relieving, anti-inflammatory medication. Brands include Advil®, Nuprin®, Ibuprin®, Medipren®, as well as generics.

ice massage Cold therapy applied by rubbing ice over an injured area.

iliotibial band A thick, fibrous band of tissue connecting the ilium (a pelvis bone) and the tibia (leg bone).

ilium The uppermost portion of the hip bone (of the pelvis).

infection Invasion of body tissues by microorganisms. Also, the toxins generated by the invasion.

inflammation Pain, heat, redness, swelling, and, sometimes, loss of function of a body part or tissue. Usually due to injury.

interdigitally Between the digits (the fingers and toes).

internal Occurring within the body.

interstitial Between the tissues or cells.

invert To turn inward.

ischemia Deficiency of blood to a body part.

ischium The lower portion of the hip bone (pelvis).

isometric Denoting contraction of a muscle without significant shortening of muscle fibers.

isotonic Denoting contraction of a muscle with marked shortening of muscle fibers.

-itis Inflammation or disease.

joint The place of union between two or more bones.

kinetic Pertaining to, or producing, motion.

kyphosis An abnormally increased convexity (outward curve) in the thoracic (upper) portion of the spine.

lateral Pertaining to a position farther from the center, or to a side.

ligament A band of tissue that connects bones or supports viscera.

lordosis An abnormally increased concavity (inward curve) of the lumbar (lower) portion of the spine.

mallet toes A contraction deformity of the toes, primarily involving the most distal joint.

march fracture A stress fracture of a bone that occurs due to extended walking, marching, or other exercise.

massage The systematic therapeutical friction, stroking, and kneading of the body.

matrix The basic material from which nail develops.

medial Closer to the middle.

meniscus A cartilage cushion, especially that within the knee.

metabolism The chemical transformations by which energy is made available to the body.

metaphysis The wider part of the long shaft of the bone.

metatarsals The five long bones in the foot extending to the base of the toes.

metatarsalgia Pain in the metatarsal area.

Morton's neuroma A painful thickening of a nerve between the toes.

Morton's syndrome A condition in which the first metatarsal is shorter than normal, and the second then needs to absorb more weight and becomes thickened.

necrosis Death of tissue.

neuroma A tumor largely made of, or growing from, nerve cells.

nodular Pertaining to a node or a localized swelling of tissue.

nonsteroidal anti-inflammatories A large group of medications that can reduce inflammation without steroids.

onychauxic nails Overgrowth of the nails.

onychomycosis A disease of the nails of the toes and fingers caused by a fungus. The nails become opaque, white, thickened, and brittle.

orthosis An externally applied device or system designed to provide control, correction, and support to joints or muscles.

osteoporosis An abnormal thinning of the bone.

over-the-counter (OTC) Denoting medication that can be bought without a prescription.

overuse syndrome Any injury that develops from repeated stress applied over a long period of time.

palpitations Unduly rapid action of the heart that is felt by the person.

paronychia   Inflammation around a nail.

pelvis   The lower portion of the trunk of the body.

periosteum   A specialized type of connective tissue covering every bone.

pes cavus   Exaggerated height of the arch of the foot.

phalanges   The bones of fingers and toes.

phenacetin (acetophenetidin)   A non-aspirin type of nonprescription pain and fever medication.

physical therapy   The utilization of one or more of various physical agents, such as light, heat, ice, diathermy, ultrasound, electrical stimulation, and mechanical techniques, to treat injury or disease.

plantar fascia   A thick, fibrous band of tissue on the bottom of the foot that inserts in the bottom of the heel and extends into the toes.

plantar warts   Warts occurring on the bottom (plantar) surface of the foot.

plica   A ridge or fold of tissue.

pronation   (a) The position of a foot turned outward (everted), upward (dorsiflexed), and away from the midline of the body (abducted). (b) The palm-down position of the hand when the elbow is flexed at 90 degrees.

proximal   Closest to any point of reference.

psoriasis   A chronic, recurring skin infection.

pubis   The bone in the pubic area.

pulse   The rate at which the heart beats.

pulse rate   The number of times per minute you can feel your heart beat.

pump bump   An enlargement on the back of the heel, generally caused by dress shoes.

quadriceps   A group of four muscles in the front of the thigh.

respiratory system   The organs performing respiration (breathing).

rheumatoid arthritis   A systemic condition resulting in an inflammation of the connective tissue structures of the body.

rhinitis   Inflammation of the mucous membrane of the nose.

RICE   First-aid treatment consisting of rest, ice, compression, and elevation.

rotator cuff   A group of muscles and their tendons around the shoulder for its movement and stabilization.

sciatica   Pain along the course of the sciatic nerve (in the lower back and hip).

scoliosis   A noticeable lateral (side-to-side) deviation in the normally straight line of the spine.

sesamoiditis   Inflammation of the sesamoid bones.

spondylolisthesis   Forward displacement of one vertebra relative to another.

sprain   A joint injury in which some of the fibers of a supporting ligament are ruptured, but the general integrity of the ligament remains intact.

stone bruise   Pain on the bottom of the heel due to hitting the heel on a hard object.

strain   To use to an extreme and harmful extent.

stress fracture   A fracture of a bone that occurs due to extended walking, marching, or other exercise.

sublux   To incompletely or partially dislocate.

supination   (a) The position of the foot when it is turned inward (inverted), downward (plantar-flexed), and toward the midline of the body (adducted). (b) The palm-up position of the hand when the elbow is flexed at 90 degrees.

syndrome   A set of symptoms that occur together.

synovitis   Inflammation of the synovial membrane.

synovium   A membrane contained in joint cavities, bursae, and tendon sheaths that secretes a viscous fluid (like egg white).

tailor's bunion   An enlargement at the base of the fifth toe (an enlarged fifth metatarsal).

tendinitis   Inflammation of any tendon.

tendon rupture   A complete break or loss of continuity of a tendon.

tenosynovitis   Inflammation of a tendon sheath.

tinea pedis   Athlete's foot.

Tinel sign   A tingling sensation felt distally when a nerve is tapped.

ulcers   Holes or open sores in the skin or mucous membrane tissue.

ultrasound   Physical therapy using sound waves to generate a deep heat effect, and more recently, a diagnostic imaging machine.

uric acid   A chemical in the body that increases with gout.

valgus   Bent outward.

varus   Bent inward.

vasoconstriction   A narrowing or constriction of the blood vessels.

vasodilation   An expansion or dilation of blood vessels.

ventricles   The two lower chambers of the heart.

verruca   Wart.

vertebrae   The bones of the spine.

virus   A microscopic organism that depends on a specific host cell for reproduction. Does not respond to antibiotics.

whirlpool   Physical therapy using air bubbles injected into water.

References

American Medical Association. (1980). *Handbook of first aid and emergency care.* Chicago: Author.

Anorexia nervosa and bulimia. (1986). *Journal of Nutrition Education,* **18**(2), 87.

Benowicz, R. (1979). *Nonprescription drugs and their side effects.* New York: Berkley Press.

Blumenthal, J.A., O'Toole, L.C., & Chang, J.L. (1984). Is running an analogue of anorexia nervosa? *Journal of the American Medical Association,* **252**(4), 520-523.

Brody, D.M. (1980). Running injuries. *Clinical Symposium,* **32**(4), 1-36.

Burke, E.R. (1981). Ulnar neuropathy in bicyclists. *The Physician and Sportsmedicine,* **9**(4), 52-56.

Cooper, K.H. (1968). *Aerobics.* New York: M. Evans and Co., in association with Lippencott, Philadelphia.

Dobyns, J.H., O'Brien, E.T., Linscheid, R.I., & Fallow, G.M. (1972). Bowler's thumb: Diagnosis and treatment. *Journal of Bone and Joint Surgery* [American], **54**, 751-755.

Graedon, J., & Graedon, T. (1985). *The people's pharmacy.* New York: St. Martin's Press.

Gugenheim, J.J. (1987, January). Are athletics safe for the immature skeleton? *AAPSM Newsletter,* p. 5.

Hellman, D.B., Helms, C.A., & Genant, H.K. (1983). Chronic repetitive trauma: A cause of atypical degenerative joint disease. *Skeletal Radiology,* **10**(4), 236-242.

Henry, S., Jr. (1982). The price of perfection. *The Runner.*

Howell, A.E., & Leach, R.E. (1970). Bowler's thumb: Perineural fibrosis of the digital nerve. *Journal of Bone and Joint Surgery* [American], **52**, 372-381.

James, S.L., Bates, B.T., & Sternig, L.R. (1978). Injuries to runners. *American Journal of Sportsmedicine,* **6**(2), 40-50.

Julsrud, M. (1985). Iliac apophysitis and a review of the osteochondrosis. *Journal of the American Podiatric Medical Association,* **75**(11), 586-589.

Kaufman, J., Rabinowitz-Dagi, L., Levin, J., McCarthy, P., Wolfe, S., Bargmann, E., & The Public Citizen Health Research Group. (1983). *Pills that don't work.* New York: Pantheon Books.

Kunz, J. (1982). *The American Medical Association family medical guide.* New York: Random House.

Lane, N.E., Bloch, D.A., Jones, H.H., Marshall, W.H., Jr., Wood, P.D., & Fries, J.F. (1986). Long-distance running, bone density, and osteoarthritis. *Journal of the American Medical Association,* **255**(9), 1147-1151.

McDermott, M., & Freyne, P. (1983). Osteoarthrosis in runners with knee pain. *British Journal of Sports Medicine,* **17**, 84-87.

Olkin, S.K. (1983). Massage for runners. *Running and Fitness,* **15**(1), 1-14.

Panush, R., Schmidt, C., Caldwell, J., Edwards, N.L., Longley, S., Yonker, R., Webster, E., Nauman, J., Stork, J., & Pettersson, H. (1986). Is running associated with degenerative joint disease? *Journal of the American Medical Association,* **255**(9), 1152-1154.

Ricciardi-Polline, P.T., Moneta, M.R., & Falez, F. (1985). The tarsal tunnel syndrome: A report of eight cases. *Foot and Ankle,* **6**(3), 146-149.

Ross, J.G., Dotson, C.O., & Gilbert, G.G. (1985, January). Are kids getting appropriate activity? *Journal of Physical Education, Recreation, and Dance,* **56**(1), 82-85.

Roy, S. (1985). Injuries of exercise. *Medical Clinicians of North America, 69*(1), 197-209.

Sachs, L. (1981). Running addictions. In M.H. Sacks & M.L. Sachs (Eds.), *Psychology of running* (pp. 116-126). Champaign, IL: Human Kinetics.

Small, D.F. (1975). Handlebar palsy. *New England Journal of Medicine, 292*(6), 322.

Sohn, R.S., & Micheli, L.J. (1985). The effect of running on the pathogenesis of osteo-arthritis of the hips and knees. *Clinical Orthopaedics and Related Research, 198*, 106-109.

Stamford, B. (1986). What are muscle cramps? *The Physician and Sportsmedicine, 14*(2), 192.

Stamford, B. (1985). A stitch in the side. *The Physician and Sportsmedicine, 13*(5), 187.

Strauss, R.H. (1984). *Sports medicine.* Philadelphia: W.B. Saunders.

U.S. Department of Commerce and National Oceanic and Atmospheric Administration. (1985). *Heatwave: A major summer killer* (NOAA/PA 85001). Washington, DC: U.S. Government Printing Office.

Yale, I. (1984). *The arthritic foot.* Baltimore: Williams & Wilkins.

Zimmerman, D. (1983). *The essential guide to nonprescription drugs.* New York: Harper & Row.

Reading List

Abel, M.S. (1985). Jogger's fracture and other stress fractures of the lumbo-sacral spine. *Skeletal Radiology, 13*(3), 221-227.

Allman, W.F. (1983, November). The knee. *Science '83*, pp. 122-123.

American Medical Association. (1980). *Handbook of first aid and emergency care.* Chicago: Author.

Anderson, B. (1975). *Stretching.* Fullerton, CA: Anderson & Anderson.

Andrews, G.C., & Domonkos, A. (1964). *Diseases of the skin.* Philadelphia: W.B. Saunders.

Andrews, J.R. (1982). Overuse syndromes of the lower extremity. *Clinical Sports Medicine, 1*(1), 137-148.

Anorexia nervosa and bulimia. (1986). *Journal of Nutrition Education, 18*(2), 87.

Apple, D. (1984, November-December). Heal thyself: At-home treatment for injuries. *Bicycling*, pp. 534-537.

Arrowsmith, S.R., Fleming, L.L., & Allman, F.L. (1983). Traumatic dislocations of the peroneal tendons. *American Journal of Sports Medicine, 11*(3), 142-146.

Baker, B.E., Peckham, A.C., Pupparo, F., & Sanborn, J.C. (1985). Review of meniscal injury and associated sports. *American Journal of Sports Medicine, 13*(1), 1-4.

Bartlett, P.C., Martin, R.J., & Cahill, B.R. (1982). Furunculosis in a high school football team. *American Journal of Sports Medicine, 10*(6), 371-374.

Basmajian, J.V. (1984). *Therapeutic exercise.* Baltimore: Williams & Wilkins.

Baxter, D.E., & Thigpen, C.M. (1984). Heel pain—Operative results. *Foot and Ankle, 5*(1), 16-25.

Beeson, P.B., & McDermott, W. (1967). *Textbook of medicine.* Philadelphia: W.B. Saunders.

Benowicz, R. (1979). *Non-prescription drugs and their side effects.* New York: Berkley Press.

Birnbaum, J. (1982). *The musculoskeletal manual.* New York: Academic Press.

Blackburn, K. (1984, May). Aerobic ailments. *Minneapolis-St. Paul*, pp. 117-119.

Blake, R.L., & Fettig, M.H. (1983). Chronic low back pain in a long-distance runner: A case report. *Journal of the American Podiatry Association, 73*(11), 598-601.

Block, S. (1982, November). Tennis elbow? Runner's knee? Golf toe? Easing the pain those fitness fads have wrought. *Los Angeles*, pp. 112-117.

Blumenthal, J.A., O'Toole, L.C., & Chang, J.L. (1984). Is running an analogue of anorexia nervosa? *Journal of the American Medical Association, 252*(4), 520-523.

Bordelon, R.L. (1985). Management of disorders of the forefoot and toenails associated with running. *Clinics in Sports Medicine, 4*(4), 717-724.

Boston Women's Health Collective. (1985). *The new our bodies, ourselves.* New York: Simon & Schuster.

Braisted, J.R., Mellin, L., Gong, E.J., & Irwin, C.E., Jr. (1985). The adolescent ballet dancer. Nutritional practices and characteristics associated with anorexia nervosa. *Journal of Adolescent Health Care, 6*(5), 365-371.

Bridges, D.A. (1984, September). Think wet! *Runner's World*, pp. 82-84.

Brody, D.M. (1980). Running injuries. *Clinical Symposium, 32*(4), 1-36.

Burke, E.R. (1981). Ulnar neuropathy in bicyclists. *The Physician and Sportsmedicine, 9*(4), 52-56.

Burton, R.M. (1980). The endurance athlete's heart: "Abnormal" is normal. *Colorado Medicine, 77*(7), 239.

Caine, D., & Linder, K. (1985). Overuse injuries of growing bones: The young female gymnast at risk? *The Physician and Sportsmedicine, 13*(12), 51-64.

Calderon, R., & Mood, E.W. (1982). An epidemiological assessment of water quality and "swimmer's ear." *Archives on Environmental Health, 37*(5), 300-305.

Canby, A. (1981, September). How women athletes can avoid injuries. *McCall's,* p. 43.

Carroll, R. (1981). Tennis elbow: Incidence in local league players. *British Journal of Sports Medicine, 15*(4), 250-256.

Cavanaugh, P. (1980, August). Advances in diagnosing the runner's injuries. *Runner's World,* pp. 67-70.

Cetti, R. (1982). Conservative treatment of injury to the fibular ligaments of the ankle. *British Journal of Sports Medicine, 16*(1), 47-52.

Chechick, A., Amit, Y., Israeli, A., & Horoszowski, H. (1982). Recurrent rupture of the Achilles tendon induced by corticosteroid injection. *British Journal of Sports Medicine, 16*(2), 89-90.

Clarke, T.E., Fredrick, E.C., & Hamill, C.L. (1983). The effects of shoe design parameters on rearfoot control in running. *Medicine and Science in Sports and Exercise, 15*(5), 376-381.

Clement, D.B., & Padmore, T. (1984, April). A complete guide to the Achilles tendon. *Runner's World,* pp. 64-70.

Clement, D.B., Taunton, J.E., & Smart, G.W. (1984). Achilles tendinitis and peritendinitis: Etiology and treatment. *American Journal of Sports Medicine, 12*(3), 179-184.

Cohen, I., Lane, S., & Koning, W. (1981). Peroneal tendon dislocations: A review of the literature. *Journal of Foot Surgery, 22*(1), 15-20.

Cole, E. (1980, August). Summer aches and pains: When to be your own doctor. *McCall's,* p. 58.

Cooney, W.P., III. (1984). Sports injuries to the upper extremity. How to recognize and deal with some problems. *Postgraduate Medicine, 76*(4), 45-50.

Cooper, K.H. (1968). *Aerobics.* New York: M. Evans & Co., in association with Lippincott, Philadelphia.

Crean, D. (1981). The management of soft tissue ankle injuries. *British Journal of Sports Medicine, 15*(1), 75-76.

Crossen, D. (1982, May). Prevention is the first step to the cure. *Runner's World,* pp. 50-53.

Dale, E., & Goldberg, D.L. (1982). Implications of nutrition in athletes' menstrual cycle irregularities. *Canadian Journal of Applied Sports Science, 7*(2), 74-78.

D'Ambrosia, R.D. (1985). Orthotic devices in running injuries. *Clinical Sports Medicine, 4*(4), 611-618.

Davis, K. (1982, June). How to avoid exercise injuries. *Mademoiselle,* pp. 80-81.

Derscheid, G.L., & Brown, W.C. (1985). Rehabilitation of the ankle. *Clinics in Sports Medicine, 4*(3), 527-544.

Dobyns, J.H., O'Brien, E.T., Linscheid, R.I., & Farrow, G.M. (1972). Bowler's thumb: Diagnosis and treatment. *Journal of Bone and Joint Surgery* [American], **54**, 751-755.

Donaldson, R. (1977). *Guidelines for successful jogging.* Washington, DC: National Jogging Association.

Epstein, E. (1956). *Skin surgery.* Philadelphia: Lea and Febiger.

Fedo, M. (1983, October). Running ailments: A hard day's night. *Runner's World,* pp. 82-84.

Ferretti, A., Ippolito, E., Mariani, P., & Puddu, G. (1983). Jumper's knee. *American Journal of Sports Medicine, 11*(2), 58-62.

Ferretti, A., Puddu, G., Mariani, P.P., & Neri, M. (1985). The natural history of jumper's knee. Patellar or quadriceps tendonitis. *International Orthopaedics, 8*(4), 239-242.

Fraser, M. (1985, March). The agony of de-feet. *WomenSports,* p. 42.

Fredrick, E.C. (1984). *Sports shoes and playing surfaces.* Champaign, IL: Human Kinetics.

Frizzell, R.T., Lans, G.H., Lowance, D.C., & Lathan, S.R. (1986). Hyponatremia and ultramarathon runners. *Journal of the American Medical Association, 255*(6), 772-774.

Garrett, W.E., Jr. (1983). Strains and sprains in athletes. *Postgraduate Medicine, 73*(3), 200-209.

Gass, G.C., Camp, E.M., Watson, J., Eager, D., Wicks, L., & Ng, A. (1983). Prolonged exercise in highly trained female endurance runners. *International Journal of Sports Medicine, 4*(4), 241-246.

Gaston, E.A. (1983, March). How do you spell relief? Preventing sports injuries. *Bicycling*, pp. 43-44.

Gaston, E.A. (1983, June). Cortisone shots and ruptured tendons. *Bicycling*, pp. 56-63.

Gerberich, S.G., & Priest, J.D. (1985). Treatment for lateral epicondylitis: Variables related to recovery. *British Journal of Sports Medicine, 19*(4), 224-227.

Goldfarb, L.A., & Plante, T.G. (1984). Fear of fat in runners: An examination of the connection between anorexia nervosa and distance running. *Psychological Report, 5*(1), 296.

Good Housekeeping. (Ed.). (1980). *Family health and medical guide*. New York: Hearst Books.

Gordon, G.M. (1984). Podiatric sports medicine. Evaluation and prevention of injuries. *Clinical Podiatry, 1*(2), 401-416.

Gould, J.A., & Davies, G.J. (1985). *Orthopaedics and sports physical therapy*. St. Louis: Mosby.

Goulet, M.J. (1984). Role of soft orthosis in treating plantar fasciitis: Suggestions from the field. *Physical Therapy, 64*, 1544.

Graedon, J., & Graedon, T. (1985). *The new people's pharmacy*. Toronto, Ontario: Bantam Books.

Grant, J.C., & Boileau, M.D. (1943). *An atlas of anatomy*. Baltimore: Williams & Wilkins.

Gray, J., Taunton, J.E., McKenzie, D.C., Clement, D.B., McConkey, J.P., & Davidson, R.G. (1985). A survey of injuries to the anterior cruciate ligament of the knee in female basketball players. *International Journal of Sports Medicine, 6*(6), 314-316.

Green, B., Daling, J., Weiss, N., Liff, J., & Koepsell, T. (1986). Exercise as a risk factor for infertility with ovulatory dysfunction. *American Journal of Public Health, 76*, 1432-1436.

Gregg, J.R., & Das, M. (1982). Foot and ankle problems in the preadolescent and adolescent athlete. *Clinics in Sports Medicine, 1*(1), 131-147.

Gugenheim, J.J. (1987, January). Are athletics safe for the immature skeleton? *AAPSM Newsletter*, p. 5.

Hagan, R.D., Smith, M.G., & Gettman, L.R. (1983). High density lipoprotein cholesterol in relation to food consumption and running distance. *Journal of Preventive Medicine, 12*(2), 287-295.

Halperin, H., Hendel, D., Fisher, S., Agasi, M., & Copeliovitch, L. (1983, October). Anterior cruciate ligament insufficiency syndrome. *Clinical Orthopaedics and Related Research, 179*, 179-184.

Harvey, J.S., Jr. (1982). Overuse syndromes in young athletes. *Pediatric Clinics of North America, 29*, 1369-1381.

Harvey, J.S., Jr. (1983). Overuse syndromes in young athletes. *Clinics in Sports Medicine, 2*, 595-607.

Hatfield, F.C. (1982). *Flexibility training for sports: PNF techniques*. New Orleans: Sports Conditioning Systems.

Hauser, A.M., Dressendorfer, R.H., Vos, M., Hashimoto, T., Gordon, S., & Timmis, G.C. (1985). Symmetric cardiac enlargement in highly trained endurance athletes: A two-dimensional echocardiographic study. *American Heart Journal, 109*, 1038-1044.

Hede, A., Hejgaard, N., Sandberg, H., & Jacobsen, K. (1985). Sports injuries of the knee ligaments—A prospective stress radiographic study. *British Journal of Sports Medicine, 19*(1), 8-10.

Hellman, D.B., Helms, C.A., & Genant, H.K. (1985). Chronic repetitive trauma: A cause of atypical degenerative joint disease. *Skeletal Radiology, 10*(4), 236-242.

Henry, S., Jr. (1982). The price of perfection. *The Runner*.

Herrick, R.T., & Herrick, S. (1983). Rupture of the plantar fascia in a middle-aged tennis player: A case report. *American Journal of Sports Medicine, 11*(2), 95.

Hlavac, H.F. (1977). *The foot book*. Mountain View, CA: World Publications.

Hockman, R. (1982, August). Body heat. *Runner's World*, pp. 70-72.

Hollander, J.L. (1974). *The arthritis handbook*. West Point, PA: Merck Sharp & Dohme.

Hopkinson, W.J., Mitchell, W.A., & Curl, W.W. (1985). Chondral fractures of the knee: Cause for confusion. *American Journal of Sports Medicine,* **13**(5), 309-312.

How much pain is normal: Knowing when to stop. (1984, January). *Runner's World,* pp. 47-48.

Howard, J. (1982, April). Combining sports can prevent injuries while providing flexibility and muscle strength. *Runner's World,* p. 64.

Howell, A.E., & Leach, R.E. (1970). Bowler's thumb: Perineural fibrosis of the digital nerve. *Journal of Bone and Joint Surgery* [American], **52**(2), 379-381.

Hunter, H.C. (1982). Injuries to the brachial plexus: Experience of a private sports medicine clinic. *Journal of the American Osteopathic Association,* **81**, 757-760.

Hutson, M.A., & Jackson, J.P. (1982). Injuries to the lateral ligament of the ankle: Assessment and treatment. *British Journal of Sports Medicine,* **16**(4), 245-249.

Irvin, C.M., Witt, C.S., & Zieldorf, L.M. (1985). Post-traumatic osteochondritis of the lateral sesamoid in active adolescents. *Journal of Foot Surgery,* **24**(3), 219-221.

Israeli, A., Ganel, A., Horoszowski, H., & Farine, I. (1981). Traumatic osteochondral lesions of the talus. *British Journal of Sports Medicine,* **15**(3), 159-162.

Jackson, M.A., & Gudas, C.J. (1982). Peroneus longus tendinitis: A possible biomechanical etiology. *Journal of Foot Surgery,* **21**(4), 344-348.

James, S.L., Bates, B.T., & Sternig, L.R. (1978). Injuries to runners. *American Journal of Sports Medicine,* **6**(2), 40-50.

Jensen, J.E., Conn, R.R., Hazelrigg, G., & Hewett, J.E. (1985). Systematic evaluation of acute knee injuries. *Clinics in Sports Medicine,* **4**(2), 295-312.

Jones, D.R., & Johnson, K.A. (1981). Diagnostic problems: Jogging and diabetes mellitus. *Foot and Ankle,* **1**(6), 362-364.

Julsrud, M. (1985). Iliac apophysitis and a review of the osteochondrosis. *Journal of the American Podiatric Medical Association,* **75**(11), 586.

Katz, J.L. (1986). Long-distance running, anorexia nervosa, and bulimia: A report of two cases. *Comprehensive Psychiatry,* **27**(1), 74-78.

Kay, D.B. (1985). The sprained ankle: Current therapy. *Foot and Ankle,* **6**(1), 22-28.

Keene, J.S. (1983). Low back pain in the athlete from spondylogenic injury during recreation or competition. *Postgraduate Medicine,* **74**(6), 209-212, 213, 217.

Kelly, D.W., Carter, V.S., Jobe, F.W., & Kerlan, R.K. (1984). Patellar and quadriceps tendon ruptures—Jumper's knee. *American Journal of Sports Medicine,* **12**(5), 375-380.

Kent, J.M. (1983). Preventing winter sports injuries. *Patient Care,* **17**(20), 145-148, 150, 159-160.

Kessler, R.M., & Hertling, D. (1983). *Management of common musculo-skeletal disorders.* Philadelphia: Harper & Row.

Kiester, E., Jr. (1985, April). Sports injuries: Treating strains and sprains at home. *Better Homes and Gardens,* pp. 56-57.

Kohn, H.S. (1985). Current status and treatment of tennis elbow. *Wisconsin Medical Journal,* **83**(3), 18-19.

Koplan, J.P., Powell, K.E., Sikes, R.K., Shirley, R.W., & Campbell, C.C. (1982). An epidemiologic study of the benefits and risks of running. *Journal of the American Medical Association,* **248**, 3118-3121.

Kotoske, K. (1983, July). Riding out a charley horse. *WomenSports,* p. 54.

Krusen, F.H., Hottke, F.J., & Ellwood, P., Jr. (1966). *Handbook of Physical Medicine and Rehabilitation.* Philadelphia: W.B. Saunders.

Kujala, U.M., Kvist, M., & Heinonen, O. (1985). Osgood-Schlatter's disease in adolescent athletes: Retrospective study of incidence and duration. *American Journal of Sports Medicine,* **13**(4), 236-241.

Kunz, J. (1982). *The American Medical Association family medical guide.* New York: Random House.

Kvist, M., & Jarvinen, M. (1982). Clinical, histochemical and biomechanical features in repair of muscle and tendon injuries. *International Journal of Sports Medicine,* **3**(1), 12-14.

Lane, N.E., Bloch, D.A., Jones, H.H., Marshall, W.H., Jr., Wood, P.D., & Fries, J.F. (1986). Long-distance running, bone density, and osteoarthritis. *Journal of the American Medical Association,* **255**(9), 1147-1151.

Laughlin, R.K., Carr, T.A., Chao, E.Y., Youdas, J.W., & Sim, F.H. (1980). Three-dimensional kinematics of the taped ankle before and after exercise. *American Journal of Sports Medicine,* **8**(6), 425-431.

Leach, R.E., DiLorio, E., & Harney, R.A. (1983, July-August). Pathologic hindfoot conditions in the athlete. *Clinical Orthopaedics and Related Research,* **177**, 116-121.

Leach, R.E., James, S., & Wasilewski, S. (1981). Achilles tendinitis. *American Journal of Sports Medicine,* **9**(2), 93-98.

Lehman, W.L., Jr. (1984). Overuse syndromes in runners. *American Family Physician,* **29**(1), 157-161.

Lillich, J., & Baxter, D. (1986). Bunionectomies and related surgery in the elite female middle-distance and marathon runner. *The American Journal of Sports Medicine,* **14**(6), 491-493.

Lipscomb, A.B., & Anderson, A.F. (1982). Tears of the anterior cruciate ligament in adolescents. *Journal of Bone and Joint Surgery,* **68**(1), 71-84.

Loomer, R.L. (1982). Elbow injuries in athletes. *Canadian Journal of Applied Sports Science,* **7**(3), 164-166.

Mack, R.P. (1982). Ankle injuries in athletics. *Clinics in Sports Medicine,* **1**(1), 71-84.

MacLellan, G.E., & Vyvyan, B. (1981). Management of pain beneath the heel and Achilles tendonitis with visco-elastic heel inserts. *British Journal of Sports Medicine,* **15**(2), 117-121.

Maddox, P.A., & Garth, W.P., Jr. (1986). Tendinitis of the patellar ligament and quadriceps (jumper's knee) as an initial presentation of hyperparathyroidism: A case report. *Journal of Bone and Joint Surgery,* **68**(2), 288-292.

Maloney, M.J. (1983). Anorexia nervosa and bulimia in dancers. Accurate diagnosis and treatment planning. *Clinics in Sports Medicine,* **2**(3), 549-555.

Marcus, R., Cann, C., Madvis, P., Minkoff, J., Goddard, M., Bayer, M., Martin, M., Gaudiani, L., Haskell, W., & Ganant, H. (1985). Menstrual function and bone mass in elite women distance runners: Endocrine and metabolic features. *Annals of Internal Medicine,* **102**, 1563-1588.

Martin, D. (1984, June). Riding the heat wave. *Runner's World,* p. 66-68.

Massimino, F., & Baxter, K. (1983, April). Injuries you can't run away from. *Runner's World,* pp. 52-59.

Mazer, E. (1983, March). Natural remedies for aching muscles: A strained muscle can mean days of pain and inconvenience. *Prevention,* pp. 71-75.

McCombs, R. (1956). *Fundamentals of internal medicine.* Chicago: Year Book Medical Publishers.

McDermott, M., & Freyne, P. (1983). Osteoarthrosis in runners with knee pain. *British Journal of Sports Medicine,* **17**(2), 84-87.

McGregor, R.R., & Devereax, S. (1982). *EEVeTeC.* Boston: Houghton Mifflin.

McKenzie, D.C., Clement, D.B., & Taunton, J.E. (1985). Running shoes, orthotics, and injuries. *Sports Medicine,* **2**(5), 334-347.

McMaster, W. (1986). Pained shoulder in swimmers: A diagnostic challenge. *The Physician and Sportsmedicine,* **14**(12), 108-122.

McMinn, R.M.H., Hutchings, R.T., & Logan, B.M. (1982). *Foot and ankle anatomy.* Connecticut: Prentice Hall.

McNicol, K., Taunton, J.E., & Clement, D.B. (1981). Iliotibial tract friction syndrome in athletes. *Canadian Journal of Applied Sports Science,* **6**(2), 76-80.

Meisel, A.D., & Bullough, P.G. (1984). *Atlas of osteoarthritis.* Philadelphia: Lea & Febiger.

Mirkin, G., & Hoffman, M. (1978). *The sportsmedicine book* (p. 141). Boston: Little, Brown.

Mirkin, G. (1981, March). Sportsmedicine: What you should know before you get hurt. *Family Health,* pp. 36-38.

Mosher, C., & Rosenbaum, J. (1984, December). Rhythm and moves: Keeping pace with aerobics. *WomenSports,* pp. 24-28.

Mozee, G., & Prokop, D. (1984, May). You can fight lower-back pain. *Runner's World,* pp. 66-70.

Murphy, P.C., & Baxter, D.E. (1985). Nerve entrapment of the foot and ankle in runners. *Clinics in Sports Medicine,* **4**(4), 753-763.

Naumetz, V.A., & Schweisel, J.F. (1980). Osteocartilagenous lesions of the talar dome. *Journal of Trauma,* **20**, 924-927.

Naveri, H., Kuoppasalmi, K., & Harkonen, M. (1985). Metabolic and hormonal changes in moderate and intense long-term running exercises. *International Journal of Sports Medicine*, **6**(5), 276-281.

Nemeth, V.A., & Thrasher, E. (1983). Ankle sprains in athletes. *Clinics in Sports Medicine*, **2**(1), 217-224.

Nicholas, J.A., & Reilly, J.P. (1985). Orthopedic problems in athletes. *Comprehensive Therapy*, **11**(1), 48-56.

Nightingale, D. (1982, May 3). Rotator cuff tear: Dr. Jobe brings hope to "dead arm." *Sporting News*, pp. 12-14.

Nightingale, D. (1982, May 17). Exercise plan may prevent torn rotator cuff ordeal. *Sporting News*, pp. 42-43.

Nirschl, R. (1980, January). Keeping fit: A top ten list to avoid. *World Tennis*, pp. 42-44.

Nirschl, R. (1981, July). The angry elbow; taming the elbow with a mind of its own: How to treat it if you've got it; how to avoid it if you haven't. *World Tennis*, pp. 38-49.

Noakes, T.D., Goodwin, N., Rayner, B.L., Branken, T., & Taylor, R.K. (1985). Water intoxication: A possible complication during endurance exercise. *Medicine and Science in Sports and Exercise*, **17**(3), 370-375.

Noyes, F.R., Paulos, L., Mooar, L.A., & Signer, B. (1980). Knee sprains and acute knee hemarthrosis: Misdiagnosis of anterior cruciate ligament tears. *Physical Therapy*, **60**, 1596-1601.

Odensten, M., Lysholm, J., & Gillquist, J. (1985). The course of partial anterior cruciate ligament ruptures. *American Journal of Sports Medicine*, **13**(3), 183-186.

Olkin, S.K. (1983). Massage for runners. American Running and Fitness Association Newsletter, *Running and Fitness*, **15**(1), 1-14.

Orava, S., & Virtanen, K. (1982). Osteochondroses in athletes. *British Journal of Sports Medicine*, **16**(3), 161-168.

Orava, S., Virtanen, K., & Typpo, T. (1982). Diffuse osteochondrosis of the patella. *British Journal of Sports Medicine*, **16**(3), 174-177.

Ottum, B. (1982, March). Injury forecasting might just help runners remain on a healthy track. *Sports Illustrated*, pp. 6-8.

Pagliano, J., & Jackson, D. (1980, November). The ultimate study of running injuries. *Runner's World*, pp. 42-49.

Pagliano, J. (1983, December). Running on the road to injuries: Common causes of typical running ailments. *Runner's World*, p. 46.

Panush, R., Schmidt, C., Caldwell, J., Edwards, N.L., Longley, S., Yonker, R., Webster, E., Naumon, J., Stork, J., & Pettersson, H. (1986). Is running associated with degenerative joint disease? *Journal of the American Medical Association*, **255**(9), 1152-1154.

Parkes, J.C., II, Hamilton, W.G., Patterson, A.H., & Rawles, J.G., Jr. (1980). The anterior impingement syndrome of the ankle. *Journal of Trauma*, **20**, 895-898.

Paulsen, J. (1983, June). Fitness injury protection and what to do when minor aches become major. *Bicycling*, pp. 56-63.

Pavlov, H., Torg, J.S., & Freiberger, R.H. (1983). Tarsal navicular stress fractures: Radiographic evaluation. *Radiology*, **148**, 641-645.

Penny, G.D., Shaver, L.G., Carlton, J., & Kendall, D.W. (1982). Comparison of serum HDL-C and HDL-total cholesterol ratio in middle-age active and inactive males. *Journal of Sports Medicine and Physical Fitness*, **22**, 432-439.

Pietschmann, D. (1983, February). Harassment on the run. *Runner's World*, pp. 26-34.

Piper, C., & Baxter, K. (1983, January). Treating injuries with aloe vera. *Runner's World*, pp. 44-47.

Pretorius, D., Noakes, T., Irving, G., & Allerton, K. (1986). Runner's knee: What is it and how effective is conservative treatment? *The Physician and Sportsmedicine*, **14**(12), 71-81.

Puddu, G., Ferretti, A., Mariani, P., & LeSpesa, F. (1984). Meniscal tears and associated anterior cruciate ligament tears in athletes: Course of treatment. *American Journal of Sports Medicine*, **12**(3), 196-198.

Raskin, R.J., & Rebecca, G.S. (1983). Posttraumatic sports-related musculoskeletal abnormalities: Prevalence in a normal population. *American Journal of Sports Medicine*, **11**(5), 336-339.

Renstrom, P., & Johnson, R.J. (1985). Overuse injuries in sports. A review. *Sports Medicine, 2*(5), 316-333.

Reynolds, G. (1987, March). Running and menstruation. *Runner's World*, pp. 36-43.

Ricciardi-Polline, P.T., Moneta, M.R., & Falez, F. (1985). The tarsal tunnel syndrome: A report of eight cases. *Foot and Ankle, 6*(3), 146-149.

Roberson, M., & Roberson, E. (1984, October). Heat or ice? *Runner's World*, pp. 56-71.

Romanes, G.J. (1964). *Cunningham's textbook of anatomy.* London: Oxford University Press.

Ross, J.G., Dotson, C.O., & Gilbert, G.G. (1985, January). Are kids getting appropriate activity? *Journal of Physical Education, Recreation and Dance, 56*(1), 82-85.

Rotkis, T., Boyden, T.W., Pamenter, R.W., Stanforth, P., & Wilmore, J. (1981). High density lipoprotein cholesterol and body composition of female runners. *Metabolism, 30*, 994-995.

Rovere, G., & Adalh, D. (1985). Medial synovial shelf plica syndrome. *American Journal of Sports Medicine, 13*(6), 382-386.

Roy, S. (1985). Injuries of exercise. *Medical Clinics of North America, 69*(1), 197-209.

Roy, S., & Irvin, J. (1983). *Sports medicine: Prevention, evaluation, management and rehabilitation.* Englewood Cliffs, NJ: Prentice Hall.

Sacks, M.H., & Sachs, M.L. (Eds.). (1981). *Psychology of running.* Champaign, IL: Human Kinetics.

Sady, S.P., Cullinane, E.M., Herbert, P.N., Kantor, M.A., & Thompson, P.D. (1984). Training, diet and physical characteristics of distance runners with low or high concentrations of high density lipoprotein cholesterol. *Atherosclerosis, 53*(3), 273-281.

Sammarco, G.J. (1982). Soft tissue conditions in athletes' feet. *Clinics in Sports Medicine, 1*(1), 149-155.

Sando, B. (1984). Injuries to the ankle. *Austrian Family Physician, 13*, 581-584.

Sauer, G.C. (1985). *Manual of skin diseases.* Philadelphia: J.B. Lippincott.

Scanlon, T. (1984, June). Questions to ask about sports safety. *Consumers Research Magazine*, pp. 18-19.

Scheller, A.D., Kasser, J.R., & Quigley, T.B. (1980). Tendon injuries about the ankle. *Orthopaedic Clinics of North America, 11*, 801-811.

Scranton, P.E., Jr. (1981). Pathologic anatomic variations in the sesamoids. *Foot and Ankle, 1*(6), 321-326.

Shangold, M. (1982, July). Women's running. *Runner's World*, p. 21.

Shangold, M. (1983, October). The best defenses against stress fractures are exercise and calcium. *Runner's World*, p. B171.

Shangold, M., & Mirkin, G. (1985). *The complete sports medicine handbook for women.* New York: Simon & Schuster.

Sheehan, G. (1978). *Running and being.* New York: Simon & Schuster.

Sheehan, G. (1982, May). How hot is it? *Runner's World*, p. 105.

Sheehan, G. (1982, July). Working out a cramp. *Runner's World*, p. 89.

Sheehan, G. (1983, January). Medical bills account for most of running's costs: The best advice is to treat your own minor injuries. *Runner's World*, pp. 83-85.

Sheehan, G. (1984, August). If one of your legs is longer than the other, you have plenty of company (and, perhaps, pain). *Runner's World*, p. 189.

Shonds, A.R., Jr., & Raney, R.B. (1967). *Handbook of orthopaedic surgery.* St. Louis: C.V. Mosby.

Sloan, D. (1980, June). Taking care of shin splints and tennis elbow. *Dallas Magazine*, pp. 44-46.

Small, D.F. (1975). Handlebar palsy. *New England Journal of Medicine, 292*(6), 322.

Smart, G.W., Taunton, J.E., & Clement, D.B. (1980). Achilles tendon disorders in runners—A review. *Medicine and Science in Sports and Exercise, 12*(4), 231-243.

Smith, R., & Reischl, S. (1986). Treatment of ankle sprains in young athletes. *The American Journal of Sports Medicine, 14*(6), 465-471.

Snider, M.P., Clancy, W.G., & McBeath, A.A. (1983). Plantar fascia release for chronic plantar fasciitis in runners. *American Journal of Sports Medicine, 11*(4), 215-219.

Sohn, R.S., & Micheli, L.J. (1985). The effect of running on the pathogenesis of osteoarthritis of the hips and knees. *Clinical Orthopaedics and Related Research,* **198,** 106-109.

Southmayd, W., & Hoffman, M. (1981). *Sports health—The complete book of athletic injuries.* New York: Putman.

Spencer, C.W., III, & Jackson, D.W. (1983). Back injuries in the athlete. *Clinics in Sports Medicine,* **2**(1), 191-215.

Stamford, B. (1985). A stitch in the side. *The Physician and Sportsmedicine,* **13**(5), 187.

Stamford, B. (1986). What are muscle cramps? *The Physician and Sportsmedicine,* **14**(2), 192.

Stanish, W.D. (1984). Overuse injuries in athletes: A perspective. *Medical Science in Sports Exercise,* **16**(1), 1-7.

The story of charley horse, turf toe, space invader's wrist, and other common maladies. (1982, November). *Current Health,* pp. 21-24.

Stover, C.N. (1980a). Air stirrup management of ankle injuries in the athlete. *American Journal of Sports Medicine,* **8**(5), 360-365.

Stover, C.N. (1980b). Recognition and management of soft tissue injuries of the ankle in the athlete. *Primary-Care,* **7**(2), 183-198.

Strauss, R.H. (1984). *Sports medicine.* Philadelphia: W.B. Saunders.

Stulberg, S.D. (1980). Sports injuries and arthritis. *Comprehensive Therapy,* **6**(9), 8-11.

Sullivan, D., Warren, R.F., Pavlov, H., & Kelman, G. (1984). Stress fractures in 51 runners. *Clinical Orthopaedics and Related Research,* **5**(1), 188-192.

Switzer, E. (1982, June). Unwelcome aspect of fitness: Chance of injury. *Vogue,* p. 106.

Symposium on ankle and foot problems in the athlete. (1982). *Clinics in Sports Medicine,* **1**(1), 1-178.

Szmukler, G.I., Eisler, I., Gillies, C., & Hayward, M.E. (1985). The implications of anorexia nervosa in a ballet school. *Journal of Psychiatry Residents,* **19**(2-3), 177-181.

Taunton, J.E., Clement, D.B., & McNicol, K. (1982). Plantar fasciitis in runners. *Canadian Journal of Applied Sports Science,* **7**(1), 41-44.

Temple, C. (1983). Sports injuries: Hazards of jogging and marathon running. *British Journal of Hospital Medicine,* **29**(3), 237-239.

Terry, G., Hughston, M., & Norwood, L. (1986). The anatomy of the iliopatellar band and iliotibial tract. *American Journal of Sports Medicine,* **14**(1), 39-45.

Thompson, J.P., & Loomer, R.L. (1984). Osteochondral lesions of the talus in a sports medicine clinic: A new radiographic technique and surgical approach. *American Journal of Sports Medicine,* **12**(6), 460-463.

Titus, K.A. (1984). Sports medicine in general with special emphasis on the prevention and treatment of injuries of the female amateur athlete. *Ohio Journal of Science,* **84**(2), 64.

Too many electrolytes spoil the drink. (1981, August 15). *Science News,* p. 104.

Tropp, H., Askling, C., & Gillquist, J. (1985). Prevention of ankle sprains. *American Journal of Sports Medicine,* **13**(4), 2562-2599.

Tursz, A., & Crost, M. (1986). Sports-related injuries in children. *American Journal of Sports Medicine,* **14**(4), 294-299.

Tuttle, W.W., & Schottelius, B. (1965). *Textbook of physiology.* St. Louis: C.V. Mosby.

Van der Meer, A. (1984, March). How to prevent sports injuries. *Weight Watchers,* pp. 14-15.

Van-Hal, M.E., Keene, J.S., Lange, T.A., & Clancy, W.G., Jr. (1982). Stress fractures of the great toe sesamoids. *American Journal of Sports Medicine,* **10**(2), 122-128.

Vesso, J.J., & Harmon, L.E., III. (1982). Nonoperative management of athletic ankle injuries. *Clinics in Sports Medicine,* **1**(1), 85-98.

Viitasalo, J.T., & Kvist, M. (1983). Some biomechanical aspects of the foot and ankle in athletes with and without shin splints. *American Journal of Sports Medicine,* **11**(3), 125-130.

Wallin, D. (1979). *An attempt to objectively evaluate the effect of stretching exercises mobility training: A comparative study of two stretching methods.* Paper presented at the Fifth Annual Meeting of the American Orthopaedic Society for Sports Medicine, Innisbrook, FL.

Wallin, D. (1985). Improvement of muscle flexibility. *American Journal of Sports Medicine,* **13**(4), 263-268.

Warren, B.L. (1984). Anatomical factors associated with predicting plantar fasciitis in long-distance runners. *Medicine and Science in Sports and Exercise,* **16**(1), 60-63.

Wasco, J. (1983, May 17). What to do when exercise hurts. *Woman's Day,* p. 8.

Wassel, A.C. (1984). Sports medicine: Acute and overuse injuries. *Orthopaedic Nursing,* **3**(2), 29-33.

Weeda-Mannak, W.L., & Drop, M.J. (1985). The discriminative value of psychological characteristics in anorexia nervosa: Clinical and psychometric comparison between anorexia nervosa patients, ballet dancers and controls. *Journal of Psychiatry Residents,* **19**(2-3), 285-290.

Weiker, G.G. (1984). Ankle injuries in the athlete. *Primary-Care,* **11**(1), 101-108.

Wellemeyer, M. (1983, June 13). Conquering sports injuries. *Fortune,* pp. 187-190.

Whiting, P.H., Maushan, R.J., & Miller, J.D. (1984). Dehydration and serum biochemical changes in marathon runners. *European Journal of Applied Physiology,* **52**(2), 183-187.

Wilkerson, G.B. (1985a). Treatment of ankle sprains with external compression and early mobilization. *The Physician and Sportsmedicine,* **13**(6), 83-87, 90.

Wilkerson, G.B. (1985b). External compression for controlling traumatic edema. *The Physician and Sportsmedicine,* **13**(6), 97-100, 103, 106.

Yale, I. (1984). *The arthritic foot.* Baltimore: Williams & Wilkins.

Yates, A., Leehey, K., & Shisslak, C. (1983). Running: An analogue of anorexia. *New England Journal of Medicine,* **308**(5), 251-255.

Zamzow, D., & Feigel, W. (1982, November). A battle of nerves. *Runner's World,* pp. 90-94.

Zucker, P. (1985). Eating disorders in young athletes. *The Physician and Sportsmedicine,* **13**(11), 89-106.

Index